Thyroid and Parathyroid Surgery

Guest Editors

RALPH P. TUFANO, MD
SARA I. PAI, MD, PhD

OTOLARYNGOLOGIC CLINICS OF NORTH AMERICA

www.oto.theclinics.com

April 2010 • Volume 43 • Number 2

SAUNDERS an imprint of ELSEVIER, Inc.

W.B. SAUNDERS COMPANY
A Division of Elsevier Inc.

1600 John F. Kennedy Boulevard ● Suite 1800 ● Philadelphia, Pennsylvania 19103-2899

http://www.theclinics.com

OTOLARYNGOLOGIC CLINICS OF NORTH AMERICA Volume 43, Number 2
April 2010 ISSN 0030-6665, ISBN-13: 978-1-4377-1850-8

Editor: Joanne Husovski

Otolaryngologic Clinics of North America (ISSN 0030-6665) is published bimonthly by Elsevier, Inc., 360 Park Avenue South, New York, NY 10010-1710. Months of issue are February, April, June, August, October, and December. Business and Editorial Offices: 1600 John F. Kennedy Blvd., Suite 1800, Philadelphia, PA 19103-2899. Customer Service Office: 6277 Sea Harbor Drive, Orlando, FL 32887-4800. Periodicals postage paid at New York, NY and additional mailing offices. Subscription prices are $290.00 per year (US individuals), $527.00 per year (US institutions), $142.00 per year (US student/resident), $382.00 per year (Canadian individuals), $662.00 per year (Canadian institutions), $429.00 per year (international individuals), $662.00 per year (international institutions), $219.00 per year (international & Canadian student/resident). Foreign air speed delivery is included in all *Clinics'* subscription prices. All prices are subject to change without notice. **POSTMASTER:** Send address changes to *Otolaryngologic Clinics of North America*, Elsevier Health Sciences Division, Subscription Customer Service, 3251 Riverport Lane, Maryland Heights, MO 63043. **Telephone: 1-800-654-2452 (U.S. and Canada); 314-447-8871 (outside U.S. and Canada). Fax: 314-447-8029. E-mail: journalscustomerservice-usa@elsevier.com (for print support); journalsonlinesupport-usa@elsevier.com (for online support).**

Reprints. For copies of 100 or more of articles in this publication, please contact the Commercial Reprints Department, Elsevier Inc., 360 Park Avenue South, New York, NY 10010-1710. Tel.: 212-633-3812; Fax: 212-462-1935; E-mail: reprints@elsevier.com.

Otolaryngologic Clinics of North America is also published in Spanish by McGraw-Hill Interamericana Editores S.A., P.O. Box 5-237, 06500 Mexico D.F., Mexico.

Otolaryngologic Clinics of North America is covered in *MEDLINE/PubMed (Index Medicus), Current Contents/Clinical Medicine, Excerpta Medica, BIOSIS, Science Citation Index,* and *ISI/BIOMED.*

Printed and bound by CPI Group (UK) Ltd, Croydon, CR0 4YY
Transferred to Digital Print 2011

Contributors

GUEST EDITORS

RALPH P. TUFANO, MD
Associate Professor, Division of Head and Neck Surgical Oncology, Department
of Otolaryngology–Head and Neck Surgery, Johns Hopkins School of Medicine,
Baltimore, Maryland

SARA I. PAI, MD, PhD
Assistant Professor, Division of Head and Neck Surgical Oncology, Department
of Otolaryngology–Head and Neck Surgery, Johns Hopkins School of Medicine;
Department of Oncology, Johns Hopkins University School of Medicine, The
Sidney Kimmel Comprehensive Cancer Center at Johns Hopkins, Baltimore,
Maryland

AUTHORS

PETER ANGELOS, MD, PhD, FACS
Professor of Surgery; Chief of Endocrine Surgery, University of Chicago; Associate
Director of the MacLean Center for Clinical Medical Ethics, University of Chicago
Medical Center, Chicago, Illinois

RIZWAN ASLAM, DO
Fellow Clinical Instructor, Head and Neck Oncology, Microvascular Reconstruction,
Department of Otolaryngology–Head and Neck Surgery, University of Cincinnati College
of Medicine, Cincinnati, Ohio

DONALD BODENNER, MD, PhD
Associate Professor, Department of Geriatrics, University of Arkansas for Medical
Sciences College of Medicine; Central Arkansas Veterans Affairs Healthcare System;
University of Arkansas for Medical Sciences Thyroid Center, Little Rock, Arkansas

STEVEN R. BOMELI, MD
Division of Head and Neck Surgery, Department of Otolaryngology, University
of Pittsburgh, Pittsburgh, Pennsylvania

DAVID CHIEN, MD
Resident in Nuclear Medicine, Division of Nuclear Medicine, The Russell H. Morgan
Department of Radiology and Radiological Science, Johns Hopkins University School
of Medicine, Baltimore, Maryland

EDMUND S. CIBAS, MD
Associate Professor of Pathology, Department of Pathology, Brigham and Women's
Hospital, Boston, Massachusetts

ALAN P.B. DACKIW, MD, PhD
Division of Endocrine and Oncologic Surgery, Department of Surgery, Section of Endocrine Surgery, Johns Hopkins Hospital, Johns Hopkins University School of Medicine, Baltimore, Maryland

GERARD M. DOHERTY, MD
Norman W. Thompson Professor of Surgery, Department of Surgery, University of Michigan, Ann Arbor, Michigan

W. CROSS DUDNEY, BS
University of Arkansas for Medical Sciences College of Medicine, Little Rock, Arkansas

VIDAS DUMASIUS, MD
General Surgery Resident, University of Chicago, Chicago, Illinois

TANYA FANCY, MD
Clinical Instructor, Department of Otolaryngology–Head and Neck Surgery, Medical University of South Carolina, Charleston, South Carolina

ERIN A. FELGER, MD
General and Endocrine Surgeon, Department of Surgery, Washington Hospital Center, Washington, DC

ROBERT L. FERRIS, MD, PhD
Vice-Chair for Clinical Operations; Chief, Division of Head and Neck Surgery, Departments of Otolaryngology and Immunology, University of Pittsburgh; Co-Leader, Cancer Immunology Program, University of Pittsburgh Cancer Institute; Eye and Ear Institute, Pittsburgh, Pennsylvania

DANIELLE FRITZE, MD
Department of Surgery, University of Michigan, Ann Arbor, Michigan

DANIEL GALLAGHER III, MD
Clinical Instructor, Department of Otolaryngology–Head and Neck Surgery, Medical University of South Carolina, Charleston, South Carolina

F. CHRISTOPHER HOLSINGER, MD
Associate Professor, Department of Head and Neck Surgery, The University of Texas MD Anderson Cancer Center, Houston, Texas

JOSHUA D. HORNIG, MD, FRSC(C)
Assistant Professor, Department of Otolaryngology–Head and Neck Surgery, Medical University of South Carolina, Charleston, South Carolina

HEATHER JACENE, MD
Assistant Professor, Division of Nuclear Medicine, The Russell H. Morgan Department of Radiology and Radiological Science, Johns Hopkins University School of Medicine, Baltimore, Maryland

EMAD KANDIL, MD
Assistant Professor of Surgery; Clinical Assistant Professor of Medicine; Adjunct Assistant Professor of Otolaryngology; Chief, Endocrine Surgery Section, Department of Surgery, Tulane Medical Center, New Orleans, Louisiana

MATTHEW KIM, MD
Instructor in Medicine, Thyroid Section, Harvard Medical School, Brigham and Women's Hospital, Boston, Massachusetts

RONALD B. KUPPERSMITH, MD, MBA
Texas Institute for Thyroid and Parathyroid Surgery, Texas ENT and Allergy, College Station, Texas

SHANE O. LEBEAU, MD
Division of Endocrinology and Metabolism, University of Pittsburgh, Pittsburgh, Pennsylvania

SARA I. PAI, MD, PhD
Assistant Professor, Division of Head and Neck Surgical Oncology, Department of Otolaryngology–Head and Neck Surgery, Johns Hopkins School of Medicine; Department of Oncology, Johns Hopkins University School of Medicine, The Sidney Kimmel Comprehensive Cancer Center at Johns Hopkins, Baltimore, Maryland

PHILLIP K. PELLITTERI, DO
Chief, Section of Head, Neck and Endocrine Surgery, Department of Otolaryngology–Head and Neck Surgery, Geisinger Health System; Clinical Professor of Otolaryngology–Head and Neck Surgery, Temple University School of Medicine, Geisinger Medical Center, Pennsylvania

AMIN SABET, MD
Instructor in Medicine, Division of Endocrinology, Diabetes and Metabolism, Harvard Medical School, Beth Israel Deaconess Medical Center, Boston, Massachusetts

MELANIE W. SEYBT, MD
MCG Thyroid Center, Department of Otolaryngology–Head and Neck Surgery, Medical College of Georgia, Augusta, Georgia

SHEILA SHETH, MD, FACR
Associate Professor of Radiology and Pathology, Division of Ultrasound and Diagnostic Imaging, The Russell H. Morgan Department of Radiology and Radiological Science, Johns Hopkins Medical Institutions, Johns Hopkins University, Baltimore, Maryland

BRENDAN C. STACK Jr, MD
Professor and Vice Chair, Department of Otolaryngology–Head and Neck Surgery; James Y. Suen, MD, Chair in Otolaryngology; Vice-Chairman of Adult Services; Director, Head and Neck Oncology; and Director of Clinical Research, Head and Neck Oncology Clinic, University of Arkansas for Medical Sciences College of Medicine; University of Arkansas for Medical Sciences Thyroid Center, Little Rock, Arkansas

DAVID STEWARD, MD
Associate Professor and Director, Division of Thyroid/Parathyroid Surgery, Department of Otolaryngology–Head and Neck Surgery, University of Cincinnati College of Medicine, Cincinnati, Ohio

DAVID J. TERRIS, MD, FACS
Porubsky Distinguished Professor and Surgical Director, MCG Thyroid Center, Department of Otolaryngology, Medical College of Georgia, Augusta, Georgia

RALPH P. TUFANO, MD
Associate Professor, Division of Head and Neck Surgical Oncology, Department of Otolaryngology–Head and Neck Surgery, Johns Hopkins School of Medicine, Baltimore, Maryland

MARK L. URKEN, MD, FACS
Director of Head - Neck Surgical Oncology, Professor of Otolaryngology, Department of Otorhinolaryngology–Head and Neck Surgery, Albert Einstein College of Medicine; Chief of Head and Neck Surgical Oncology, Department of Otolaryngology, Beth Israel Medical Center, Continuum Cancer Centers of New York; Phillips Ambulatory Care Center, Institute for Head and Neck and Thyroid Cancer, New York, New York

ADVISORS TO OTOLARYNGOLOGIC CLINICS 2010:

SAMUEL BECKER, MD
Becker Nose and Sinus Center; Voorhees, New Jersey

DAVID HAYNES, MD
Vanderbilt University; Nashville, Tennessee

BRIAN KAPLAN, MD
Ear, Nose, and Throat Associates; Baltimore, Maryland

JOHN KROUSE, MD, PhD
Temple University Medicine; Philadelphia, Pennsylvania

ANIL KUMAR LALWANI, MD
New York University Langone Medical Center; New York, New York

ARLEN MEYERS, MD, MBA
University of Colorado; Denver, Colorado

MATTHEW RYAN, MD
University of Texas Southwestern, Dallas

RALPH P. TUFANO, MD
Johns Hopkins Medicine; Baltimore, Maryland

Contents

a patient can be followed with repeated examinations or referred for surgery. The value of FNA can be enhanced by attention to technical details. Communication between operator and pathologist is essential. A pathologist's interpretation is aided if essential clinical information is provided on a requisition form. Although reporting terminology has been varied and confusing in the past, a proposal for a uniform reporting system provides 6 clearly defined and clinically relevant reporting categories and promises to standardize the reporting of thyroid FNA results.

The surgical management of thyroid disease and its indications continue to evolve. Selecting the appropriate management can often be challenging to both physician and patient. This article describes the surgical management of various thyroid pathologies. Using contemporary guidelines and clinical experience a framework for selecting appropriate surgical treatment is provided.

Well-differentiated thyroid cancer (DTC) carries an excellent prognosis. Although long-term survival rates are high, regional lymph node metastases are common. Surgical management of cervical lymph nodes is integral to the comprehensive treatment of DTC, but data from large randomized trials do not exist to define optimal treatment. Therapy is thus guided by observational data, and founded on an understanding of the behavior of lymphatic metastases in DTC. This article focuses on the significance of lymph node metastases in thyroid cancer, and the strategy for surgical management.

Invasive thyroid cancer is often asymptomatic and can take the surgeon and the patient by surprise. Maintenance of a high level of suspicion in patients who present with symptoms, an abnormal examination, recurrent disease, or documented metastatic disease lead the clinician to obtain appropriate cross-sectional imaging that helps to define the full extent of the disease. Specific guidelines are provided for the management of the various structures in the neck that are at risk for involvement by disease extension outside the gland or extracapsular extension outside a lymph node with involvement by metastatic disease. This article reviews the prognosis, diagnosis, management, and implications of invasive thyroid cancer affecting the various structures of the central and lateral compartments of the neck.

Differentiated thyroid cancer is increasing in prevalence. This article discusses various aspects of the postoperative management of differentiated thyroid cancer including cancer staging, treatment, and monitoring. Treatment options discussed include radioactive iodine remnant ablation and levothyroxine suppression therapy. Recommendations are given for monitoring based on thyroglobulin determination and available imaging modalities.

Reoperative surgery in the neck for recurrent/persistent well-differentiated thyroid cancer is associated with increased morbidity compared with primary surgery. Reoperative surgery is technically more challenging because of the presence of scar tissue and disruption of the normal fascial planes and anatomy, which may result in a greater risk of injury to nerves and other vital structures. When performing reoperative surgery, an algorithm should be followed that allows for safe and effective removal of recurrent/persistent disease. This algorithm should include a systematic review of prior operative and pathology notes, imaging studies appropriate for localization of disease, an understanding of reoperative central and lateral neck anatomy, along with an appreciation for disease behavior.

Medullary thyroid cancer (MTC), accounts for approximately 5% to 10% of all thyroid cancers. Significant advances in the understanding of the biology and clinical outcomes of MTC have been made over the last decade, culminating most recently in the publication of treatment guidelines by the American Thyroid Association that follow an evidence-based approach that is summarized in this presentation. Prognosis, genetic testing, surgical technique, and re-operation are also discussed.

After nearly a century of performing thyroidectomy essentially the way it was described by Theodore Kocher in the nineteenth century, the technique has quickly evolved. Parathyroidectomy has advanced as biochemical assays and physiologic imaging have become available. Minimally invasive and endoscopic thyroidectomy and parathyroidectomy can now be performed in many patients who benefit from the reduced dissection and smaller incisions associated with these approaches. Although many of the cosmetic, quality of life, and functional improvements have been proved, a better understanding of the procedure and the appropriate indications for its application will continue to develop even as the technique itself evolves, and as new approaches emerge.

In the last 20 years, there has been a significant increase in the diagnosis of benign and malignant thyroid tumors. With improved ultrasound technology and better access to sonographic imaging, many tumors are identified at earlier stages. Consequently, there has been an evolution in surgical technique, moving toward minimally invasive approaches. This article describes the technique of robotic thyroidectomy via transaxillary endoscopic approach without CO_2 insufflation.

Hypercalcemia, which results from the rate of calcium influx into the extracellular fluid exceeding the rate of calcium efflux from the extracellular fluid, has been reported as occurring in approximately 1% to 4% of the adult population in general, and anywhere from 0.5% to 3% of hospitalized adult populations. Hypercalcemia associated with primary hyperparathyroidism has frequently resulted in the development of pancreatitis and peptic ulcer disease; however, the pathophysiologic mechanism of this association remains uncertain. This article examines the etiology and differential diagnosis of hypercalcemia, in particular regarding its association with primary hyperparathyroidism.

Preoperative imaging studies have an important role in facilitating successful localization of adenomas for surgeons. Their use has increased and parallels the recent growth of minimally invasive parathyroidectomy. Based on findings that scintigraphy is reported to have the highest accuracy for localization of adenomas when compared with anatomic imaging techniques, this article discusses the current role and limitations of imaging, with a focus on scintigraphy, in the evaluation of patients before surgery for hyperparathyroidism.

Primary hyperparathyroidism is the most common cause of hypercalcemia in the outpatient setting. Phenotypically, it has evolved from a disease of overt symptomatology to one of vague complaints and biochemical diagnosis. Preoperative localization and intraoperative parathyroid hormone have revolutionized the surgical management of these patients. Minimally invasive operations are now common worldwide with low morbidity and high patient satisfaction.

The treatment of hyperparathyroidism secondary to renal failure is a complex clinical dilemma. No simple optimal approach to patient selection and stratification for surgical intervention is available at this time. The goals of this publication are to review the pathophysiology of parathyroid gland function in patients with impaired renal function, make recommendations for how to proceed with a parathyroidectomy in these patients, and to provide some guidelines for preoperative and postoperative management.

Parathyroid carcinoma is a rare tumor that is prone to recurrence and poor local-regional control. Despite advances in technologies that have shown promise for accurate diagnosis, the mainstay of initial diagnosis remains pathologic analysis and clinical assessment. A surgeon's intraoperative analysis is important in managing patients with parathyroid carcinoma. If parathyroid carcinoma is suspected intraoperatively, a more aggressive surgical strategy should be implemented. This article presents a case series and summary of the existing parathyroid carcinoma literature.

THE CLINICS ARE NOW AVAILABLE ONLINE!

Access your subscription at:
www.theclinics.com

Preface

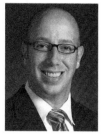 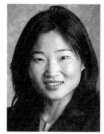

Ralph P. Tufano, MD   Sara I. Pai, MD, PhD
Guest Editors

It's an exciting time for all involved in the care of patients with thyroid and parathyroid disease processes. Novel diagnostic, therapeutic and prognostic tools are being developed and implemented to provide personalized medicine. New technology is developing at an incredible pace to enable safe and effective surgery with the potential for an improved quality of life. These advances require that surgeons, endocrinologists, radiologists and nuclear medicine physicians effectively communicate so that patients achieve the best outcomes possible. Patients not only expect that of us as clinicians, but we demand it upon ourselves as caregivers.

These communications are evident in societies like the American Thyroid Association where practitioners from all training backgrounds work together to formulate treatment guidelines. They are evident in the National Institutes of Health Guidelines for surgical treatment of asymptomatic primary hyperparathyroidism. The era of siloed health care is in the past as we move forward in treating these disease processes as a health care team.

The collection of authors contributing to this issue of *Otolaryngologic Clinics of North America* have been some of the main thought leaders in forging multidisciplinary relationships and programs on a local and national level to improve the care of patients with thyroid and parathyroid disease processes. Their contributions to this volume highlight the importance of multidisciplinary care and provide a detailed overview of state of the art concepts in managing thyroid and parathyroid disorders. We hope this volume helps to inspire open, educated communication among all practitioners who care for thyroid and parathyroid disease so that we can realize our shared goal of achieving the best possible care for our patients.

Ralph P. Tufano, MD
Sara I. Pai, MD, PhD

Otolaryngol Clin N Am 43 (2010) xiii–xiv
doi:10.1016/j.otc.2010.04.001
0030-6665/10/$ – see front matter © 2010 Elsevier Inc. All rights reserved.

oto.theclinics.com

Ralph P. Tufano, MD
Division of Head and Neck Surgical Oncology
Department of Otolaryngology-Head and Neck Surgery
Johns Hopkins School of Medicine
601 North Caroline Street
JHOC 6th Floor
Baltimore, MD 21287, USA

Sara I. Pai, MD, PhD
Division of Head and Neck Surgical Oncology
Departments of Otolaryngology-Head and Neck Surgery and Oncology
Johns Hopkins School of Medicine
601 North Caroline Street
JHOC 6th Floor
Baltimore, MD 21287, USA

E-mail addresses:
rtufano@jhmi.edu (R.P. Tufano)
spai@jhmi.edu (S.I. Pai)

Surgical Anatomy of the Thyroid and Parathyroid Glands

Tanya Fancy, MD, Daniel Gallagher III, MD, Joshua D. Hornig, MD, FRSC(C)*

KEYWORDS

- Anatomy • Thyroid • Parathyroid • Embryology
- Recurrent laryngeal nerve • Superior laryngeal nerve

EMBRYOLOGY OF THE THYROID GLAND

During the fourth week of development, the foramen cecum develops as an endodermal thickening in the floor of the primitive pharynx at the junction between the first and second pharyngeal pouches, immediately dorsal to the aortic sac. The medial thyroid primordium derives as a ventral diverticulum at the foramen cecum. During the fourth to seventh week of gestation, this primitive thyroid tissue penetrates the underlying mesenchymal tissue and descends anterior to the hyoid bone and the laryngeal cartilages to reach its final adult pretracheal position. During its descent, it is first spherical, and then enlarges and becomes bilobed as it grows caudally. The proximal portion of the diverticulum (connecting the gland and the foramen cecum) retracts and forms a solid fibrous stalk early in the fifth week. This thyroglossal duct ultimately atrophies, but any portion of it may persist to become the site of a thyroglossal duct cyst. The distal portion of this duct gives rise to the pyramidal lobe and levator superioris thyroideae in adults.[1] The lateral thyroid primordia (from the fourth and fifth pharyngeal pouches) descend to join the central component during the fifth week of gestation.

Calcitonin-secreting parafollicular C cells arise within the ultimobranchial bodies (recognized within the lateral thyroid primordia) from neural crest cells of the fourth pharyngeal pouch. They fuse to the medial thyroid anlage during the fifth week of gestation. These cells are therefore restricted to a zone deep within the middle to upper third of the lateral lobes.

The thyroid primordium initially consists of a solid mass of endodermal cells, which later break up into a network of cords with the invasion of the surrounding mesenchyme.[2] The epithelial cords organize into clusters of cells with a central lumen.

Department of Otolaryngology-Head & Neck Surgery, Medical University of South Carolina, 135 Rutledge Avenue, PO Box 250550, Charleston, SC 29425, USA
* Corresponding author.
E-mail address: hornigjd@musc.edu

Otolaryngol Clin N Am 43 (2010) 221–227
doi:10.1016/j.otc.2010.01.001
0030-6665/10/$ – see front matter © 2010 Elsevier Inc. All rights reserved.

Follicles begin to appear at the beginning of the second month, and most follicles have been formed by the end of the fourth prenatal month.[1] Thereafter, additional growth is by enlargement of existing follicles. By the end of the third month the gland begins to function, and is able to concentrate radioiodine and synthesize iodothyronines.[3]

Thyroid Ectopia

During the course of its development, the gland (or parts of it) may fail to reach its definitive adult position. Ectopic thyroid tissue can be found at any level along the pathway of its embryological descent. The entire gland may ascend with embryonic growth and lie close to its point of origin at the foramen cecum, giving rise to a lingual thyroid. Lingual thyroid masses have been found in as many as 10% of autopsies, although not all are clinically relevant.[2] Alternatively, the tissue may be sublingual or prelaryngeal in location, and often may be mistaken for a thyroglossal duct cyst. It is essential to determine the presence or absence of functional thyroid tissue at this ectopic location before removal. About 70% of patients with lingual thyroid glands have no thyroid tissue in the neck.[3,4] In many cases the lingual thyroid does not function normally.[4]

In some patients the thyroid gland may be in its normal anatomic location but accessory ectopic tissue may also be present. Although this tissue may be functional, it is often of insufficient size to maintain normal function if the main gland is removed. Nodules of thyroid tissue found within lymph nodes were initially believed to be ectopic foci, but now all such deposits are regarded as metastatic. Agenesis of the thyroid gland is a rare anomaly. When hemiagenesis occurs, the left lobe is more commonly absent.[2]

EMBRYOLOGY OF THE RECURRENT LARYNGEAL NERVE

The recurrent laryngeal nerve is originally associated with the sixth branchial arch. It supplies the region of the future larynx that lies caudal to the fifth pharyngeal pouch. The primordium of the vagus nerve is appreciated by the end of the fifth week, whereas the recurrent branch is apparent by the end of the sixth week. Initially, all of the aortic arches are cranial to the larynx, and so the recurrent nerve passes directly to the larynx.[1] As the pharyngeal pouches disappear and the neck elongates, the aortic arch and associated system of vessels remain in the thorax, whereas the larynx moves craniad in the neck. As a result, the recurrent nerve located lateral to the arches must pass medially under the last arch to reach the larynx. This pathway creates a looplike configuration for which the nerve is named. On the left, the sixth arch persists until birth as the ductus arteriosus, and then regresses to form the ligamentum arteriosum. The recurrent laryngeal nerve must pass under it and reascend to reach the larynx.[1] On the right, because the distal part of the sixth aortic arch degenerates, the right nerve is able to ascend as high as the right subclavian artery (part of the right fourth aortic arch). The recurrent nerves therefore become asymmetric.

The course of the recurrent nerves is determined largely by the pattern of the developing arteries. The most frequent variation occurs when the right subclavian artery arises from the distal aortic arch and passes to the right, posterior to the esophagus.[1] The right recurrent nerve now arises from the vagus nerve at the level of the superior pole of the thyroid gland, and enters the larynx directly without forming a recurrent loop. This nonrecurrent nerve is present in about 0.5% to 1% of the population.[1,5] The main danger to the nonrecurrent nerve is in mistaking it for the inferior thyroid artery during thyroidectomy, or in including it in ligation of the superior pole.

Another variation involves a reversal of the asymmetry between the two recurrent laryngeal nerves. This reversal occurs when a right-sided aortic arch is present, with a right ligamentum arteriosum, causing the right recurrent nerve to loop around the right-sided arch, whereas the left nerve loops around the left subclavian artery. Rarely, a nonrecurrent left nerve may be present in these patients, if the left sublcavian artery is retroesophageal.

ANATOMY OF THE THYROID GLAND

The thyroid gland derives its name from its resemblance to a shield (Greek: thyreos, shield; eidos, form).[3] The thyroid gland weighs between 15 and 25 g in adults, and comprises 2 lateral lobes connected by a central isthmus. Each lobe is approximately 4 cm in length, 2 cm in width, and 2 to 3 cm in thickness. The isthmus measures about 2 cm in width, 2 cm in height, and 2 to 6 mm in thickness.[3,6] The gland lies on the anterolateral aspect of the cervical trachea, with the isthmus related to the second, third, and fourth tracheal rings posteriorly. The superior pole lies lateral to the inferior constrictor muscle, and posterior to the sternothyroid muscle. The inferior pole extends to the levels of the fifth or sixth tracheal ring. Posterolaterally the gland overlaps the carotid sheath and its contents. A pyramidal lobe may be present in about 50% of patients, arising from either lobe or the isthmus, and is directed upward, usually to the left. If present, the levator glandulae thyroideae extends from the isthmus or lateral lobe to the hyoid bone or thyroid cartilage. It may be innervated by a branch of the ansa cervicalis or the superior laryngeal nerve.[3]

The thyroid is enveloped by the layers of the deep cervical fascia, and is covered by the strap muscles anteriorly and the sternocleidomastoid muscle more laterally. The true thyroid capsule is tightly adherent to the gland, and continues into the parenchyma to form fibrous septae separating the gland into lobules. Posteriorly, the middle layer of the deep cervical fascia condenses to form the posterior suspensory ligament of Berry, connecting the lobes of the thyroid to the cricoid cartilage and the first two tracheal rings.[6]

The blood supply to the thyroid gland is derived from two pairs of arteries. The superior thyroid artery which is described as the first branch of the external carotid artery, travels along the inferior constrictor muscle with the superior thyroid vein to supply the upper pole of the gland. In this position, the artery lies superficial to the external branch of the superior laryngeal nerve as it courses to supply the cricothyroid muscle. In 16% of cases, the superior thyroid artery may be a branch of the common carotid artery.[4] After passing deep to the infrahyoid strap muscles, the artery divides into anterior and posterior branches at the level of the superior pole to supply their respective surfaces of the lobe.[3] Before branching at the superior pole, each artery gives off a superior laryngeal artery which travels across the thyrohyoid membrane with the superior laryngeal nerve to enter the larynx, and a cricothyroid artery which lies on the cricothyroid membrane near the lower border of the thyroid cartilage.[4] The larger inferior thyroid artery is a branch of the thyrocervical trunk that arises from the subclavian artery. It courses along the anterior scalene muscle, turns medially behind the common carotid artery to descend on the posterior aspect of the lateral lobes before entering the inferior thyroid pole. In its course behind the common carotid artery, the artery exhibits a variable relationship to the sympathetic chain.[3] This vessel may be absent in 6% of patients.[5,7] The thyroid ima artery is inconsistently present, and arises from the innominate artery, either subclavian artery, right common carotid artery, internal mammary, or aortic arch to supply the thyroid gland near the midline. It may occasionally replace the inferior thyroid artery as one of the principle vessels supplying the gland.[3,4] It is more common on the right side. Because of its relation to the anterior aspect of the trachea, the thyroid ima artery is in danger of injury during a tracheotomy.

There is a dense network of connecting vessels within the thyroid capsule, with branches passing into the connective tissue between the lobules to form extensive capillary plexuses around individual follicles. The veins draining the capillary plexuses give rise to the inferior, middle, and superior thyroid veins. These join the internal jugular or innominate veins. The paired inferior thyroid veins lie on the anterior aspect of the trachea and anastomose freely with each other before draining into the innominate veins. They represent a potential source of bleeding during thyroidectomy or tracheotomy.[4]

The lymphatics of the gland generally drain with the veins. Those traveling with the superior and middle thyroid vessels drain into the upper and middle deep cervical chain nodes respectively. Lymphatics draining with the inferior thyroid vessels empty into the lower deep cervical chain nodes and the supraclavicular, pretracheal, and prelaryngeal nodes. In addition, lymphatics have been identified that drain directly into the subclavian vein without traveling through lymph nodes.[3]

The thyroid gland has a predominantly sympathetic innervation, from the superior, middle, and inferior cervical ganglia.

ANATOMY OF THE RECURRENT LARYNGEAL NERVE

As described earlier, the recurrent laryngeal nerves are asymmetric. The nerve on the left arises from the vagus where it crosses the arch of aorta. The recurrent nerve then loops around the aorta to ascend in the tracheoesophageal groove posterior to the thyroid gland on that side to enter the larynx. The right recurrent laryngeal nerve arises from the vagus as this nerve crosses anterior to the right subclavian artery. The recurrent nerve then loops around the artery and ascends in the tracheoesophageal groove, posterior to the thyroid gland, to enter the larynx behind the cricothyroid articulation and the inferior cornu of the thyroid cartilage.[8]

As the nerve ascends, it is covered by a layer of fascia that also encloses the trachea and the inferior thyroid vein. The left recurrent nerve is generally more closely applied to the trachea in the lower part of its ascending course than is the right nerve. At the level of the lower pole of the thyroid gland, the right nerve is slightly more anterior than the left.[8,9] The connective tissue surrounding the nerve is usually thicker on the right.[8] The nerve runs at a slight angle across the tracheoesophageal groove and then becomes parallel and closely applied to the trachea. During the middle part of its course, the nerve is found within the tracheoesophageal groove in about half of the population.[8] In the other half of patients it may be found anterior or posterior to the groove (within the suspensory ligament of Berry, anterolateral to the trachea in the substance of the thyroid gland, or lateral to the esophagus).

As the recurrent laryngeal nerves ascend toward the middle of the thyroid gland, they are intimately associated with the inferior thyroid artery. Multiple variations have been described in the relationship of the nerve to the inferior thyroid artery and its branches. The 3 basic configurations include nerve anterior to the artery, nerve between branches of the artery (found in about 50% of patients on the right), and nerve posterior to the artery (found in about 50% of patients on the left).[4,8,9]

The recurrent laryngeal nerve may divide before entering the larynx. It is believed that only one of these branches is motor, and the others are sensory. It innervates all the intrinsic muscles of the larynx except the cricothyroid, and provides sensory innervation to the subglottic area and proximal trachea. An ascending branch of the recurrent laryngeal anastomoses with a branch of the superior laryngeal to form the Galen anastomosis. Branches from this anastomosis pierce the transverse arytenoid muscle to reach the mucosa of the posterior laryngeal wall.[10,11]

Classically, the recurrent laryngeal nerve is found intraoperatively in the Simon triangle, formed by the common carotid artery laterally, the esophagus medially, and the inferior thyroid artery superiorly. The nerve can also be reliably found where it enters the larynx just behind the inferior cornu of the thyroid cartilage.

ANATOMY OF THE SUPERIOR LARYNGEAL NERVE

The superior laryngeal nerve originates at the inferior ganglion of the vagus nerve (nodose ganglion) near the jugular foramen. It courses posterior and medial to the internal carotid artery and descends anterior and inferior toward the larynx. At the level of the greater cornu of the hyoid it divides into a large internal branch and a smaller external branch. The internal branch courses between the thyrohyoid muscle and the thyrohyoid membrane, piercing the latter along with the superior laryngeal artery and vein. The internal branch supplies sensation to the supraglottis and pyriform sinus.[12]

At the level of the superior horn of the thyroid cartilage, the external branch turns medially and runs posterior and parallel to the oblique line. It can penetrate the inferior constrictor and run along its deep surface at any point along this course, or remain on its surface.[13]

The external branch is typically deep to the superior thyroid artery, but can cross anterior or between branches as the artery enters the gland 14% to 18% of the time.[14] The nerve is variable in its relationship to the highest point of the superior pole of the thyroid gland. A classification of the external branch with respect to the superior pole, described by Cernea and colleagues,[15] places 37% of external branches at risk of injury during thyroid surgery, passing below the level of the upper pole of the thyroid gland or within 1 cm above it.

The external branch of the superior laryngeal nerve supplies motor input to the inferior constrictor and the cricothyroid muscles.[12] Iatrogenic injury is possible during thyroid, parathyroid, carotid, or cervical spine surgery.[16] The reported incidence of superior laryngeal nerve injury after thyroidectomy ranges from 0% to 58%, and is most likely underdiagnosed.[17] Injury typically presents with symptoms of hoarseness, huskiness, decreased pitch or volume, and early voice fatigue. The consequences are significantly worse in the setting of bilateral injury.[18] Video stroboscopy of unilateral injury reveals posterior glottic rotation to the affected side, vocal cord bowing, and decreased mucosal wave with inferior displacement of the ipsilateral vocal cord.[19] Laryngeal electromyography is the gold standard evaluation of injury to the external branch of the superior laryngeal nerve, as shown by an absence of interference patterns with high-pitched vocalization and electrical silence.[17]

Prevention of injury to the external branch of the superior laryngeal nerve has historically been underemphasized in thyroid and parathyroid surgery. Steps to maximize identification and preservation of the nerve are division of the sternothyroid muscle, careful dissection in the cricothyroid space that lies between the medial surface of the thyroid lobe and the cricothyroid muscle, and meticulous isolation and division of superior thyroid vessels.[16]

EMBRYOLOGY AND ANATOMY OF THE PARATHYROID GLANDS

The parathyroid glands derive from the endoderm of the third and fourth pharyngeal pouches, starting in the fifth week of development.[20] Their function is the production of parathyroid hormone, which regulates the distribution of calcium in the bloodstream and bone. Typically, paired superior and inferior glands develop for a total of four, although up to 13% incidence of supernumerary glands has been described, up to

11 glands in large autopsy series.[21] Each gland typically weighs 35 to 40 mg, measures 3 to 8 mm in all 3 dimensions, and can vary in color from light yellow to reddish brown.

The inferior parathyroid glands arise from the third pharyngeal pouch endoderm and have a common origin and migration with the thymus. Starting at the region of the pharyngeal wall, they migrate inferior and medially in the neck, eventually separating from thymus tissue before it enters the anterior mediastinum.[22] This long course of descent can lead to a large area of possible ectopic inferior parathyroid glands that can be found anywhere from the level of the mandibular angle to the pericardium.[23] The most common ectopic location for an inferior gland is in the anterior mediastinum; this is found in 5% of ectopic cases.[23]

The inferior parathyroid gland can be found within 1 cm inferior, lateral, or posterior to the inferior pole of the thyroid in 50% of cases, and is typically anterior to a plane drawn along the course of the recurrent laryngeal nerve.[22] In an autopsy series of 503 cases,[21] 17% could be found on or within the capsule of the thyroid gland, whereas 26% could be found within the cervical part of the thymus. Rarely (2.8%), the inferior gland was found superior to the intersection of the recurrent nerve and the inferior thyroid artery. Two-thirds of supernumerary cases in this series revealed the fifth gland inferior to the lower pole of the thyroid associated with the thyrothymic ligament or the thymus, whereas one third had the supernumerary gland in the vicinity of the thyroid between the orthotopic superior and inferior parathyroids.

The fourth pharyngeal pouch gives rise to the superior parathyroid glands, which have a much shorter embryologic descent than their inferior counterparts. After losing contact with the pharynx in the sixth week of development,[20] it attaches to the caudally migrating thyroid, and remains in contact with the posterior midportion of the thyroid lobe. This limited course leads to a smaller variability in location compared with the inferior gland, and in 85% of cases the superior parathyroid can be found at the posterior aspect of the thyroid lobe in a 2-cm diameter area centered 1 cm above the crossing of the inferior thyroid artery and the recurrent nerve.[21,22] In the large autopsy series mentioned earlier, 2% of ectopic superior thyroid glands were found at the level of the superior pole of the thyroid, and less than 1% were superior to it.[21]

Because the embryologic descent of the inferior parathyroid crosses that of the superior gland, they can rarely be found at the same level, above or below the crossing of the inferior thyroid artery and recurrent laryngeal nerve. In this instance, it may not be possible to differentiate the superior and inferior glands. Symmetry in the approximate location of the glands when comparing right with left has been reported at 80% for the superior and 70% for the inferior glands.[21] Thus, when unable to locate a missing parathyroid, contralateral dissection for comparison may be useful. Given their variable topography in the neck, keeping the embryology of the parathyroid glands in mind is critical when planning parathyroid surgery.

REFERENCES

1. Gray SW, Skandalakis JE, Akin JT. Embryological considerations of thyroid surgery: developmental anatomy of the thyroid, parathyroids and the recurrent laryngeal nerve. Am Surg 1976;42(9):621–8.
2. Moore KL, Persaud TVN. The pharyngeal (branchial apparatus). In: The developing human: clinically oriented embryology. 6th edition. Philadelphia: WB Saunders; 1998. p. 230–3.
3. Hoyes AD, Kershaw DR. Anatomy and development of the thyroid gland. Ear Nose Throat J 1985;64(10):318–32.

4. Hollinshead WH. Anatomy of the endocrine glands. Surg Clin North Am 1958;39: 1115–40.
5. Henry J, Audiffret J, Denizot A, et al. The nonrecurrent inferior laryngeal nerve: review of 33 cases, including two on the left side. Surgery 1988;104:977–84.
6. Lai SY, Mandel SJ, Weber RS. Management of thyroid neoplasms. In: Cummings otolaryngology: head and neck surgery. 4th edition. Philadelphia: Mosby; 2005. p. 2687–718, Chapter 119.
7. Faller A, Schärer O. Uber die variabilität der arteriae thyroideae [On the variability of the thyroid arteries]. Acta Anat 1947;4(Suppl):119–22 [in German].
8. Skandalakis JE, Droulias C, Harlaftis N, et al. The recurrent laryngeal nerve. Am Surg 1976;42(9):629–34.
9. Berlin DD. The recurrent laryngeal nerves in total ablation of the normal thyroid gland. Surg Gynecol Obstet 1935;60:19–26.
10. Janfaza P, Montgomery WW, Randolph GW. Anterior regions of the neck. In: Janfaza P, Nadol JB Jr, Galla R, et al, editors. Surgical anatomy of the head and neck. Philadelphia: Lippincott Williams & Wilkins; 2001. p. 664–7.
11. Droulias C, Tzinas S, Harlaftis N, et al. The superior laryngeal nerve. Am Surg 1976;42(9):635–8.
12. Janfaza P, Nadol JB, Fabian RL, et al. Surgical anatomy of the head and neck. Philadelphia: Lippincott Williams & Wilkins; 2001.
13. Ozlugedik S, Acar H, Apaydin N, et al. Surgical anatomy of the external branch of the superior laryngeal nerve. Clin Anat 2007;20:387–91.
14. Lennquist S, Cahlin C, Smeds S. The superior laryngeal nerve in thyroid surgery. Surgery 1987;102:999–1008.
15. Cernea C, Ferraz A, Nishio S, et al. Surgical anatomy of the external branch of the superior laryngeal nerve. Head Neck 1992;14:380–3.
16. Morton RP, Whitfield P, Al-Ali S. Anatomical and surgical considerations of the external branch of the superior laryngeal nerve: a systematic review. Clin Otolaryngol 2006;31:368–74.
17. Aluffi P, Policarpo M, Chevorac C, et al. Post-thyroidectomy superior laryngeal nerve injury. Eur Arch Otorhinolaryngol 2001;258:451–4.
18. Naidoo D, Boon JM, Mieny CJ, et al. Relation of the external branch of the superior laryngeal nerve to the superior pole of the thyroid gland: an anatomical study. Clin Anat 2007;20:516–20.
19. Stojadinovic A, Shaha A, Orlikoff R, et al. Prospective functional voice assessment in patients undergoing thyroid surgery. Ann Surg 2002;236(6):823–32.
20. Moore K, Persaud T. The developing human. 6th edition. Philadelphia: WB Saunders; 1998.
21. Akerström G, Malmaeus J, Bergström R. Surgical anatomy of human parathyroid glands. Surgery 1984;95(1):14–21.
22. Randolph G. Surgery of the thyroid and parathyroid glands. Philadelphia: WB Saunders; 2003.
23. Wang C. The anatomic basis of parathyroid surgery. Ann Surg 1976;183(3): 271–5.

Evaluation of a Thyroid Nodule

Steven R. Bomeli, MD[a], Shane O. LeBeau, MD[b],
Robert L. Ferris, MD, PhD[a,c,d,e,*]

KEYWORDS

- Thyroid nodule • Thyroidectomy • BRAF • RAS • Papillary
- Follicular • Fine-needle aspiration biopsy • Thyroid cancer

The thyroid nodule is a common entity. Although autopsy data indicate a 50% prevalence of thyroid nodules larger than 1 cm in patients without clinical evidence of thyroid disease, the prevalence of palpable nodules is only 4% to 7%.[1,2] Ultrasonography is far more sensitive than palpation because it detects nodules of any size in up to 67% of the general population.[3] Thyroid nodules warrant removal when they are large enough to be symptomatic or if there is a concern for malignancy. The majority of nodules are asymptomatic, and with only 5% to 10% of nodules being malignant, the decision to operate is made on therapeutic or diagnostic grounds.[4,5] Ultrasound imaging studies and cytology from fine-needle aspiration (FNA) are the main tools used by the clinician to decide whether surgical excision of a thyroid nodule is warranted. Molecular genetic biomarker analyses are now being used to increase the accuracy of fine-needle aspiration biopsies (FNAB), and appear to substantially alter the clinical decision-making process as they become more widely available and more thoroughly evaluated.

CLINICAL ASSESSMENT

Patients most often present with a large palpable nodule in the neck or report of an incidental nodule found on imaging studies performed for another reason. A single dominant or solitary nodule is more likely to represent carcinoma than a single nodule within a multinodular gland, with an incidence of malignancy from 2.7% to 30% and

The authors have no conflicts of interest or sources of funding to disclose.

[a] Division of Head and Neck Surgery, Department of Otolaryngology, University of Pittsburgh, PA, USA

[b] Division of Endocrinology and Metabolism, University of Pittsburgh, Pittsburgh, PA, USA

[c] Department of Immunology, University of Pittsburgh, Pittsburgh, PA, USA

[d] Cancer Immunology Program, University of Pittsburgh Cancer Institute, Pittsburgh, PA, USA

[e] Eye & Ear Institute, Suite 500, 203 Lothrop Street, Pittsburgh, PA 15213, USA

* Corresponding author. Eye & Ear Institute, Suite 500, 203 Lothrop Street, Pittsburgh, PA 15213.

E-mail address: ferrrl@upmc.edu

Otolaryngol Clin N Am 43 (2010) 229–238

doi:10.1016/j.otc.2010.01.002

0030-6665/10/$ – see front matter © 2010 Elsevier Inc. All rights reserved.

1.4% to 10% respectively.[6] Yet, the overall risk for malignancy within a gland with a solitary nodule is approximately equal to that of a multinodular gland because of the additive risk of each nodule.[7] Important elements in patients' history that increase the likelihood of malignancy include prior head and neck irradiation (especially during childhood, with a relative risk of 8.7 at 1 Gy for X rays and gamma radiation); reports of rapid growth, dysphagia, dysphonia, male gender, presentation at extremes of age (less than 20 years or more than 70 years); and a family history of medullary thyroid carcinoma or multiple endocrine neoplasia.[8,9]

Physical examination findings that increase the concern for malignancy include

- Nodules larger than 4 cm in size (19.3% risk of malignancy)[10]
- Firmness to palpation
- Fixation of the nodule to adjacent tissues
- Cervical lymphadenopathy
- Vocal fold immobility.

Physical examination may be limited by patients' body habitus and an inherent variation between physicians and their assessment of nodules such that more precise measurements are obtained through imaging.[11] Positive predictive values of 100% for thyroid malignancy in the setting of a nodule have been reported for the physical examination findings of cervical lymphadenopathy (greater than 1 cm) and vocal fold immobility.[12] Assessment of a patient's voice is not adequately sensitive at detecting vocal fold immobility when compared with flexible laryngoscopy.[13] A thorough head and neck examination with visualization of vocal fold movement is therefore of utmost importance on initial presentation.

LABORATORY STUDIES

Most patients presenting with a solitary thyroid nodule are euthyroid, and the simplest way to verify this is a serum thyrotropin (TSH) level. If below normal, the workup proceeds with total or free thyroxine (T4) and total triiodothyronine (T3) to better evaluate the hyperthyroid state. This result occurs in approximately 10% of patients with a solitary thyroid nodule and is suggestive of a benign hyperfunctioning adenoma.[14] Serum calcitonin levels should be obtained in any patient with a family history of medullary thyroid carcinoma, multiple endocrine neoplasia types 2a or b, pheochromocytoma, or hyperparathyroidism. Because only 1 in 250 nodules represent medullary thyroid carcinoma, serum calcitonin testing is reserved for high-risk patients.[15] Furthermore, calcitonin levels alone are unable to distinguish between benign and malignant disease.[16]

IMAGING STUDIES
Ultrasonography

Ultrasonography is the imaging study of choice for thyroid nodules. It can identify nodules too small to be palpated, the presence of multiple nodules, central or lateral neck lymphadenopathy, and provides accurate measurements of nodule diameter for interval monitoring. Additionally, it allows characterization of nodules by sonographic features that suggest malignancy. Solid appearance (or hypoechogenicity); increased vascularity; microcalcifications;, irregular margins; and the absence of a halo are features that have been consistently associated with malignancy (**Table 1**).[4,17] There is certainly some subjectivity to these features, and characteristics vary depending on the histology such that ultrasound alone cannot reliably distinguish malignant and benign lesions.[18] Although they do not obviate the need for biopsy, these features

Table 1
Reported sensitivities and specificities of sonographic characteristics for detection of thyroid cancer

	Median Sensitivity (%)	Median Specificity (%)
Microcalcifications	52	83
Absence of halo	66	54
Irregular margins	55	79
Hypoechoic	81	53
Increased intranodular flow	67	81

Data from Fish SA, Langer JE, Mandel SJ. Sonographic imaging of thyroid nodules and cervical lymph nodes. Endocrinol Metab Clin North Am 2008;37(2):401–17.

are extremely useful in selecting the site within a nodule for FNAB to improve diagnostic yield or to select appropriate nodules to aspirate within a multinodular thyroid.[4]

Radioisotope Imaging

Radioisotope scanning can be used to determine if a thyroid nodule is functioning but it does not provide an accurate measurement of size. Radioisotopes that have been used are technetium (^{99m}Tc), ^{123}I, and ^{131}I, and though similar information is obtained with similar amounts of radiation exposure, radioiodine is preferred.[19] About 80% to 85% of thyroid nodules are cold, and about 10% of these nodules represent a malignancy. Hot nodules account for 5% of all nodules, and the likelihood of malignancy is less than 1% for these nodules. Taken together, the sensitivity for the diagnosis of thyroid cancer is 89% to 93%, specificity is 5%, and the positive predictive value of malignancy is only 10%.[20] Except for obviating the need to perform an FNAB on a hyperfunctioning nodule in patients who are thyrotoxic, the use of radioisotope scanning has been nearly abandoned in the initial workup of a thyroid nodule.

CT and MRI

Both of these imaging modalities have almost no role in the initial evaluation of a thyroid nodule and are rarely indicated in the initial workup. However, they are both excellent (100% sensitivities) for evaluating the extent of large substernal goiters that may be compressing nearby structures.[21] Iodinated contrast material utilized for CT scan should be avoided because its use prevents scintigraphy or administration of radioactive iodine therapy for a period of 1 to 2 months. Gadolinium contrast used with MRI does not interfere with thyroid uptake of radiotracer, but it is significantly more expensive than CT or ultrasound.

^{18}F-fluorodeoxyglucose Positron Emission Tomography-CT

^{18}F-fluorodeoxyglucose positron emission tomography-CT (^{18}FDG-PET/CT) is used extensively in oncology for staging, evaluation of treatment response, and detecting recurrences on the principle that malignant cells have a higher uptake of ^{18}FDG because of increased metabolic demands when compared with normal tissues.[22] Generally, the appearance of the images and maximum standard uptake value (SUV_{max}) can be used to distinguish between malignant and benign lesions. This does not appear to be the case with thyroid nodules because there is no significant difference in SUV_{max} between benign and malignant ^{18}FDG-avid nodules.[23] Some have suggested that ^{18}FDG-PET/CT may play a role in reducing the need for diagnostic thyroid lobectomy for FNAB indeterminate lesions because it has negative predictive values 95% to 100%.[24,25] Although such preliminary studies are promising, further research is needed before observation could universally be recommended over surgery for non-[18]FDG–avid thyroid nodules with indeterminate FNA cytology. Although [18]FDG-PET/CT does not play a role in the workup of a nodule, any [18]FDG-avid thyroid nodule found incidentally deserves a thorough workup for malignancy.[26]

FNAB

FNAB is the most important step in the workup of the thyroid nodule, as cytology is the primary determinant in whether thyroidectomy is indicated. FNAB is widely available and well tolerated, with a low risk for complications. Its use has dramatically decreased the number of thyroidectomies performed and improved the yield of malignancy in glands that have been extirpated.[27] FNAB can be performed with or without ultrasound guidance, but diagnostic accuracy is improved using sonographic needle localization because of a decreased number of inadequate specimens and false-negative results.[28]

The pathology report from FNAB may be read as benign, malignant, indeterminate, or nondiagnostic. The exact terminology may vary between institutions as there is currently no standard means of reporting FNAB cytology specimens, especially with regard to indeterminate specimens. The latest proposal from the National Cancer Institute is that cytology should universally be reported under six categories that more accurately predict the risk for malignancy (**Table 2**).[29] Benign lesions on FNAB have an approximate 3% risk for malignancy (although this will vary with patient population), and may be followed clinically with ultrasound or with a repeat FNAB which, if also benign, decreases the risk for a false negative to 1.3%.[30]

The only malignant pathology reliably diagnosed through FNA is papillary thyroid carcinoma because features, such as Orphan Annie nuclei, nuclear grooves, intranuclear inclusions, and psammoma bodies, can be sufficient for a diagnosis. Medullary carcinoma, anaplastic carcinoma, lymphoma, poorly differentiated carcinoma, and metastatic disease have also been reported to be classified on the basis of cytology.[29] Benign and malignant follicular neoplasms and oncocytic (formerly called Hurthle cell) adenomas and carcinomas cannot be distinguished on the basis of cytology alone, because tissue architecture is required to make the diagnosis of malignancy through observation of capsular or angiolymphatic invasion. Although this has historically been

Table 2
National Cancer Institute Thyroid Fine-Needle Aspiration State of the Science Conference

Proposed Categories	Risk of Malignancy (%)
Benign	<1
Follicular lesion of undetermined significance	5–10
Neoplasm (follicular or oncocytic)	20–30
Suspicious for malignancy	50–75
Malignant	100
Nondiagnostic	N/A

Abbreviation: NA, not applicable.

Data from Baloch ZW, LiVolsi VA, Asa SL, et al. Diagnostic terminology and morphologic criteria for cytologic diagnosis of thyroid lesions: a synopsis of the National Cancer Institute Thyroid Fine-Needle Aspiration State of the Science Conference. Diagn Cytopathol 2008;36(6):425–37.

true, recent advances in the application of molecular markers to FNAB are changing these principles.

MOLECULAR MARKERS IN FNAB

Although still early in clinical application, the use of genetic biomarkers to assist in interpretation of FNAB samples is likely to greatly enhance the ability to distinguish benign from malignant thyroid nodules in conjunction with cytology. The current algorithms for the extent of thyroid surgery based upon these results are evolving. This evolution stands in distinct contrast to immunohistochemical staining techniques, such as HBME-1, galectin-3, and cytokeratin, that may assist with indeterminate FNAB specimens, but have not dramatically changed clinical practice because of difficulties with the amount of tissue needed and subjective interpretation of stains.[31]

Genetic mutations implicated in the development of differentiated thyroid carcinoma alter the DNA sequence encoding tyrosine kinase receptors (RET/PTC, NTRK), nuclear proteins (PAX-8-PPARγ), and signaling proteins (RAS, BRAF). RET/PTC rearrangements occur only in papillary thyroid carcinoma, but NTRK and BRAF mutations are also common. Greater than 70% of papillary thyroid carcinomas will have mutations in the BRAF, RAS, or RET/PTC genes.[32] The BRAF V600E mutation is associated with more aggressive forms of papillary carcinoma.[33,34] The mutations in the RAS proto-oncogenes (HRAS, NRAS, KRAS) or PAX-8-PPARγ rearrangement are found in approximately 70% of follicular carcinomas.[35] Finding the BRAF mutation, RET/PTC, or PAX-8-PPARγ rearrangements in an indeterminate FNAB specimen has been correlated with a 100% specificity of thyroid cancer in a recent prospective study, and RAS mutation similarly correlated with a 83% to 87% risk for malignancy in any FNAB sample.[36] A false-positive BRAF mutation has been described and the RET/PTC rearrangement can be found in benign conditions, such as trabecular adenoma and Hashimoto thyroiditis, so all clinical and cytologic data must be interpreted in addition to mutation analyses.[37,38] BRAF and RAS are currently the most widely prevalent and studied mutations utilized for making clinical decisions. Although preliminary data for RET/PTC and PAX-8-PPARγ mutations appears promising, the numbers of published cases are too sparse to assist with clinical decisions at the present time.[36,39] Although the exact indications for mutation analysis are under investigation, it appears that most clinical utility lies in helping to make the decision between thyroid lobectomy and total thyroidectomy when the cytology is characterized as follicular neoplasm or suspicious for malignancy. Treatment algorithms will change as more data accumulates and these assays become more widely available.

NODULE SIZE

Sampling error of a FNAB increases as the size of a thyroid nodule increases. A 17% false-negative rate for solid thyroid nodules 3 cm or larger and a 30% false-negative rate for cystic nodules 3 cm or larger led to a recommendation of diagnostic lobectomy for any nodule 3 cm or larger.[40] More recent research has reported that this measurement may be increased to 4 cm with the increased diagnostic yield of modern ultrasound guidance for FNAB. The rate of cancer for 4 cm nodules is 19% with a false-negative rate for FNAB of 12.7%.[10] Recommendations of surgery based on size alone are controversial, but patients' risk factors and concerns often guide the management of nodules this large. The age of patients must also be considered, because a definitive lobectomy is often preferred to the multiple FNABs required to follow a nodule in younger patients. A single preoperative FNAB is still useful in nodules 3 to 4 cm in diameter that are destined for surgical excision, because a malignant biopsy allows planning for total thyroidectomy without the need for frozen-section analysis.

FROZEN-SECTION ANALYSIS

For FNAB indeterminate specimens, a diagnostic thyroid lobectomy is often performed with intraoperative frozen-section analysis to prevent a return trip to the operating room for completion thyroidectomy. There is certainly variation in the confidence at which a pathologist will read a frozen section, as the result will be deferred in any instances of uncertainty. The true utility of this practice has long been debated. Proponents for routine use of intraoperative frozen section have demonstrated cost effectiveness and a reduced number of completion thyroidectomies when it is utilized for follicular lesions.[41] Others disagree on the basis that increased costs from additional operating time and pathologists needed to read the specimens are not justified by a significant benefit in patient outcomes.[42] Frozen-section analysis often complements the FNA cytology in cases with cytologic atypia or suspicious appearance, and is most useful at making a diagnosis of papillary thyroid carcinoma.[43] Its efficacy, and therefore use, will vary between institutions, surgeons, and pathologists.

WORKUP AND SURGICAL RECOMMENDATIONS

The authors have proposed the algorithm in **Fig. 1** for the thyroid surgeon's workup of a thyroid nodule. It is based upon the 2006 American Thyroid Association guidelines for the workup of a thyroid nodule with incorporation of mutational analysis.[44] One indication for surgery is whether the nodule is symptomatic because of compression of nearby structures. These patients are typically evaluated with CT or MRI and loop spirometry, and a lobectomy is typically performed to remove the compressive lesion. In rare instances, a total thyroidectomy is indicated if both lobes of the thyroid are

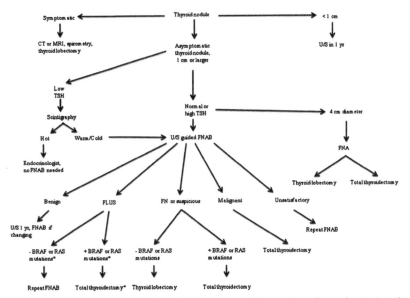

Fig. 1. Workup of a thyroid nodule. *Based on unpublished data from the University of Pittsburgh Medical Center, 2009.

problematic. Any asymptomatic thyroid nodule should be evaluated with a diagnostic ultrasound and a TSH level. Often times, these tests have been completed prior to a patient's arrival in the surgeon's office. Nodules smaller than 1 cm in diameter should be followed with a yearly ultrasound, with FNAB indicated for any concerning changes in appearance or growth. A biopsy of sub-centimeter nodules may be indicated if there is a significant history of radiation exposure, a strong family history of thyroid carcinoma, or worrisome sonographic features.

A subnormal TSH level increases suspicion for a hyperfunctioning nodule, and only in this circumstance should a thyroid uptake scan be ordered. If the nodule is hot, patients can be managed by their endocrinologist without further workup because there is less than 1% risk for malignancy.[20] This situation is rather rare in the clinical practice of a thyroid surgeon, because the majority of patients with nodules are euthyroid and patients with hyperthyroidism are typically referred to the endocrinologist's office for medical management.

Unless easily palpable, an ultrasound-guided FNAB is the first diagnostic step for an asymptomatic thyroid nodule with a diameter of 1 cm or larger in patients who are euthyroid. Even if the nodule is symptomatic or in the 4 cm size range, which alone warrants surgical excision, an FNAB is recommended because it may preoperatively determine whether a total thyroidectomy is to be performed over a lobectomy. FNAB cytology will return as unsatisfactory, benign, intermediate, or malignant.

The intermediate group has been sub-classified into follicular lesion of undetermined significance (FLUS), follicular neoplasm, or suspicious for malignancy according to the 2007 Bethesda thyroid cytology classification from the National Cancer Institute.[29]

FNAB specimens read as unsatisfactory should be sent for a repeat biopsy so that useful diagnostic information may be obtained. Samples read as FLUS are generally sent for repeat FNAB, as the risk for malignancy is only 5% to 10%. Yet, if the FLUS sample is positive for BRAF or RAS mutations, unpublished data from more than 900 cases at the University of Pittsburgh Medical Center suggests that a total thyroidectomy is indicated (Nikiforov, Y, et al, unpublished data, 2009). The portion of **Fig. 1** designated with an asterisk reflects this practice, but it is not fully validated or universally accepted at this point in time.

Benign lesions can safely be followed with yearly ultrasound examinations, with a repeat FNA with any increase in size or development of concerning sonographic features. Efforts to shrink the size of a benign nodule with TSH suppression are not generally useful.[44]

A malignant lesion identified by FNAB is an indication for total thyroidectomy, and ultrasonography should assess central or lateral nodal status.

Patients with lesions classified as follicular or oncocytic neoplasm, or suspicious for malignancy should be offered a diagnostic lobectomy in situations where molecular testing is not available. Where diagnostic testing with BRAF and RAS mutations is available, finding one of these mutations in an indeterminate FNA specimen predicts malignancy with a 100% specificity and positive predictive value according to a recent prospective study.[36] A 100% specificity for BRAF has been confirmed by a second prospective study.[39] Finding one of these mutations in an indeterminate FNA specimen may be considered an indication for total thyroidectomy in some medical centers. Caution is advised, as a false-positive BRAF mutation has been described. In this case, the final pathology was of atypical nodular hyperplasia which may be a premalignant lesion.[37] Surgical excision of any RAS mutated cytology specimen in the form of lobectomy regardless of cytopathology must also be considered because it has an 87.5% risk for malignancy.[36] Even when histologically benign, RAS-positive follicular adenomas are likely precursors to follicular carcinoma.[35] The use of molecular testing is unlikely to be routinely performed on all FNA specimens because of cost, but their role in the indeterminate FNA appears to be invaluable. Further clinical studies are required to determine the cytology and imaging characteristics of nodules where molecular markers are beneficial while cost efficient, and whether these markers have any prognostic information about the status of lymphatic spread into the neck.

SUMMARY

Thyroid nodules are common entities that a thyroid surgeon must evaluate. Nodules are found through physical examination or incidentally through imaging modalities performed for other reasons. The majority of thyroid nodules are benign, but they warrant surgical excision when they are large enough to be symptomatic or if there is concern for malignancy. Ultrasound is the primary study by which the thyroid gland is imaged. Nodules 1 cm or larger or sonographically suspicious sub-centimeter nodules warrant cytologic analysis through FNAB to determine the risk for malignancy. Molecular biomarkers have shown great promise in their ability to detect malignancy in FNAB specimens, and are serving as a powerful adjunct to cytology where they are available. Detecting malignancy preoperatively allows total thyroidectomy in a single operation without the need for frozen section or removal of the thyroid remnant in a second surgery. Cytology and molecular biomarkers are the primary diagnostic modalities a surgeon utilizes to determine the extent of thyroid surgery.

REFERENCES

1. Mortensen JD, Woolner LB, Bennett WA. Gross and microscopic findings in clinically normal thyroid glands. J Clin Endocrinol Metab 1955;15(10):1270–80.
2. Singer PA. Evaluation and management of the solitary thyroid nodule. Otolaryngol Clin North Am 1996;29(4):577–91.
3. Ezzat S, Sarti DA, Cain DR, et al. Thyroid incidentalomas. Prevalence by palpation and ultrasonography. Arch Intern Med 1994;154(16):1838–40.
4. Papini E, Guglielmi R, Bianchini A, et al. Risk of malignancy in nonpalpable thyroid nodules: predictive value of ultrasound and color-Doppler features. J Clin Endocrinol Metab 2002;87(5):1941–6.
5. Nam-Goong IS, Kim HY, Gong G, et al. Ultrasonography-guided fine-needle aspiration of thyroid incidentaloma: correlation with pathological findings. Clin Endocrinol (Oxf) 2004;60(1):21–8.
6. Barroeta JE, Wang H, Shiina N, et al. Is fine-needle aspiration (FNA) of multiple thyroid nodules justified? Endocr Pathol 2006;17(1):61–5.
7. Frates MC, Benson CB, Doubilet PM, et al. Prevalence and distribution of carcinoma in patients with solitary and multiple thyroid nodules on sonography. J Clin Endocrinol Metab 2006;91(9):3411–7.
8. Ferrone S, Marincola FM. Loss of HLA class I antigens by melanoma cells: molecular mechanisms, functional significance and clinical relevance. Immunol Today 1995;16(10):487–94.
9. Hegedus L. Clinical practice. The thyroid nodule. N Engl J Med 2004;351(17):1764–71.
10. McCoy KL, Jabbour N, Ogilvie JB, et al. The incidence of cancer and rate of false-negative cytology in thyroid nodules greater than or equal to 4 cm in size. Surgery 2007;142(6):837–44 [discussion: 844 e1–3].

11. Jarlov AE, Nygaard B, Hegedus L, et al. Observer variation in the clinical and laboratory evaluation of patients with thyroid dysfunction and goiter. Thyroid 1998;8(5):393–8.
12. Raza SN, Shah MD, Palme CE, et al. Risk factors for well-differentiated thyroid carcinoma in patients with thyroid nodular disease. Otolaryngol Head Neck Surg 2008;139(1):21–6.
13. Hanna BC, Brooker DS. A preliminary study of simple voice assessment in a routine clinical setting to predict vocal cord paralysis after thyroid or parathyroid surgery. Clin Otolaryngol 2008;33(1):63–6.
14. Wong CK, Wheeler MH. Thyroid nodules: rational management. World J Surg 2000;24(8):934–41.
15. Elisei R, Bottici V, Luchetti F, et al. Impact of routine measurement of serum calcitonin on the diagnosis and outcome of medullary thyroid cancer: experience in 10,864 patients with nodular thyroid disorders. J Clin Endocrinol Metab 2004; 89(1):163–8.
16. Gleich LL, Gluckman JL, Nemunaitis J, et al. Clinical experience with HLA-B7 plasmid DNA/lipid complex in advanced squamous cell carcinoma of the head and neck. Arch Otolaryngol Head Neck Surg 2001;127(7):775–9.
17. Fish SA, Langer JE, Mandel SJ. Sonographic imaging of thyroid nodules and cervical lymph nodes. Endocrinol Metab Clin North Am 2008;37(2):401–17, ix.
18. Hegedus L. Thyroid ultrasound. Endocrinol Metab Clin North Am 2001;30(2): 339–60, viii–ix.
19. Shibuya TY, Kim S, Nguyen K, et al. Covalent linking of proteins and cytokines to suture: enhancing the immune response of head and neck cancer patients. Laryngoscope 2003;113(11):1870–84.
20. Cases JA, Surks MI. The changing role of scintigraphy in the evaluation of thyroid nodules. Semin Nucl Med 2000;30(2):81–7.
21. Mazzaferri EL. Management of a solitary thyroid nodule. N Engl J Med 1993; 328(8):553–9.
22. Rohren EM, Turkington TG, Coleman RE. Clinical applications of PET in oncology. Radiology 2004;231(2):305–32.
23. Bogsrud TV, Karantanis D, Nathan MA, et al. The value of quantifying 18F-FDG uptake in thyroid nodules found incidentally on whole-body PET-CT. Nucl Med Commun 2007;28(5):373–81.
24. Mitchell JC, Grant F, Evenson AR, et al. Preoperative evaluation of thyroid nodules with 18FDG-PET/CT. Surgery 2005;138(6):1166–74 [discussion: 1174–5].
25. de Geus-Oei LF, Pieters GF, Bonenkamp JJ, et al. 18F-FDG PET reduces unnecessary hemithyroidectomies for thyroid nodules with inconclusive cytologic results. J Nucl Med 2006;47(5):770–5.
26. Razfar A, Christopoulos, A, Lebeau, SO, et al. Clinical utility of PET-CT in recurrent thyroid carcinoma. Arch Otolaryngol 2010;136(2):120–5.
27. Sidawy MK, Del Vecchio DM, Knoll SM. Fine-needle aspiration of thyroid nodules: correlation between cytology and histology and evaluation of discrepant cases. Cancer 1997;81(4):253–9.
28. Danese D, Sciacchitano S, Farsetti A, et al. Diagnostic accuracy of conventional versus sonography-guided fine-needle aspiration biopsy of thyroid nodules. Thyroid 1998;8(1):15–21.
29. Baloch ZW, LiVolsi VA, Asa SL, et al. Diagnostic terminology and morphologic criteria for cytologic diagnosis of thyroid lesions: a synopsis of the National Cancer Institute Thyroid Fine-Needle Aspiration State of the Science Conference. Diagn Cytopathol 2008;36(6):425–37.

30. Chehade JM, Silverberg AB, Kim J, et al. Role of repeated fine-needle aspiration of thyroid nodules with benign cytologic features. Endocr Pract 2001;7(4): 237–43.
31. Franco C, Martinez V, Allamand JP, et al. Molecular markers in thyroid fine-needle aspiration biopsy: a prospective study. Appl Immunohistochem Mol Morphol 2009;17(3):211–5.
32. Adeniran AJ, Zhu Z, Gandhi M, et al. Correlation between genetic alterations and microscopic features, clinical manifestations, and prognostic characteristics of thyroid papillary carcinomas. Am J Surg Pathol 2006;30(2):216–22.
33. Xing M, Westra WH, Tufano RP, et al. BRAF mutation predicts a poorer clinical prognosis for papillary thyroid cancer. J Clin Endocrinol Metab 2005;90(12): 6373–9.
34. Elisei R, Ugolini C, Viola D, et al. BRAF(V600E) mutation and outcome of patients with papillary thyroid carcinoma: a 15-year median follow-up study. J Clin Endocrinol Metab 2008;93(10):3943–9.
35. Nikiforova MN, Lynch RA, Biddinger PW, et al. RAS point mutations and PAX8-PPAR gamma rearrangement in thyroid tumors: evidence for distinct molecular pathways in thyroid follicular carcinoma. J Clin Endocrinol Metab 2003;88(5): 2318–26.
36. Nikiforov YE, Steward DL, Robinson-Smith TM, et al. Molecular testing for mutations in improving the fine-needle aspiration diagnosis of thyroid nodules. J Clin Endocrinol Metab 2009;94(6):2092–8.
37. Chung KW, Yang SK, Lee GK, et al. Detection of BRAFV600E mutation on fine needle aspiration specimens of thyroid nodule refines cyto-pathology diagnosis, especially in BRAF600E mutation-prevalent area. Clin Endocrinol (Oxf) 2006; 65(5):660–6.
38. Salvatore G, Giannini R, Faviana P, et al. Analysis of BRAF point mutation and RET/PTC rearrangement refines the fine-needle aspiration diagnosis of papillary thyroid carcinoma. J Clin Endocrinol Metab 2004;89(10):5175–80.
39. Sapio MR, Posca D, Raggioli A, et al. Detection of RET/PTC, TRK and BRAF mutations in preoperative diagnosis of thyroid nodules with indeterminate cytological findings. Clin Endocrinol (Oxf) 2007;66(5):678–83.
40. Meko JB, Norton JA. Large cystic/solid thyroid nodules: a potential false-negative fine-needle aspiration. Surgery 1995;118(6):996–1003 [discussion: 1003–4].
41. Miller MC, Rubin CJ, Cunnane M, et al. Intraoperative pathologic examination: cost effectiveness and clinical value in patients with cytologic diagnosis of cellular follicular thyroid lesion. Thyroid 2007;17(6):557–65.
42. Richards ML, Chisholm R, Bruder JM, et al. Is thyroid frozen section too much for too little? Am J Surg 2002;184(6):510–4 [discussion: 514].
43. Cheng MS, Morgan JL, Serpell JW. Does frozen section have a role in the intra-operative management of thyroid nodules? ANZ J Surg 2002;72(8):570–2.
44. Cooper DS, Doherty GM, Haugen BR, et al. Management guidelines for patients with thyroid nodules and differentiated thyroid cancer. Thyroid 2006;16(2): 109–42.

Role of Ultrasonography in Thyroid Disease

Sheila Sheth, MD

KEYWORDS

• Thyroid ultrasound • Thyroid cancer • Thyroid nodules

Thyroid nodules are very common; autopsy studies show that nearly half the population of the United States harbors thyroid nodules.[1] However, only 4% to 8% of these nodules are palpable and detected clinically. Many more are discovered incidentally on a computed tomographic scan, magnetic resonance imaging, or ultrasound of the neck performed for an indication unrelated to thyroid disease.[2] In recent years, there has been an explosion of investigation generated by the discovery of these incidental thyroid nodules. Despite the high prevalence of thyroid nodules in the general population, only 5% to 10% of nodules are malignant. The overwhelming majority of thyroid nodules are not true neoplasms but rather represent nodular hyperplasia (also called adenomatoid or colloid nodule). Thyroid cancer is uncommon: in 2008, there were 37,340 new cases diagnosed and 1590 patients died from the disease.[3] Well-differentiated papillary thyroid carcinomas (PTCs) account for 75% to 90% of all thyroid cancers. It is clear from these statistics that one of the important challenges for imagers and clinicians is to identify potentially cancerous lesions and reassure the vast majority of patients harboring benign nodules.

Ultrasonography (US) is the single-most valuable imaging modality in the evaluation of the thyroid gland. Indications for thyroid US include evaluation for a palpable thyroid nodule or suspected thyroid enlargement and workup of thyroid nodules discovered incidentally. It should not be used as a screening test for the detection of nodules.[4] In addition to nodule detection and characterization, US provides optimal guidance for fine-needle aspiration biopsy (FNAB), which, despite some limitations, remains the gold standard for the characterization of thyroid nodules.

This review discusses the US appearances of thyroid nodules, emphasizing sonographic features associated with potentially malignant or, at the other end of the spectrum, likely benign nodules. Diffuse thyroid abnormalities have also been reviewed. The technique of ultrasound-guided FNAB and the emerging role of elastography in characterizing thyroid nodules have also been addressed.

Division of Ultrasound and Diagnostic Imaging, The Russell H. Morgan Department of Radiology and Radiological Science, Johns Hopkins Medical Institutions, Johns Hopkins University, 600 North Wolfe Street, Baltimore, MD 21287, USA
E-mail address: ssheth@jhmi.edu

Otolaryngol Clin N Am 43 (2010) 239–255
doi:10.1016/j.otc.2010.02.001
0030-6665/10/$ – see front matter © 2010 Elsevier Inc. All rights reserved.

TECHNIQUE AND NORMAL APPEARANCE

The thyroid gland is imaged using high-frequency linear transducers, 8 to 15 MHz, depending on the thickness of the patient's neck. Gray-scale transverse and sagittal images are recorded for each lobe. Occasionally, in large patients, additional scanning with a 6-MHz linear transducer may prove beneficial. If the thyroid gland is enlarged, a curvilinear transducer may be used for better measurements.

The normal thyroid has a homogeneous, medium gray echotexture (**Fig. 1**). Anatomic landmarks are best defined on transverse sections: the thyroid gland is found between the common carotid artery laterally and the trachea medially.

Measurements of any detected thyroid nodule should be performed in sagittal, transverse, and anteroposterior dimensions with electronic calipers placed outside any visible halo.

US EVALUATION OF THYROID NODULES

Once a thyroid nodule is discovered, the single-most important next step is to decide whether an FNAB should be recommended. Although this procedure is relatively noninvasive, it is desirable to limit its use for nodules that are suspicious or indeterminate to minimize unnecessary costs and anxiety to the patient. In addition, there is a documented 5% false-negative rate for FNAB.[5]

US CHARACTERISTICS OF THYROID NODULES: A SYSTEMATIC ANALYSIS

To encourage a rationale approach to the management of thyroid nodules detected on US, several medical societies, including the American Thyroid Association (ATA), the Society of Radiologists in Ultrasound (SRU), and the American Association of Clinical Endocrinologists (AACE), have recently published a series of guidelines.[4,6,7] The US features of thyroid nodules that should be analyzed are summarized in the Consensus Statement on thyroid nodules from the SRU[7] and the AACE.[4] They include nodule size and content (solid, complex, or cystic). For solid thyroid nodules, the following parameters should be evaluated: nodule echotexture, shape, borders (smooth or nodular), the presence and quality of intranodular calcifications, and the presence of a perinodular halo. **Table 1** compares the sensitivity, specificity, positive predictive values, and negative predictive values of each of these sonographic criteria from 6 large studies, including a large retrospective study of 849 thyroid nodules recently conducted by the

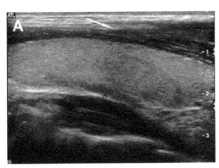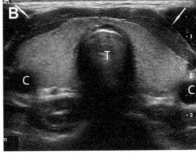

Fig. 1. Normal thyroid gland. (*A*) Sagittal US right thyroid lobe shows a homogeneous gland with medium gray echogenicity. (*B*) Transverse US shows both thyroid lobes. Note the hypoechoic strap muscle anteriorly (*arrows*). C, common carotid artery; T, trachea.

Table 1
Comparison of sonographic criteria from 6 studies

Study	Number of Nodules	Clinical	Hypoecho-genicity (%)				Shape Spherical/ Taller Than Wide (%)				Spiculated Margins (%)				Microcalcifications (%)			
			Sensitivity	Specificity	PPV	NPV	Sensitivity	Specificity	PPV	NPV	Sensitivity	Specificity	PPV	NPV	Sensitivity	Specificity	PPV	NPV
Takashima et al[8]	259	P & NonP	83	49	40	89	—	—	—	—	72	63	44	85	36	93	70	78
Kim et al[10,a]	155	NonP	26.5	94.3	68.4	73.5	32.7	92.5	66.7	74.8	55.1	83	60	80	55.1	83	60	80
Papini et al[13,b]	402	NonP	87.1	43.4	11.4	—	—	—	—	—	77.5	85	30		—	—	—	—
Nam-Goong et al[12]	317	NonP	68.2	52.9	27	—	—	—	—	—	—	—	—	—	36.4	85.5	39	—
Capelli et al[9,b]	701	NonP	79.1	53.3	15.1	96	83.6	81.5	32.4	97.9	47.8	74.3	16.4	93	73.1	69.2	20	96
Moon et al[11]	849	P & NonP	87.2	58.5	60.7	86.1	40	91.4	77.4	67.4	48.3	91.8	81.3	70.7	44.2	90.8	77.9	68.8

Abbreviations: NonP, nonpalpable; NPV, negative predictive value; P, palpable; PPV, positive predictive value.
[a] Marked hypoechogenicity.
[b] Clustered blurred and spiculated margins together.

Korean Society of Neuro and Head and Neck Radiology Thyroid study group. Many of the statistics listed below stem from these articles and are summarized in **Table 1**.[9–13]

Nodule Content: Cystic Versus Solid Nodules

Before the availability of high-resolution high-frequency transducers, the role of US was limited to distinguishing between cystic and solid nodules. Purely cystic nodules are anechoic. They are almost invariably benign and represent colloid cysts. Some colloid cysts contain echogenic foci with posterior reverberation or comet tail artifact (**Fig. 2**). A subset of cystic nodules shows a lacelike or honeycomb pattern of multiple small cysts separated by thin septations (**Fig. 3**). This pattern is strongly associated with a benign hyperplastic nodule[11,14,15] and has been dubbed the "leave me alone" lesion.[15] Consequently, purely cystic nodules, with or without comet tails, and cystic nodules with a honeycomb appearance do not need FNAB.[14]

However, many cystic thyroid nodules have a solid-appearing component. Although these complex nodules are often referred for biopsy for concern that they represent a cystic papillary cancer, their most common underlying cause is a degenerated colloid nodule (**Fig. 4**). Because these nodules contain avascular debris and fibrosis, they tend to yield scant or no follicular cells and are associated with a higher number of inconclusive FNAB.[14,16]

Careful analysis of any solid area within cystic nodules is imperative to identify the rare papillary thyroid cancer (approximately 2.5%) with a large cystic component. Hatabu and colleagues[17] described the "calcified nodule within a cyst," a sign of papillary excrescences with microcalcifications protruding into the cyst, as specific for papillary thyroid cancer (**Fig. 5**). Such an area should be specifically targeted during fine-needle aspiration.

Echotexture

The echotexture (or shade of gray) of solid nodules is another important criterion taken into consideration when analyzing nodules. The echotexture of the nodule is compared with that of the surrounding thyroid parenchyma and the strap muscle (**Fig. 6**). Nodules are described as isoechoic (same shade of gray as the thyroid), hypo-echoic (darker than the thyroid) or markedly hypoechoic (darker than the strap muscle). Hypoechoic and very hypoechoic nodules are classified as suspicious and

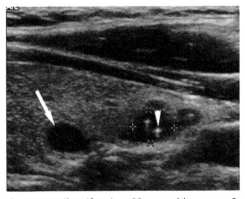

Fig. 2. Colloid cyst with comet tail artifact in a 33-year-old woman. Sagittal US of the right thyroid lobe demonstrates a 7-mm cystic nodule (*between calibers*) with 2 echogenic foci with comet tail artifact (*arrowhead*). This is a benign lesion. Note the second purely cystic nodule (*arrow*).

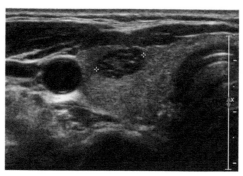

Fig. 3. Cystic nodule with a honeycomb pattern in a 54-year-old woman with hyperparathyroidism. Transverse US of the right thyroid lobe shows a 9-mm nodule (*between calibers*) with multiple small cysts separated by thin echogenic septa, a classic honeycomb pattern associated with benign hyperplastic nodules.

referred for FNAB.[10] Kim and colleagues[10] found that 26.5% of malignant nodules were markedly hypoechoic (see **Fig. 6**) compared with only 5.6% of benign nodules. The underlying histology for these nodules is usually PTC, and it is postulated that the dense cellularity of PTC produces very few interfaces to the sound beam and hence the hypoechoic appearance. Follicular neoplasms, whether benign adenomas or follicular carcinomas, contain colloid, have a microfollicular structure, and usually display an echogenic or mixed echotexture. Pathologically, they are typically encapsulated and tend to be sharply demarcated from the surrounding thyroid parenchyma on US.[14]

Shape

Moon and colleagues[11] reported that an elongated shape as compared with a wide shape, defined as an anteroposterior to transverse ratio of 1 or greater, is highly specific (91.4%) for malignancy. These results confirmed the reports published earlier.[9,10] In another series, nodules with a spherical shape (ratio of long to short axis <1.5) were found to be associated with an 18% risk of cancer.[18] By contrast, a ratio of long to short axis greater than 2.5 was found to have a 100% negative

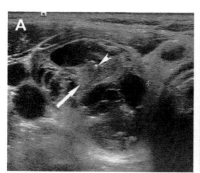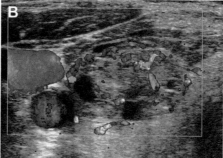

Fig. 4. Adenomatoid nodule presenting as a complex cystic nodule in a 49-year-old woman. (*A*) Transverse US of the right thyroid lobe demonstrates a 3.5-cm complex cystic nodule (*between calibers*). The nodule is predominantly cystic with septations and a solid appearing component (*arrow*). Note echogenic foci with comet tail artifact (*arrowhead*). (*B*) Transverse US of the right thyroid lobe with color Doppler shows vascularity within the solid component. The diagnosis of adenomatoid nodule was confirmed with US-guided FNAB.

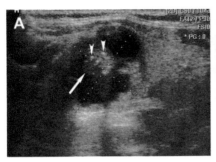
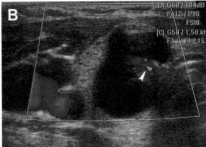

Fig. 5. Cystic PTC in a 51-year-old woman who presented with right neck swelling. (*A*) Sagittal US of the right thyroid lobe shows a 2-cm complex cystic nodule (*between calibers*). There is a large solid component (*arrow*) with tiny echogenic foci suspicious for microcalcifications (*arrowhead*). The solid component was specifically targeted during the FNAB procedure. (*B*) Transverse US of the right thyroid lobe with color Doppler shows some vascularity (*arrowheads*) within the solid component. The diagnosis of PTC was confirmed with US-guided FNAB and surgery.

predictive value for malignancy. It is speculated that cancers tend to grow across tissue planes and assume a spherical shape to maximize their oxygen supply, whereas benign lesions respect normal thyroid parenchyma.

Borders

Predictably, a spiculated or nodular border is associated with a higher probability of malignancy (see **Fig. 6**). Classically, PTC invades the surrounding thyroid tissue and is poorly encapsulated. In the series published by Moon and colleagues,[11] 48.3% of thyroid cancers had spiculated margins and 32.5% had smooth borders, whereas 75.9% of benign nodules had smooth margins and only 8.2% were spiculated. These results confirm findings from previous studies.[10] Demonstration of a refractive shadow from the edge of a solid nodule is another suspicious finding that warrants fine-needle aspiration.[14]

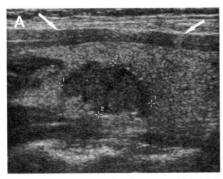
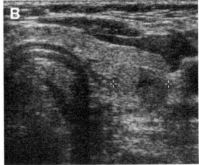

Fig. 6. Right PTC and left adenomatoid nodule in a 37-year-old woman. (*A*) Sagittal US of the right thyroid lobe shows a 1.6-cm markedly hypoechoic nodule (between calibers). Note that the nodule is more hypoechoic than the strap muscle (*arrows*) and that its borders are spiculated. The diagnosis of PTC was confirmed by FNAB. (*B*) Transverse US of the left thyroid lobe shows a 1-cm nodule that is nearly isoechoic to the thyroid gland (between calibers). The diagnosis of adenomatoid nodule was confirmed by fine-needle aspiration.

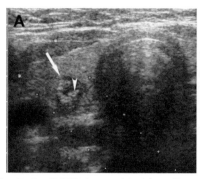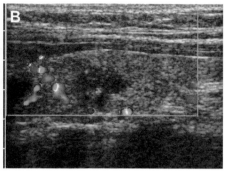

Fig. 7. Small PTC detected incidentally in a 32-year-old woman. (*A*) Transverse US of the right thyroid lobe shows an 8-mm hypoechoic nodule that is taller than is wide (*arrow*). Note tiny echogenic foci compatible with microcalcifications (*arrowhead*). The diagnosis of PTC was confirmed with US-guided FNAB. Despite the small size of this lesion, metastatic cancer was found in 1 node at surgery. (*B*) Sagittal US of the right thyroid lobe with color Doppler shows that the lesion is avascular.

Perinodular Halo

Some thyroid nodules are surrounded by a distinct hypoechoic halo. Although it was initially speculated that this hypoechoic rim represents thyroid parenchyma compressed by a slow-growing and therefore presumably benign process, correlation with histology has shown that follicular adenomas and carcinomas are well encapsulated and may display a well-defined thick hypoechoic rim.[19] In fact, adenomatous (colloid) nodules can be incompletely encapsulated or poorly demarcated from the rest of the thyroid parenchyma.[20] Therefore, the presence of a halo is not a particularly useful sonographic criterion to suggest a benign process.

Calcifications

Calcifications are detected in almost one-third of thyroid nodules. Microcalcifications are defined as punctuate echogenic foci measuring less than 2 mm. Because of their small size, they do not produce acoustic shadowing. Microcalcifications are thought

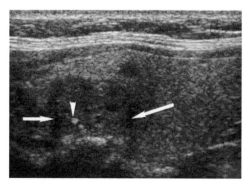

Fig. 8. Classic appearance of PTC in a 52-year-old woman. Sagittal US of the right thyroid lobe shows a well-defined hypoechoic nodule. The nodule contains a few foci of microcalcifications (*arrowhead*). Notice the refracting shadow from the edge of the nodule, another indication that the nodule may be malignant.

to represent the psammoma bodies or calcified laminated nidus that are frequently found in PTC. The presence of microcalcifications in a solid nodule has a high specificity of 91.3% to 96.3% and a positive predictive value of 74.8% for malignancy; unfortunately, the sensitivity is only 29% to 51.4% (**Figs. 7** and **8**).[11,13]

Coarse larger calcifications are caused by areas of degeneration and necrosis within thyroid nodules. On US, these calcifications appear as echogenic foci associated with distal acoustic shadowing. These larger calcifications are found in both benign and malignant nodules, particularly in long-standing goiter and in medullary thyroid cancer (MTC). Thus the presence of coarse calcifications within a hypoechoic solid nodule warrants FNAB.[14]

Vascularity

Color or power Doppler US provides useful additional information in the characterization of solid nodules by depicting nodular vascularity. It is postulated that malignant nodules are more likely to have disorganized internal vascularity and generally thyroid cancers tend to be hypervascular compared with the adjacent thyroid parenchyma (**Fig. 9**). Papini and colleagues[13] defined an intranodular vascular pattern on color Doppler US as most suspicious, with sensitivity of 74.2% and specificity of 80.8%. Benign nodules tend to be avascular or demonstrate only perinodular vascularity. It has also been postulated that power Doppler may be useful because it measures the amplitude of the Doppler signal rather than the mean velocity and is thus more sensitive to slow flow that may be present in small vessels.[21] However, Frates and colleagues[22] found that 14% of malignant nodules were iso- or hypovascular to the rest of the gland (see **Fig. 7**). We have observed that benign nodules may harbor internal vascularity and thus believe that the gray-scale appearance of nodules is more helpful than their internal vascularity in predicting malignancy.

ULTRASOUND DIAGNOSIS OF THYROID NODULES: SUMMARY, CONTROVERSIES, AND CHALLENGES

In spite of the invaluable contribution of thyroid US in the assessment of thyroid nodules, there are many challenges, pitfalls, and controversies that need to be considered.

Multiple Suspicious Sonographic Findings

As shown in **Table 1**, individual sonographic signs are only moderately sensitive and specific for predicting malignancy in solid thyroid nodules, as there can be significant

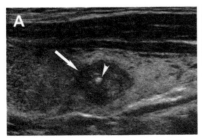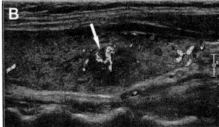

Fig. 9. Vascular MTC in a 36-year-old man with a family history of medullary cancer. (*A*) Sagittal US of the right thyroid lobe shows a hypoechoic nodule (*arrow*) with a coarse central calcification (*arrowhead*). (*B*) Sagittal US of the right thyroid lobe with color Doppler shows a hypervascular hypoechoic nodule (*arrow*). The diagnosis of MTC was confirmed by FNAB of an adjacent node.

overlap with benign processes because almost 70% of histologically proved benign nodules may exhibit 1 suspicious sonographic sign.[23] However, malignant nodules tend to harbor multiple suspicious findings, for example, a mean of 2.6 abnormalities in the study by Kim and colleagues[10] and the additional presence of microcalcifications in a solid hypoechoic nodule that increased the odds ratio of this nodule being malignant from 6.5 to 13.1 in the series published by Nam-Goong and colleagues.[12]

Does Number Matter?

Even in patients referred for a palpable lesion, US can detect additional nodules in 45% of cases.[24] However, the prevalence of thyroid cancer is similar in patients with solitary nodules or multinodular thyroid: in a large population of 1985 patients with single or multiple nodules greater than 1 cm, the prevalence of thyroid cancer was 14.8% in the solitary nodule group and 14.9% in the multinodular group.[25]

Too Small to Biopsy?

There is no correlation between the size of a thyroid nodule and the risk of underlying cancer. The prevalence of thyroid cancer is similar in palpable and nonpalpable nodules, including incidentally discovered nodules measuring 10 mm or less.[13] However, it is unclear whether diagnosis of micro-PTC affects life expectancy or whether microcarcinomas as defined by a size smaller than 1 cm is less aggressive.[26] In a series published by Nam-Goong and colleagues,[12] 69% of patients with incidental PTC had extrathyroidal extension of the tumor or nodal metastases (see **Fig. 7**). Both the ATA and the SRU recommend further workup of nodules greater than 1 cm and careful analysis of the US characteristics listed earlier before formulating a decision to perform FNAB.[6,7] The AACE/Associazione Medici Endocrinologi (AME) guidelines argue against an arbitrary cut off number to avoid missing very small but potentially aggressive tumors.[4] Ultimately, the decision should be individualized, taking into consideration the age of the patient and the presence of comorbidity and risk factors for thyroid cancer, such as a positive family history, multiple endocrine neoplasia type 2 syndrome, or previous head and neck irradiation.

The Special Case of Follicular Neoplasms

The suspicious sonographic appearances described earlier are usually associated with PTC, which represent approximately 70% of all thyroid malignancies. However, follicular neoplasms, which are less common, often do not exhibit classic malignant sonographic features. When comparing PTC with follicular carcinomas, Jeh and colleagues[19] found that 65.2% of follicular cancers were isoechoic to the thyroid parenchyma, 72.7% were oval, and 86.6% had a thin or thick hypoechoic rim. None of the cancers had microcalcifications. Benign follicular adenomas demonstrate similar sonographic findings on gray-scale US. Because a solid, homogeneous oval nodule with a hypoechoic capsule may represent a follicular neoplasm, such a lesion should be referred for fine-needle aspiration (**Fig. 10**).[14] Although some have suggested that follicular carcinomas may exhibit more internal vascularity[27] as compared with follicular adenomas, there is considerable overlap and it is not possible to differentiate the two radiographically or based on cytologic specimen (see **Fig. 10**). Hürthle cell neoplasms are considered to be a variant of follicular cell neoplasms by some investigators, although more recent molecular analyses suggest that they are likely a distinct group of tumors. Their sonographic appearance is similar to that of follicular neoplasms.[28] The follicular variant of PTC, which represents 9% to 22% of PTC, may have a sonographic appearance similar to follicular neoplasms (**Fig. 11**).[29]

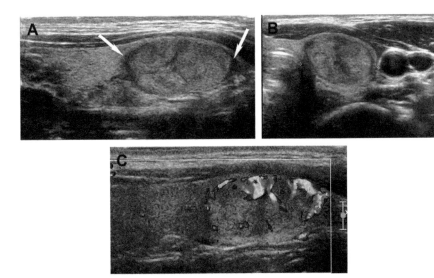

Fig. 10. Follicular neoplasm in a 38-year-old woman. (*A*) Sagittal US of the left thyroid lobe shows an isoechoic solid nodule with well-defined borders and a hypoechoic rim (*arrows*). This appearance is suggestive of a follicular neoplasm and should prompt recommendation for FNAB. (*B*) Transverse US of the left thyroid lobe confirms the findings. (*C*) Sagittal US of the left thyroid lobe with color Doppler shows increased vascularity in the nodule. Fine-needle aspiration yielded the diagnosis of "suspicious for a follicular neoplasm." Final pathology after surgical removal was follicular adenoma.

ULTRASOUND APPEARANCE OF RARE THYROID MALIGNANCIES
Medullary Thyroid Cancer

MTC arises from the calcitonin-secreting C cells and account for approximately 5% of thyroid malignancies. There is a familial form of medullary cancer, and it also affects patients with multiple endocrine neoplasia type II. On US, the appearance of MTC is difficult to differentiate from PTC; most present as a hypoechoic nodule. When calcifications are present, they tend to be coarse and centrally located and may be related to underlying fibrosis and amyloid deposits (see **Fig. 9**).[14] However, MTC can mimic

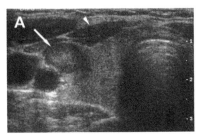
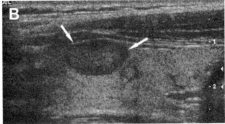

Fig. 11. Follicular variant of PTC in a 47-year-old woman with a history of hyperparathyroidism. (*A*) Transverse US of the right thyroid lobe shows a well-defined oval nodule (*arrow*). The nodule is hypoechoic to the thyroid gland but less hypoechoic than the strap muscle (*arrowhead*). (*B*) Sagittal US of the right thyroid lobe shows that the nodule has a hypoechoic halo (*arrows*). The diagnosis of papillary thyroid cancer, follicular variant was made after surgical removal.

the far more common PTC with internal microcalcifications or appear as a solid non-calcified mass.

Anaplastic Thyroid Cancer

Anaplastic thyroid cancer accounts for 2% of all thyroid cancers, usually affects elderly patients, and is the most aggressive and lethal form of thyroid cancer, with a 5-year mortality of more than 95%. It often presents as a large hypoechoic mass, and invasion of adjacent muscles or the trachea is not uncommon.

Lymphoma and Metastases

Non-Hodgkin lymphoma represents approximately 4% of thyroid cancers and is often associated with Hashimoto thyroiditis. Patients typically present with an enlarging neck mass. On US, it appears as a large hypoechoic, often relatively homogeneous and vascular mass (**Fig. 12**).[30]

Metastases to the thyroid gland are uncommon, with melanoma, breast carcinoma, and renal cell carcinoma being the most common primary tumors.

US EVALUATION OF DIFFUSE THYROID DISEASES

In the evaluation of diffuse thyroid abnormalities, the role of US is generally limited to differentiating multinodular thyroid from other diffuse processes affecting the gland. However, some of these conditions, particularly Hashimoto thyroiditis can be mistaken for nodular diseases by novice imagers.

Hashimoto Thyroiditis

Hashimoto thyroiditis, an autoimmune inflammatory condition, affects 4% of women and is the most common cause of hypothyroidism in the United States.[31] Antibodies to thyroglobulin and to thyroid peroxidase develop and cause gradual thyroid failure. The sonographic appearance of the affected gland reflects the underlying histopathologic changes of diffuse infiltration of the thyroid parenchyma with lymphocytes and fibrosis. The thyroid parenchyma is heterogeneous, peppered with innumerable small hypoechoic nodules measuring a few millimeters and separated by echogenic septae.[14,32] Depending on the stage and duration of the disease, the thyroid may be normal in size, enlarged, or small and vascularity can also be variable. This characteristic sonographic appearance has a 95% positive predictive value for Hashimoto

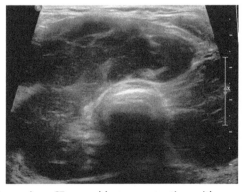

Fig. 12. B-cell lymphoma in a 67-year-old man presenting with a rapidly enlarging neck mass. Transverse US of the thyroid gland shows that the gland is markedly enlarged with hypoechoic parenchyma. The diagnosis of B-cell lymphoma was made by FNAB.

thyroiditis and should not be confused with a multinodular thyroid (**Fig. 13**). The diagnosis is usually confirmed by measuring the levels of serum antithyroglobulin and antithyroid peroxidase antibodies.

However, there are some challenges associated with Hashimoto thyroiditis. Because of the underlying heterogeneity of the thyroid parenchyma, it is more difficult to characterize discrete nodules in these patients. It is, however, imperative to be vigilant and carefully assess any discrete nodules in patients with Hashimoto thyroiditis, particularly women, because of an apparent increased incidence of PTC[31] and lymphoma.

Graves Disease

The diagnosis of Graves disease is based on clinical and laboratory abnormalities, and the role of US is limited to the detection of associated nodules. It is important to carefully evaluate any nodule in these patients, as recent studies seem to indicate an increased incidence of thyroid cancer in patients with Graves disease. In a multicenter study of 557 patients with the disease, 3.8% had PTC.[33]

ULTRASOUND-GUIDED THYROID FINE-NEEDLE ASPIRATION BIOPSY

FNAB of the thyroid plays a crucial role in the characterization of suspicious or indeterminate thyroid nodules. Traditionally, FNAB of a thyroid nodule was performed by palpation; however, FNAB of thyroid nodules is now increasingly being performed with US guidance. Carmeci and colleagues[34] found that the rate of obtaining a nondiagnostic sample was decreased to 7% when using US guidance as compared with 16% when using the palpation technique. The following advantages justify the current shift toward US guidance.[35]

1. Nodules discovered incidentally on imaging are often nonpalpable and can only be accessed with US.
2. Even in palpable nodules, it may be beneficial to target specific areas; this is particularly important in partially cystic nodules, in which case it is critical to biopsy the solid component to improve diagnostic yield.
3. In large solid nodules, US guidance ensures that different areas of the nodule are sampled.
4. The accuracy of US-guided FNAB reported in the literature varies from 85% to 94%.

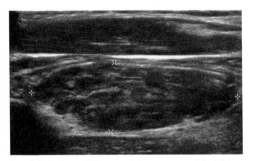

Fig. 13. Hashimoto thyroiditis in a 38-year-old woman with history of hypothyroidism. Sagittal US of the right thyroid lobe demonstrates a heterogeneous echotexture of the right lobe with innumerable hypoechoic nodules separated by echogenic septa.

Technique

Several techniques of US guidance and tissue sampling are used in standard practice. Once the appropriate nodule is identified, some operators use the freehand technique, whereby the US transducer is placed over the nodule and the needle is inserted next to the transducer, whereas others use a fixed needle guide attached to the transducer to introduce the needle (needle guide technique). Once the needle is inserted, the stylet is removed and the needle is moved rapidly within the target. Typically, 7 to 10 incursions are made till a flash of bloody fluid is seen within the needle hub.

In addition to the various techniques used for needle insertion, 2 aspiration techniques can be used. In the capillary method, no suction is applied and the sample is obtained by capillary action. Theoretically, this method minimizes trauma to the tissue and may decrease contamination by blood, especially if the nodule is very vascular. Some operators favor the suction technique, applying 3 to 5 mL of suction via a syringe attached to the FNAB needle. This method may be slightly more cumbersome and allow slightly less control over needle motion but may yield more cells if the nodule is fibrotic. A recent study compared both techniques in 180 samples and found no statistically significant difference in diagnostic accuracy between the 2 methods.[36]

At our institution, we favor the needle guide technique and capillary sampling method. We use a 25-gauge 9-cm long needle and infiltrate the skin with 1% buffered lidocaine before FNAB to minimize any patient discomfort, anticipating that a minimum of 3 samples will be required from each site. A trained cytopathologist or cytopathology technician is always available on-site to evaluate the adequacy of the sample at the time of biopsy.

NEW HORIZONS: ELASTOGRAPHY AND THE ROLE OF PREOPERATIVE NECK US IN PATIENTS WITH THYROID CANCER

In recent years, 2 additional techniques have emerged in the armamentarium of evaluating thyroid nodules and their utility is currently being debated in the literature.

Role of Preoperative Neck US in Patients with Thyroid Cancer

The value of neck US in the detection of local recurrences and cervical nodal metastases after total thyroidectomy for well-differentiated thyroid cancer is well established. Although PTC is a relatively indolent malignancy, it is associated with a relatively high incidence of local recurrences occurring in 30% of patients after initial thyroidectomy. In an attempt to diminish the risk of cervical metastases, several additions to standard thyroidectomy have been proposed, including central compartment nodal dissection and lateral neck dissection in patients with biopsy-proven cervical node metastases at the time of initial diagnosis. Thus, preoperative neck US has a role in surgical planning, as was documented in 6% of patients in the series by Kouvaraki and colleagues.[37] In addition, patients with positive nodes at the time of initial surgery are at higher risk of recurrences in the future.[38] Patients with MTC have an even higher incidence of nodal metastases at the time of diagnosis, reported to reach 32% to 80%.[39] Based on these data, the ATA has recommended preoperative neck US in patients with MTC in its most recent guidelines.[40]

The sonographic appearance of suspicious cervical nodes include a lack of the normal echogenic hilum, a round shape, the presence of intranodular microcalcification or cystic areas, and increased vascularity by color Doppler (**Fig. 14**).[41]

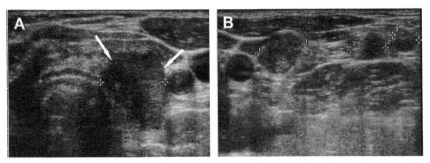

Fig. 14. Lateral compartment nodal metastases in a 64-year-old patient with a suspicious thyroid nodule. (*A*) Transverse US of the left thyroid lobe shows a large hypoechoic mass (*arrows*). The mass is taller than is wide, has nodular borders, and thus is highly suspicious for malignancy. (*B*) Transverse US of the left neck, level III shows 3 round heterogeneous nodes without a fatty hilum. FNAB of the thyroid nodule and one of the nodes yielded cells diagnostic for medullary thyroid carcinoma.

Elastography

Ultrasound elastography is used to evaluate tissue stiffness noninvasively. As a steady pressure is applied to the thyroid gland, the degree of deformity of the underlying tissue is measured. This technique takes advantage of the fact that malignant nodules tend to be harder than benign nodules and thus deform less compared with the surrounding normal thyroid parenchyma (**Fig. 15**). Two recent studies have shown a statistically significant higher tissue stiffness index in malignant nodules as compared with normal tissue and benign nodules, with a sensitivity of approximately 88% and specificity of 77.5% to 90%.[42,43] Applications of this technique may be limited to papillary thyroid cancer, which was the primary tumor evaluated in the prior studies; thus, the findings may not be applicable to other thyroid tumor types. Another limitation to this technique is that it is operator dependent and requires operator expertise. Larger studies are warranted before elastography can be routinely included in the evaluation of thyroid nodules.

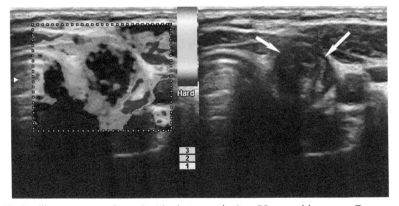

Fig. 15. Papillary cancer evaluated with elastography in a 56-year-old woman. Transverse US of the left thyroid lobe shows a hypoechoic nodule. Elastography shows that the nodule displays predominantly a blue shade indicating that it is stiffer then the surrounding normal thyroid. FNAB of the thyroid nodule yielded cells diagnostic for papillary thyroid cancer.

SUMMARY

US remains the optimal imaging modality for the detection and characterization of thyroid nodules. Careful analysis of key sonographic features as described earlier allow for more appropriate selection of indeterminate or suspicious nodules that should be referred for FNAB. US is also being increasingly used to guide FNAB, as it has been shown to improve diagnostic yield and is indispensable when obtaining biopsies of an increasing number of nodules which are subcentimeter in size.

The larger question remains, however, as to whether the exhaustive workup of incidentally detected thyroid nodules leading to the diagnosis and treatment of asymptomatic micropapillary thyroid cancers ultimately affects survival and justifies the costs and associated potential risks. With regards to thyroid incidentaloma, it is unclear if we have moved beyond, in the words of Dr Topliss, "the ignorant in the pursuit of the impalpable."[44]

REFERENCES

1. Mortensen JD, Woolner LB, Bennett WA. Gross and microscopic findings in clinically normal thyroid glands. J Clin Endocrinol Metab 1955;15(10):1270–80.
2. Hegedus L. Clinical practice. The thyroid nodule. N Engl J Med 2004;351(17): 1764–71.
3. Jemal A, Siegel R, Ward E, et al. Cancer statistics, 2008. CA Cancer J Clin 2008; 58(2):71–96.
4. Gharib H, Papini E, Valcavi R, et al. American Association of Clinical Endocrinologists and Associazione Medici Endocrinologi medical guidelines for clinical practice for the diagnosis and management of thyroid nodules. Endocr Pract 2006;12(1):63–102.
5. Gharib H, Goellner JR. Fine-needle aspiration biopsy of the thyroid: an appraisal. Ann Intern Med 1993;118(4):282–9.
6. Cooper DS, Doherty GM, Haugen BR, et al. Management guidelines for patients with thyroid nodules and differentiated thyroid cancer. Thyroid 2006;16(2): 109–42.
7. Frates MC, Benson CB, Charboneau JW, et al. Management of thyroid nodules detected at US: Society of Radiologists in Ultrasound consensus conference statement. Radiology 2005;237(3):794–800.
8. Takashima S, Fukuda H, Nomura N, et al. Thyroid nodules: re-evaluation with ultrasound. J Clin Ultrasound 1995;23:179–84.
9. Cappelli C, Castellano M, Pirola I, et al. Thyroid nodule shape suggests malignancy. Eur J Endocrinol 2006;155(1):27–31.
10. Kim EK, Park CS, Chung WY, et al. New sonographic criteria for recommending fine-needle aspiration biopsy of nonpalpable solid nodules of the thyroid. AJR Am J Roentgenol 2002;178(3):687–91.
11. Moon WJ, Jung SL, Lee JH, et al. Benign and malignant thyroid nodules: US differentiation–multicenter retrospective study. Radiology 2008;247(3): 762–70.
12. Nam-Goong IS, Kim HY, Gong G, et al. Ultrasonography-guided fine-needle aspiration of thyroid incidentaloma: correlation with pathological findings. Clin Endocrinol (Oxf) 2004;60(1):21–8.
13. Papini E, Guglielmi R, Bianchini A, et al. Risk of malignancy in nonpalpable thyroid nodules: predictive value of ultrasound and color-Doppler features. J Clin Endocrinol Metab 2002;87(5):1941–6.

14. Reading CC, Charboneau JW, Hay ID, et al. Sonography of thyroid nodules: a "classic pattern" diagnostic approach. Ultrasound Q 2005;21(3):157–65.
15. Moon WJ, Kwag HJ, Na DG. Are there any specific ultrasound findings of nodular hyperplasia ("leave me alone" lesion) to differentiate it from follicular adenoma? Acta Radiol 2009;50(4):383–8.
16. Layfield LJ, Cibas ES, Gharib H, et al. Thyroid aspiration cytology: current status. CA Cancer J Clin 2009;59(2):99–110.
17. Hatabu H, Kasagi K, Yamamoto K, et al. Cystic papillary carcinoma of the thyroid gland: a new sonographic sign. Clin Radiol 1991;43(2):121–4.
18. Alexander EK, Marqusee E, Orcutt J, et al. Thyroid nodule shape and prediction of malignancy. Thyroid 2004;14(11):953–8.
19. Jeh SK, Jung SL, Kim BS, et al. Evaluating the degree of conformity of papillary carcinoma and follicular carcinoma to the reported ultrasonographic findings of malignant thyroid tumor. Korean J Radiol 2007;8(3):192–7.
20. Mazzaferri EL. Management of a solitary thyroid nodule. N Engl J Med 1993; 328(8):553–9.
21. Cerbone G, Spiezia S, Colao A, et al. Power Doppler improves the diagnostic accuracy of color Doppler ultrasonography in cold thyroid nodules: follow-up results. Horm Res 1999;52(1):19–24.
22. Frates MC, Benson CB, Doubilet PM, et al. Can color Doppler sonography aid in the prediction of malignancy of thyroid nodules? J Ultrasound Med 2003;22(2): 127–31 [quiz: 132–4].
23. Wienke JR, Chong WK, Fielding JR, et al. Sonographic features of benign thyroid nodules: interobserver reliability and overlap with malignancy. J Ultrasound Med 2003;22(10):1027–31.
24. Mandel SJ. Diagnostic use of ultrasonography in patients with nodular thyroid disease. Endocr Pract 2004;10(3):246–52.
25. Frates MC, Benson CB, Doubilet PM, et al. Prevalence and distribution of carcinoma in patients with solitary and multiple thyroid nodules on sonography. J Clin Endocrinol Metab 2006;91(9):3411–7.
26. Kim JY, Lee CH, Kim SY, et al. Radiologic and pathologic findings of nonpalpable thyroid carcinomas detected by ultrasonography in a medical screening center. J Ultrasound Med 2008;27(2):215–23.
27. Fukunari N, Nagahama M, Sugino K, et al. Clinical evaluation of color Doppler imaging for the differential diagnosis of thyroid follicular lesions. World J Surg 2004;28(12):1261–5.
28. Maizlin ZV, Wiseman SM, Vora P, et al. Hurthle cell neoplasms of the thyroid: sonographic appearance and histologic characteristics. J Ultrasound Med 2008; 27(5):751–7 [quiz: 759].
29. Yoon JH, Kim EK, Hong SW, et al. Sonographic features of the follicular variant of papillary thyroid carcinoma. J Ultrasound Med 2008;27(10):1431–7.
30. Kwak JY, Kim EK, Ko KH, et al. Primary thyroid lymphoma: role of ultrasound-guided needle biopsy. J Ultrasound Med 2007;26(12):1761–5.
31. Repplinger D, Bargren A, Zhang YW, et al. Is Hashimoto's thyroiditis a risk factor for papillary thyroid cancer? J Surg Res 2008;150(1):49–52.
32. Yeh HC, Futterweit W, Gilbert P. Micronodulation: ultrasonographic sign of Hashimoto thyroiditis. J Ultrasound Med 1996;15(12):813–9.
33. Kraimps JL, Bouin-Pineau MH, Mathonnet M, et al. Multicentre study of thyroid nodules in patients with Graves' disease. Br J Surg 2000;87(8):1111–3.
34. Carmeci C, Jeffrey RB, McDougall IR, et al. Ultrasound-guided fine-needle aspiration biopsy of thyroid masses. Thyroid 1998;8(4):283–9.

35. Tublin ME, Martin JA, Rollin LJ, et al. Ultrasound-guided fine-needle aspiration versus fine-needle capillary sampling biopsy of thyroid nodules: does technique matter? J Ultrasound Med 2007;26(12):1697–701.
36. Schoedel KE, Tublin ME, Pealer K, et al. Ultrasound-guided biopsy of the thyroid: a comparison of technique with respect to diagnostic accuracy. Diagn Cytopathol 2008;36(11):787–9.
37. Kouvaraki MA, Shapiro SE, Fornage BD, et al. Role of preoperative ultrasonography in the surgical management of patients with thyroid cancer. Surgery 2003;134(6):946–54 [discussion: 954–5].
38. Davidson HC, Park BJ, Johnson JT. Papillary thyroid cancer: controversies in the management of neck metastasis. Laryngoscope 2008;118(12):2161–5.
39. Ball DW. American Thyroid Association guidelines for management of medullary thyroid cancer: an adult endocrinology perspective. Thyroid 2009;19(6):547–50.
40. Kloos RT, Eng C, Evans DB, et al. Medullary thyroid cancer: management guidelines of the American Thyroid Association. Thyroid 2009;19(6):565–612.
41. Sheth S, Hamper UM. Role of sonography after total thyroidectomy for thyroid cancer. Ultrasound Q 2008;24(3):147–54.
42. Hong Y, Liu X, Li Z, et al. Real-time ultrasound elastography in the differential diagnosis of benign and malignant thyroid nodules. J Ultrasound Med 2009; 28(7):861–7.
43. Dighe M, Bae U, Richardson ML, et al. Differential diagnosis of thyroid nodules with US elastography using carotid artery pulsation. Radiology 2008;248(2): 662–9.
44. Topliss D. Thyroid incidentaloma: the ignorant in pursuit of the impalpable. Clin Endocrinol (Oxf) 2004;60(1):18–20.

Fine-Needle Aspiration in the Work-Up of Thyroid Nodules

Edmund S. Cibas, MD

KEYWORDS

- Thyroid • Fine-needle aspiration • Cytology
- Indications • Terminology

Fine-needle aspiration (FNA) plays an essential role in the evaluation of patients with a thyroid nodule. It helps to minimize unnecessary thyroid surgery for patients with benign nodules and appropriately triages patients with thyroid cancer to surgery. Before the routine use of thyroid FNA, the percentage of surgically resected thyroid nodules that were malignant was 14%.[1] With current thyroid FNA practice, the percentage of resected nodules that are malignant exceeds 50%.[2]

In October 2007, the National Cancer Institute (NCI) sponsored a multidisciplinary conference in Bethesda, Maryland, to review the state of the science of FNA in the management of thyroid nodules. After the meeting, several summary documents were published.[3–6] This article draws heavily on the conclusions reached at that conference.

INDICATIONS FOR FNA

Thyroid nodules are identified by palpation or by an imaging study. Every patient with a palpable thyroid nodule is a candidate for FNA and should undergo further evaluation to determine if an FNA is warranted.[7–9] Before the decision is made to perform an FNA, a serum thyrotropin level and thyroid ultrasound (US) should be obtained.[7,9–12] Patients with a normal or elevated serum thyrotropin level should proceed to a thyroid US to determine if an FNA needs to be performed. Those with a depressed serum thyrotropin level should have a radionuclide thyroid scan, the results of which should be correlated with sonographic findings.[7,9–11,13] In general, functioning thyroid nodules in the absence of significant clinical findings do not require an FNA because the incidence of malignancy is exceedingly low.[14] A nodule that appears iso- or

Department of Pathology, Brigham and Women's Hospital, 75 Francis Street, Boston, MA 02115, USA
E-mail address: ecibas@partners.org

Otolaryngol Clin N Am 43 (2010) 257–271
doi:10.1016/j.otc.2010.01.003
0030-6665/10/$ – see front matter © 2010 Elsevier Inc. All rights reserved.

hypofunctioning on radionuclide scan should be considered for FNA based on US findings.[7–9]

Incidental thyroid nodules (incidentalomas) are detected by fluorodeoxyglucose–positron emission tomography ([18]FDG-PET), sestamibi, US, CT, and MRI scans. Incidentalomas detected by [18]FDG-PET are unusual (2%–3% of all PET scans) but have a higher risk of cancer (14%–50%) compared with the background incidence.[15–23] A focally [18]FDG-PET–avid thyroid nodule is more likely to be a primary thyroid cancer than metastatic disease to the thyroid, even in patients with an extrathyroidal malignancy. Therefore, a focal nodule that is [18]FDG-PET avid is an indication for FNA. This applies only to focal lesions. Diffuse increased uptake on [18]FDG-PET does not warrant FNA unless thyroid sonography detects a discrete nodule.

All focal hot nodules detected on sestamibi scans and confirmed by US to be a discrete nodule should undergo FNA. Thyroid incidentalomas detected on sestamibi scans have a higher risk of cancer (22%–66%).[24–28]

Incidentalomas detected by US (such as carotid Doppler scans or scans done for parathyroid disease) have a cancer risk of approximately 10% to 15% (range 0%–29%)[29–40] and should undergo dedicated thyroid sonographic evaluation. Lesions with a maximum diameter greater than 1.0 to 1.5 cm should be considered for biopsy unless they are simple cysts or septated cysts with no solid elements. FNA may also occasionally be replaced by periodic follow-up for nodules of borderline size (between 1.0 and 1.5 cm in maximum diameter) if they have sonographic features that are strongly associated with benign cytology.

A nodule of any size with sonographically suspicious features should also be considered for FNA. Sonographically suspicious features include microcalcifications, hypoechoic solid nodules, irregular/lobulated margins, intranodular vascularity, and nodal metastases (or signs of extracapsular spread). This recommendation is controversial because it includes patients with microcarcinomas, in whom a survival benefit after an FNA diagnosis has not been documented. Nevertheless, the American Thyroid Association,[7] the Academy of Clinical Thyroidologists,[29] and a collaborative effort of the American Association of Clinical Endocrinologists and the Associazione Medici Endocrinologi[41] have outlined this recommendation.[3] There are several reasons for this. If a sonographically suspicious nodule is benign by FNA, a patient can be reassured and subsequent follow-up can be less frequent.[42] On the contrary, if an FNA reveals that a nodule is malignant, surgery is generally recommended. The natural history of micropapillary carcinomas, however, is not well understood. Most remain indolent, as implied by the 13% prevalence of micropapillary cancers in the United States diagnosed at autopsy examination.[43] A minority follow a more aggressive course; this subgroup might be identified by sonographic evidence of lateral cervical node metastases, tumor multifocality, extrathyroidal invasion, or cytopathologic features that suggest a high-grade malignancy.[44] The development and application of even more sensitive and specific markers of aggressive potential (including molecular and genetic markers) may one day facilitate the triage of patients with a microcarcinoma.

There are few direct data on the cancer risk of thyroid incidentalomas detected by CT or MRI. Thyroid incidentalomas are seen in at least 16% of patients evaluated by neck CT or MRI.[45] The risk of cancer in one study was predicted at 10%, but it included only a few patients who went on to FNA.[46] CT and MRI features cannot determine the risk of malignancy, except in advanced cases that are unlikely to be incidental. Until more data are available, incidentalomas seen on CT or MRI should undergo dedicated thyroid sonographic evaluation. Any nodule with sonographically suspicious features (discussed previously) should be considered for FNA. In addition, lesions that have a maximum diameter greater than 1.0 to 1.5 cm should also be considered for FNA (discussed previously).

PERFORMING THE FNA

FNA can be performed using palpation or US for guidance. The benefits of palpation-guided FNA of thyroid nodules are reduced cost in comparison with US-guided FNA and logistical efficiency: a practitioner can perform the procedure without a US machine or assistance from other practitioners. US evaluation and US guidance, however, can reduce the rates of nondiagnostic and false-negative aspirates and can change the management in 63% of patients with palpable thyroid nodules.[47–52] US also allows sampling from solid areas of partially cystic lesions, accounting for some increase in adequacy.[53]

In general, US guidance is an equally adequate or at times superior alternative to palpation guidance because it ensures that a discrete nodule or solid component of a cystic lesion is present before aspiration, permits operators to be certain that a nodule of interest is aspirated by direct imaging, and avoids passing the needle into critical structures in the neck. In particular, US guidance should be used to aspirate nodules that are not palpable and nodules that have an appreciable (>25%) cystic component. US guidance should also be used if a prior aspiration contained insufficient cells/colloid for interpretation (nondiagnostic result).

TECHNIQUE

The principles of thyroid FNA technique are identical whether or not the needle is inserted using palpation or US for guidance.[54] Commonly available 22- to 27-gauge needles are used for thyroid FNA, but 25- to 27-gauge needles are preferred because the specimens obtained with them tend to be less bloody and are just as cellular (if not more so). A variety of syringe holders are available (Cameco Syringe Pistol, Tao instrument, and Inrad Aspiration Biopsy Syringe Gun), but the intrinsic suction provided by surface tension with smaller diameter needles often makes devices for additional suction unnecessary.

When visualized with US imaging, different areas of large masses should be sampled. If the nodule is complex, the wall, solid elements, and suspicious calcified areas should be sampled while avoiding cystic areas. As a starting point, a dwell time of 2 to 5 seconds within the nodule, with 3 forward and back oscillations per second, usually maximizes cell yield, minimizes blood contamination, and efficiently produces 1 to 2 slides per biopsy pass. The relatively short dwell time (2–5 seconds) per pass that is recommended is not intuitive, but experience has shown that longer dwell times do not offer any significant advantage and often merely dilute the sample with excessive blood. Between 2 and 5 passes per nodule seems reasonable number to optimize the likelihood of obtaining an adequate sample.

Most thyroid FNAs are well tolerated and are not associated with significant patient discomfort or pain. The use of local anesthesia, however, assures that the procedure is not painful and offers peace of mind, resulting in an overall more comfortable experience. For this reason, some experienced FNA physicians use local anesthesia for all thyroid FNAs. Local anesthetic may cause difficulty in subsequent sample evaluation, however. For deep, nonpalpable thyroid nodules that may require more time and probing to reach the nodule, and for all biopsies using needles other than a fine needle, local anesthesia is recommended. The local anesthetic of choice is 1% lidocaine or lidocaine 2% with 1:100,000 epinephrine. Approximately 0.5 mL of anesthetic should be injected into the subcutaneous tissue overlying the area of directed needle place-ment for biopsy.[54]

Aspirated tissue or cyst fluid may be directly smeared on glass slides for air-dried or alcohol-fixed preparations stained by the Romanowsky or Papanicolaou technique, respectively. Liquid-based cytology (LBC) processing can be used alone or as a supplement to direct smears. For LBC, the aspiration needle should be flushed with a small amount (approximately 0.5 mL) of liquid (CytoLyt, CytoRich Red, balanced saline, or Hanks solution) and placed in a Falcon tube for transport to a laboratory. For remote transport or for specimens expected to have delayed processing, a fixative, such as PreservCyt, is necessary for optimal cell preservation. Cell-rich liquid speci-mens can also be used for cell block preparation when needed. Residual cyst fluid may be submitted to a laboratory fresh or fixed for further processing by LBC or cell block. Direct smears, however, are essential for immediate assessment.

INFORMATION REQUIRED ON THE REQUISITION FORM THAT ACCOMPANIES A THYROID FNA

Federal regulations in the United States require that certain identifying information be provided to laboratories with all specimens submitted for laboratory testing,[55] including

- Name and address of person requesting the test
- Patient's name or unique identifier
- Patient's gender
- Patient's age or date of birth
- Name of the test to be performed
- Specimen source
- Date of specimen collection
- Any additional relevant information.

The additional relevant information that a laboratory needs to properly evaluate a thyroid FNA specimen was considered at the 2007 NCI conference.[3] To facilitate cytologic interpretation or histologic correlation (in the case of a subsequent surgical specimen), it was concluded that, at a minimum, the following data should appear on the requisition form that accompanies a thyroid FNA to a laboratory:

1. Usual required data for laboratory test submission (discussed previously)
2. Location of the nodule
3. Size of the nodule
4. History of hypothyroidism, autoimmune thyroiditis, or a positive test for antithy-roid antibodies
5. History of Graves disease
6. History of ^{131}I or external radiation therapy
7. Personal history of cancer
8. Family history of thyroid cancer.

REPORTING TERMINOLOGY—THE BETHESDA SYSTEM

It is critical that pathologists communicate thyroid FNA interpretations to referring physicians in terms that are succinct, unambiguous, and clinically helpful. Historically, terminology for thyroid FNA has varied significantly from one laboratory to another, creating confusion and hindering the sharing of clinically meaningful data among multiple institutions.

The 2007 NCI Thyroid Fine Needle Aspiration State of the Science Conference participants acknowledged the importance of developing a uniform terminology for reporting thyroid FNA results. The discussions and conclusions regarding terminology and morphologic criteria from the NCI meeting, summarized in the publications by Baloch and colleagues,[4,6] form the framework of the terminology presented in this article and in atlas form, called The Bethesda System for Reporting Thyroid Cytopathology (TBSRTC).[56] It is intended as a flexible framework that can be modified to suit the needs of the particular laboratory and the patients it serves.

Format of TBSRTC

For clarity of communication, TBSRTC recommends that each report begin with 1 of 6 general diagnostic categories (**Table 1**). Some categories have 2 options as names; a consensus was not reached at the NCI conference on a single name for these categories. Each of the categories has an implied cancer risk (ranging from 0% to 3% for the benign category to virtually 100% for the malignant category) that links it to a rational clinical management guideline (**Table 2**).

For some of the general categories, some degree of subcategorization can be informative and is often appropriate; recommended terminology is shown in **Table 1**.

Table 1
The Bethesda System for Reporting Thyroid Cytopathology: recommended diagnostic categories

I. Nondiagnostic or unsatisfactory
  CFO
  Virtually acellular specimen
  Other (obscuring blood, clotting artifact, etc)

II. Benign
  Consistent with a BFN (includes adenomatoid nodule, colloid nodule, etc)
  Consistent with lymphocytic (Hashimoto) thyroiditis in the proper clinical context
  Consistent with granulomatous (subacute) thyroiditis
  Other

III. Atypia of undetermined significance or follicular lesion of undetermined significance

IV. Follicular neoplasm or suspicious for a follicular neoplasm
  Specify if Hürthle cell (oncocytic) type

V. Suspicious for malignancy
  Suspicious for papillary carcinoma
  Suspicious for medullary carcinoma
  Suspicious for metastatic carcinoma
  Suspicious for lymphoma
  Other

VI. Malignant
  PTC
  Poorly differentiated carcinoma
  Medullary thyroid carcinoma
  Undifferentiated (anaplastic) carcinoma
  Squamous cell carcinoma
  Carcinoma with mixed features (specify)
  Metastatic carcinoma
  Non-Hodgkin lymphoma
  Other

From Ali SZ, Cibas ES, editors. The Bethesda System for Reporting Thyroid Cytopathology: definitions, criteria and explanatory notes. New York: Springer; 2009; with permission.

Table 2
The Bethesda System for Reporting Thyroid Cytopathology: implied risk of malignancy and recommended clinical management

Diagnostic Category	Risk of Malignancy (%)	Usual Management[a]
I. Nondiagnostic or unsatisfactory	—[b]	Repeat FNA with US guidance
II. Benign	0%–3%	Clinical follow-up
III. Atypia of undetermined significance or follicular lesion of undetermined significance	~5%–15%[c]	Repeat FNA
IV. Follicular neoplasm or suspicious for a follicular neoplasm	15%–30%	Surgical lobectomy
V. Suspicious for malignancy	60%–75%	Near-total thyroidectomy or surgical lobectomy[d]
VI. Malignant	97%–99%	Near-total thyroidectomy[d]

[a] Actual management may depend on other factors (eg, clinical or sonographic) besides the FNA interpretation.
[b] See text for discussion.
[c] Estimate extrapolated from histopathologic data from patients with repeated atypicals. (*Data from* Yang J, Schnadig V, Logrono R, et al. Fine-needle aspiration of thyroid nodules: a study of 4703 patients with histologic and clinical correlations. Cancer 2007;111:306–15; and Yassa L, Cibas ES, Benson CB, et al. Long-term assessment of a multidisciplinary approach to thyroid nodule diagnostic evaluation. Cancer 2007;111:508–16.)
[d] In the case of suspicious for metastatic tumor or a malignant interpretation indicating metastatic tumor rather than a primary thyroid malignancy, surgery may not be indicated.
Modified from Ali SZ, Cibas ES, editors. The Bethesda System for Reporting Thyroid Cytopathology: definitions, criteria and explanatory notes. New York: Springer; 2009; with permission.

Additional descriptive comments (beyond such subcategorization) are optional and left to the discretion of the cytopathologist.

Nondiagnostic or Unsatisfactory

Every thyroid FNA must be evaluated for adequacy. Inadequate samples are reported as nondiagnostic (ND) or unsatisfactory (UNS). This category applies to specimens that are UNS due to obscuring blood, overly thick smears, air-drying of alcohol-fixed smears, or an inadequate number of follicular cells. For a thyroid FNA specimen to be satisfactory for evaluation (and benign), at least 6 groups of benign follicular cells are required, each group composed of at least 10 cells.[57,58]

There are several exceptions to the numerical requirement of benign follicular cells. Any specimen that contains abundant colloid is considered adequate (and benign), even if 6 groups of follicular cells are not identified: a sparsely cellular specimen with abundant colloid is, by implication, a predominantly macrofollicular nodule and, therefore, almost certainly benign. Whenever a specific diagnosis (eg, lymphocytic thyroiditis) can be rendered and whenever there is any atypia, the specimen is, by definition, adequate for evaluation. ND/UNS results occur in 2% to 20% of cases but ideally should be limited to no more than 10% of thyroid FNAs, excluding samples exclusively composed of macrophages.[8,59,60]

Specimens that consist only of cyst contents (macrophages) are problematic. Many laboratories have traditionally considered a macrophages-only sample UNS and included them in the ND/UNS category, with the understanding that, because the parenchyma of the nodule has not been sampled, a cystic papillary carcinoma cannot be excluded. In such laboratories, macrophages-only samples often constituted the great majority of ND/UNS cases, with rates that ranged from 15% to 30%.[2,59,61,62] Other laboratories considered the risk of a false-negative result negligible and reported macrophages-only samples as benign.[60,61] At the 2007 NCI conference, it was decided that cyst fluid–only (CFO) cases should be considered a clearly identified subset of ND/UNS. The significance (and clinical value) of a CFO result depends in large part on sonographic correlation. If the nodule is almost entirely cystic with no worrisome sonographic features, an endocrinologist might proceed as if the CFO were a benign result. On the other hand, it might be clinically equivalent to a ND result if the sonographic features are worrisome and an endocrinologist is not convinced that the sample is representative. In a study that segregated CFO cases and analyzed them separately, the risk of malignancy for a CFO sample was 4%.[59] The risk of malignancy for ND/UNS (not including CFO) is 1% to 4%.[8,59,60]

A repeat aspiration with US guidance is recommended for ND/UNS, including the clinically/sonographically worrisome CFO cases, and is diagnostic in 50% to 88% of cases,[2,57,59,61,63,64] but some nodules remain persistently ND/UNS. Surgical excision is considered for persistently ND/UNS nodules because approximately 10% prove malignant.[63]

Unless specified as ND/UNS, the FNA is considered adequate for evaluation; an explicit statement of adequacy is optional.

Benign

The benefit of a thyroid FNA derives in large part from the ability to make a reliably benign interpretation that avoids unnecessary surgery. A benign result is obtained in 60% to 70% of thyroid FNAs. Descriptive comments that follow are used to subclassify the benign interpretation. The term, *benign follicular nodule (BFN)*, applies to the most common benign pattern: an adequately cellular specimen comprised of varying proportions of colloid and benign follicular cells arranged as macrofollicles and macrofollicle fragments (**Fig. 1**). If resected, virtually all BFNs turn out to be nodules of a multinodular goiter (MNG) or follicular adenomas (FAs). This distinction cannot be made by FNA and is of no consequence to patients. The false-negative rate of a benign interpretation is low (0%–3%),[2,62] but patients are nevertheless followed with repeat assessment by palpation or US at 6- to 18-month intervals.[42] If a nodule shows significant growth or suspicious sonographic changes, a repeat FNA is considered.

Other benign subcategories include consistent with lymphocytic (hashimoto) thyroiditis in the proper clinical context and consistent with granulomatous (subacute) thyroiditis. This is a partial list and does not include a variety of other benign conditions, such as infections and amyloid goiter, that are occasionally sampled by FNA. Additional benign findings (eg, black thyroid, reactive changes, radiation changes, or cyst-lining cells) can be mentioned as descriptive diagnoses at the discretion of pathologists.

Atypia of Undetermined Significance or Follicular Lesion of Undetermined Significance

Some thyroid FNAs are not easily classified into the benign, suspicious, or malignant categories. Such cases represent a minority of thyroid FNAs and in TBSRTC are reported as atypia of undetermined significance (AUS) or follicular lesion of undetermined significance (FLUS). The necessity for this category was debated at the NCI conference, after which a vote (limited to the clinicians in attendance) was taken, and the majority voted in favor of this category.

The heterogeneity of this category precludes outlining all scenarios for which an AUS interpretation is appropriate. The most common scenarios are described in the TBSRTC atlas.[56]

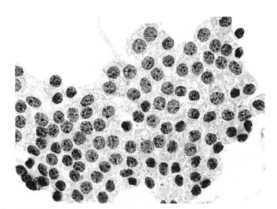

Fig. 1. Benign. The follicular cells in a BFN (eg, MNG and some FAs) are often arranged in a flat sheet that represents a fragmented macrofollicle. Note the even spacing of the cells, the uniformly round nuclei, and the coarsely textured chromatin, all characteristic features of a benign thyroid nodule.

An AUS result is obtained in 3% to 6% of thyroid FNAs.[2,60] Higher rates likely represent an overuse of this category when other interpretations are more appropriate. The recommended management is clinical correlation and a repeat FNA at an appropriate interval.[2,42] In most cases, a repeat FNA results in a more definitive interpretation; only about 20% of nodules are repeatedly AUS.[2] In some cases, however, a physician may choose not to repeat the FNA but follow the nodule clinically or, alternatively, refer a patient for surgery because of concerning clinical or sonographic features.

The risk of malignancy for an AUS nodule is difficult to ascertain because only a minority of cases in this category have surgical follow-up. Those that are resected represent a selected population of patients with repeatedly AUS results or patients with worrisome clinical or sonographic findings. In this selected population, 20% to 25% of patients with AUS prove to have cancer after surgery, but this is undoubtedly an overestimate of the risk for all AUS interpretations.[2,60] The risk of malignancy is certainly lower and probably closer to 5% to 15%. An effort should be made to use this category as a last resort and limit its use to approximately 7% or fewer of all thyroid FNAs.

Follicular Neoplasm or Suspicious for Follicular Neoplasm

The purpose of this diagnostic category is to identify a nodule that might be a follicular carcinoma (FC) and triage it for surgical lobectomy. FNA is diagnostic of many thyroid conditions (eg, papillary carcinoma or lymphocytic thyroiditis), but, with regard to FC, it is better considered a screening test. FCs have cytomorphologic features that distinguish them from BFNs. Although these cytomorphologic features do not permit distinction from a FA, they are reportable as follicular neoplasm (FN) or suspicious for a follicular neoplasm (SFN), leading to a definitive diagnostic procedure, usually lobectomy.[42,62,65] SFN is preferred by some laboratories over FN for this category because a significant proportion of cases (up to 35%) prove not to be neoplasms but rather hyperplastic proliferations of follicular cells, most commonly those of MNG.[60,66–69] About 15% to 30% of cases called FN/SFN prove to be malignant.[2,60,67,70] The majority of SFN cases turn out to be FAs or adenomatoid nodules of MNG, both of which are more common than FC. Of those that prove malignant, many are FCs, but a significant proportion are follicular variants of papillary carcinoma.[2,8,61,67]

Cytologic preparations typically have high cellularity, and colloid is scant or absent. The hallmark of this diagnostic category is an altered cytoarchitecture: follicular cells are arranged predominantly in microfollicular or trabecular arrangements (**Fig. 2**). Cases that demonstrate the nuclear features of papillary carcinoma are excluded from this category. Cellular crowding and overlapping are conspicuous, and the follicular cells are usually larger than normal. Nuclear atypia/pleomorphism and mitoses are uncommon. A minor population of macrofollicles (intact spheres and fragments) can be present. Conspicuous cellularity alone does not qualify the nodule for a suspicious interpretation.[71] If a sample is cellular but mostly macrofollicular (intact spheres and flat fragments of evenly spaced follicular cells), a benign interpretation is appropriate. BFNs often have a small population of microfollicles and crowded groups. If these compose the minority of the follicular cells, they have little significance and the FNA can be interpreted as benign. A suspicious interpretation is rendered only when the majority of the follicular cells are arranged in abnormal architectural groupings (such as microfollicles or crowded trabeculae).

The general category FN/SFN is a self-sufficient interpretation; narrative comments that follow are optional.

In the World Health Organization classification, Hürthle cell adenoma (HA) and Hürthle cell carcinoma are considered oncocytic variants of FA and FC, respectively.[72] Studies suggest, however, that follicular and Hürthle cell tumors have different underlying genetics.[6,73] For this reason, and because they have such distinctive morphologic features, it is helpful to specify that a sample raises the possibility of a Hürthle cell rather than a follicular neoplasm. This interpretation applies to cellular samples that are composed exclusively (or almost exclusively) of Hürthle cells. Oncocytic cells with nuclear features of papillary carcinoma are excluded from this interpretation. A significant proportion of these cases (16%–25%) prove not to be neoplasms but rather hyperplastic proliferations of Hürthle cells in nodular goiter or lymphocytic thyroiditis.[74,75] Fifteen percent to 45% nodules are malignant, and the remainder of the neoplasms prove to be HAs.[70,74,75]

Suspicious for Malignancy

Many thyroid cancers, especially papillary thyroid carcinoma (PTC), can be diagnosed with certainty by FNA. The nuclear and architectural changes of some

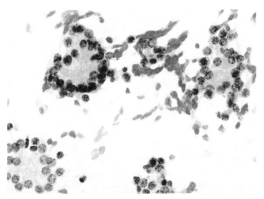

Fig. 2. FN/SFN. This aspirate shows significant architectural atypia of the follicular cells. Rather than arranged in a flat sheet (ie, a fragmented macrofollicule), the follicular cells are crowded into ring-like structures called microfollicles.

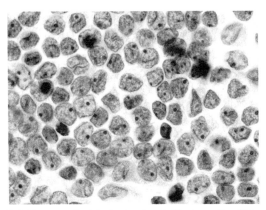

Fig. 3. Malignant: PTC. Compared with the benign follicular cells of **Fig. 1**, these malignant follicular cells have crowded, enlarged nuclei. Their chromatin is pale, the nuclei are irregular in contour, and nuclear grooves are prominent. These features are characteristic of PTC.

PTCs, however, are subtle and focal. This is particularly true of the follicular variant of PTC, which can be difficult to distinguish from a BFN.[76] Other PTCs may be incompletely sampled and yield only a few abnormal cells.[77] If only 1 or 2 characteristic features of PTC are present, if they are only focal and not widespread throughout the follicular cell population, or if the sample is sparsely cellular, a malignant diagnosis cannot be made with certainty. Such cases occur with some regularity and they are best classified as suspicious for malignancy, qualified as suspicious for papillary carcinoma. Nodules called suspicious for papillary carcinoma are resected by lobectomy or thyroidectomy. Most (60%–75%) prove to be papillary carcinomas and the rest are usually FAs.[2,60,62,78]

The same principle applies to other thyroid malignancies, such as medullary carcinoma and lymphoma, but these are encountered less frequently than PTC.

Malignant

The general category, malignant, is used whenever cytomorphologic features are conclusive for malignancy (**Fig. 3**). Descriptive comments that follow are used to subclassify the malignancy and summarize the results of special studies, if any. Approximately 3% to 7% of thyroid FNAs have conclusive features of malignancy, and most are papillary carcinomas.[2,60–62] Malignant nodules are usually removed by thyroidectomy, with some exceptions (eg, metastatic tumors, non-Hodgkin lymphomas, and anaplastic carcinomas). The positive predictive value of a malignant FNA interpretation is 97% to 99%.

SUMMARY

Given the considerable clinical value of thyroid FNA, it is important to understand its indications, some principles of optimal technique, the need for communicating relevant clinical information to pathologists on the requisition form, and the advantages of a reporting framework linked to management guidelines. The value of thyroid FNA is maximized when it is used for the appropriate indications, performed with good technique, and reported with terminology that is unambiguous and clinically useful.

REFERENCES

1. Hamberger B, Gharib H, Melton LJ 3rd, et al. Fine-needle aspiration biopsy of thyroid nodules. Impact on thyroid practice and cost of care. Am J Med 1982; 73(3):381–4.
2. Yassa L, Cibas ES, Benson CB, et al. Long-term assessment of a multidisciplinary approach to thyroid nodule diagnostic evaluation. Cancer 2007; 111(6):508–16.
3. Cibas ES, Alexander EK, Benson CB, et al. Indications for thyroid FNA and pre-FNA requirements: a synopsis of the National Cancer Institute Thyroid Fine-Needle Aspiration State of the Science Conference. Diagn Cytopathol 2008;36(6): 390–9.
4. Baloch ZW, Cibas ES, Clark DP, et al. The National Cancer Institute Thyroid fine needle aspiration state of the science conference: a summation. Cytojournal 2008;5:6.
5. Layfield LJ, Cibas ES, Gharib H, et al. Thyroid aspiration cytology: current status. CA Cancer J Clin 2009;59(2):99–110.
6. Baloch ZW, LiVolsi VA, Asa SL, et al. Diagnostic terminology and morphologic criteria for cytologic diagnosis of thyroid lesions: a synopsis of the National Cancer Institute Thyroid Fine-Needle Aspiration State of the Science Conference. Diagn Cytopathol 2008;36(6):425–37.
7. Cooper DS, Doherty GM, Haugen BR, et al. Management guidelines for patients with thyroid nodules and differentiated thyroid cancer. Thyroid 2006; 16:109–40.
8. Ravetto C, Columbo L, Dottorini ME. Usefulness of fine-needle aspiration in the diagnosis of thyroid carcinoma: a retrospective study in 37,895 patients. Cancer Cytopathol 2000;90:357–63.
9. Hegedus L. The thyroid nodule. N Engl J Med 2004;351:1764–71.
10. Sherman SI, Angelos P, Ball D, et al. Thyroid carcinoma. J National Compr Canc Netw 2005;3:404–57.
11. Ross DS. Evaluation and nonsurgical management of the thyroid nodule. In: Randolph G, editor. Surgery of the thyroid and parathyroid glands. Philadelphia: Saunders; 2003. p. 139–48.
12. Wong CK, Wheeler MH. Thyroid nodules: rational management. World J Surg 2000;24:934–41.
13. Burch HB. Evaluation and management of the thyroid nodule. Endocrinol Metab Clin North Am 1995;24:663.
14. Ashcraft MW, Van Herle AJ. Management of thyroid nodules. II: scanning techniques, thyroid suppressive therapy, and fine needle aspiration. Head Neck Surg 1981;3(4):297–322.
15. Are C, Hsu JF, Schoder H, et al. FDG-PET detected thyroid incidentalomas: need for further investigation? Ann Surg Oncol 2007;14:239–47.
16. Chen YK, Ding HJ, Chen KT, et al. Prevalence and risk of cancer of focal thyroid incidentaloma identified by 18F-fluorodeoxyglucose positron emission tomography for cancer screening in healthy subjects. Anticancer Res 2005;25:1421–6.
17. Choi JY, Lee KS, Kim HJ, et al. Focal thyroid lesions incidentally identified by integrated 18F-FDG PET/CT: clinical significance and improved characterization. J Nucl Med 2006;47:609–15.
18. Chu QD, Connor MM, Lilien DL, et al. Positron emission tomography (PET) positive thyroid incidentaloma: the risk of malignancy observed in a tertiary referral center. Am Surg 2006;72:272–5.

19. Cohen MS, Arslan N, Dehdashti F, et al. Risk of malignancy in thyroid incidentalomas identified by fluorodeoxyglucose-positron emission tomography. Surgery 2001;130:941–6.
20. Kang KW, Kim SK, Kang HS, et al. Prevalence and risk of cancer of focal thyroid incidentaloma identified by 18F-fluorodeoxyglucose positron emission tomography of metastasis evaluation and cancer screening in healthy subjects. J Clin Endocrinol Metab 2003;88:4100–4.
21. Kim TY, Kim WB, Ryu JS, et al. 18F-fluorodeoxyglucose uptake in thyroid from positron emission tomogram (PET) for evaluation in cancer patients: high prevalence of malignancy in thyroid PET incidentaloma. Laryngoscope 2005;115: 1074–8.
22. Kresnik E, Gallowitsch HJ, Mikosch P, et al. Fluorine-18-fluorodeoxyglucose positron emission tomography in the preoperative assessment of thyroid nodules in an endemic goiter area. Surgery 2003;133:294–9.
23. Yi JG, Marom EM, Munden RF, et al. Focal uptake of fluorodeoxyglucose by the thyroid in patients undergoing initial disease staging with combined PET/CT for non-small cell lung cancer. Radiology 2005;236:271–5.
24. Alonso O, Lago G, Mut F, et al. Thyroid imaging with Tc-99m MIBI in patients with solitary cold single nodules on pertechnetate imaging. Clin Nucl Med 1996;21: 363–7.
25. Hurtado-Lopez LM, Arellano-Montano S, Torres-Acosta EM, et al. Combined of fine-needle aspiration biopsy, MIBI scans and frozen section biopsy offers and the best diagnostic accuracy in the assessment of the hypofunctioning solitary thyroid nodule. Eur J Nucl Med Mol Imaging 2004;31:1273–9.
26. Kresnik E, Gallowitsch HJ, Mikosch P, et al. Technetium-99M-MIBI scintigraphy of thyroid nodules in an endemic goiter area. J Nucl Med 1997;38:62–5.
27. Mezosi E, Bajnok L, Gyory F, et al. The role of technetium-99m methoxyisobutylisonitrile scintigraphy in the differential diagnosis of cold thyroid nodules. Eur J Nucl Med 1999;26:798–803.
28. Sathekge MM, Mageza RB, Muthuphei MN, et al. Evaluation of thyroid nodules with technetium-909m MIBI and technetium-99m pertechnetate. Head Neck 2001;23:305–10.
29. Academy of Clinical Thyroidologists. Position paper on FNA for non-palpable thyroid nodules. Available at: http://www.thyroidologists.com/papers.html. Accessed February 16, 2010.
30. Brander AE, Viikinkoski VP, Nickels JI, et al. Importance of thyroid abnormalities detected in US screening: a 5-year follow-up. Radiology 2000;215:801–6.
31. Chung WY, Chang HS, Kim EK, et al. Ultrasonographic mass screening for thyroid carcinoma: a study in women scheduled to undergo a breast examination. Surg Today 2001;31:763–7.
32. Frates MC, Benson CB, Charboneau JW, et al. Management of thyroid nodules detected at US: Society of Radiologists in Ultrasound Consensus Conference Statement. Radiology 2005;237:794–800.
33. Kang HW, No JH, Chung JH, et al. Prevalence, clinical and ultrasonographic characteristics of thyroid incidentalomas. Thyroid 2004;14:29–33.
34. Kim EK, Park CS, Chung WY, et al. New sonographic criteria for recommending fine-needle aspiration biopsy of nonpalpable solid nodules of the thyroid. AJR Am J Roentgenol 2002;178:687–91.
35. Leenhardt L, Hejblum G, Franc B, et al. Indications and limits of ultrasound-guided cytology in the management of nonpalpable thyroid nodules. J Clin Endocrinol Metab 1999;84:24–8.

36. Liebeskind A, Sikora AG, Komisar A, et al. Rates of malignancy in incidentally discovered thyroid nodules evaluated with sonography and fine-needle aspiration. J Ultrasound Med 2005;24:629–34.
37. Nabriski D, Ness-Abramof R, Brosh T, et al. Clinical relevance of non-palpable thyroid nodules as assessed by ultrasound-guided fine needle aspiration biopsy. J Endocrinol Invest 2003;26:61–4.
38. Nan-Goong IS, Kim HY, Gong G, et al. Ultrasonography-guided fine-needle aspiration of thyroid incidentaloma: correlation with pathological findings. Clin Endocrinol 2004;60:21–8.
39. Papini E, Guglielmi R, Bianchini A, et al. Risk of malignancy in nonpalpable thyroid nodules: predictive value of ultrasound and color-Doppler features. J Clin Endocrinol Metab 2002;87(5):1941–6.
40. Steele SR, Martin MJ, Mullenix PS, et al. The significance of incidental thyroid abnormalities identified during carotid duplex ultrasonography. Arch Surg 2005;140:981–5.
41. AACE/AME Task Force on Thyroid Nodules. American Association of Clinical Endocrinologists and Associazione Medici Endocrinologi: medical guidelines for clinical practice for the diagnosis and management of thyroid nodules. Endocr Pract 2006;12:63–101.
42. Layfield LJ, Abrams J, Cochand-Priollet B, et al. Post thyroid FNA testing and treatment options: a synopsis of the National Cancer Institute Thyroid Fine Needle Aspiration State of the Science Conference. Diagn Cytopathol 2008; 36:442–8.
43. Harach HR, Franssila KO, Wasenius VM. Occult papillary carcinoma of the thyroid. A "normal" finding in Finland. A systematic autopsy study. Cancer 1985;56(3):531–8.
44. Ito Y, Miyauchi A. A therapeutic strategy for incidentally detected papillary microcarcinoma of the thyroid. Nat Clin Pract Endocrinol Metab 2007;3(3):240–8.
45. Yousem DM, Huang T, Loevner LA, et al. Clinical and economic impact of incidental thyroid lesions found with CT and MR. AJNR Am J Neuroradiol 1997;18: 1423–8.
46. Shetty SK, Maher MM, Hahn PF, et al. Significance of incidental thyroid lesions detected on CT: correlation among CT, sonography, and pathology. AJR Am J Roentgenol 2006;187:1349–56.
47. Marqusee E, Benson CB, Frates MC, et al. Utility of ultrasound in the management of nodular thyroid disease. Ann Intern Med 2000;133:696–700.
48. Carmeci C, Jeffrey RB, McDougall IR, et al. Ultrasound-guided fine-needle aspiration biopsy of thyroid masses. Thyroid 1998;8(4):283–9.
49. Cesur M, Corapcioglu D, Bulut S, et al. Comparison of palpation-guided fine-needle aspiration biopsy to ultrasound-guided fine-needle aspiration biopsy in the evaluation of thyroid nodules. Thyroid 2006;16(6):555–61.
50. Danese D, Sciacchitano S, Farsetti A, et al. Diagnostic accuracy of conventional versus sonography-guided fine-needle aspiration biopsy of thyroid nodules. Thyroid 1998;8(1):15–21.
51. Yokozawa T, Fukata S, Kuma K, et al. Thyroid cancer detected by ultrasound-guided fine-needle aspiration biopsy. World J Surg 1996;20(7):848–53.
52. Yokozawa T, Miyauchi A, Kuma K, et al. Accurate and simple method of diagnosing thyroid nodules the modified technique of ultrasound-guided fine needle aspiration biopsy. Thyroid 1995;5(2):141–5.
53. Court-Payen M, Nygaard B, Horn T, et al. US-guided fine-needle aspiration biopsy of thyroid nodules. Acta Radiol 2002;43(2):131–40.

54. Pitman MB, Abele J, Ali SZ, et al. Techniques for thyroid FNA: a synopsis of the National Cancer Institute Thyroid Fine-Needle Aspiration State of the Science Conference. Diagn Cytopathol 2008;36(6):407–24.
55. Centers for Medicare and Medicaid Services. Laboratory requirements. Available at: http://www.cdc.gov/clia/pdf/42cfr493_2003.pdf. Accessed November 27, 2007.
56. Ali SZ, Cibas ES. The Bethesda system for reporting thyroid cytopathology. New York: Springer; 2009.
57. Goellner JR, Gharib H, Grant CS, et al. Fine-needle aspiration cytology of the thyroid, 1980 to 1986. Acta Cytol 1987;31:587–90.
58. Grant CS, Hay ID, Gough IR, et al. Long-term follow-up of patients with benign thyroid fine-needle aspiration cytologic diagnoses. Surgery 1989;106:980–5.
59. Renshaw AA. Accuracy of thyroid fine-needle aspiration using receiver operator characteristic curves. Am J Clin Pathol 2001;116:477–82.
60. Yang J, Schnadig V, Logrono R, et al. Fine-needle aspiration of thyroid nodules: a study of 4703 patients with histologic and clinical correlations. Cancer 2007; 111(5):306–15.
61. Amrikachi M, Ramzy I, Rubenfeld S, et al. Accuracy of fine-needle aspiration of thyroid: a review of 6226 cases and correlation with surgical or clinical outcome. Arch Pathol Lab Med 2001;125:484–8.
62. Gharib H, Goellner JR, Johnson DA. Fine-needle aspiration cytology of the thyroid: a 12-year experience with 11,000 biopsies. Clin Lab Med 1993;13:699–709.
63. McHenry CR, Walfish PG, Rosen IB. Non-diagnostic fine-needle aspiration biopsy: a dilemma in management of nodular thyroid disease. Am Surg 1993; 59:415–9.
64. van Hoeven KH, Gupta PK, LiVolsi VA. Value of repeat fine needle aspiration (FNA) of the thyroid [abstract]. Mod Pathol 1994;7:43A.
65. Mazzaferri EL. NCCN thyroid carcinoma practice guidelines. Oncology 1999;13: 391–442.
66. Deveci MS, Deveci G, LiVolsi VA, et al. Fine-needle aspiration of follicular lesions of the thyroid. Diagnosis and follow-Up. Cytojournal 2006;3:9.
67. Baloch ZW, Fleisher S, LiVolsi VA, et al. Diagnosis of "follicular neoplasm": a gray zone in thyroid fine-needle aspiration cytology. Diagn Cytopathol 2002;26(1): 41–4.
68. Schlinkert RT, van Heerden JA, Goellner JR, et al. Factors that predict malignant thyroid lesions when fine-needle aspiration is "suspicious for follicular neoplasm". Mayo Clin Proc 1997;72(10):913–6.
69. Kelman AS, Rathan A, Leibowitz J, et al. Thyroid cytology and the risk of malignancy in thyroid nodules: importance of nuclear atypia in indeterminate specimens. Thyroid 2001;11(3):271–7.
70. Gharib H, Goellner JR. Fine-needle aspiration biopsy of the thyroid: an appraisal. Ann Intern Med 1993;118:282–9.
71. Suen KC. How does one separate cellular follicular lesions of the thyroid by fine-needle aspiration biopsy? Diagn Cytopathol 1988;4:78–81.
72. DeLellis RA, Lloyd RV, Heitz PU, et al. World Health Organization classification of tumours. Pathology and genetics of tumours of endocrine organs. Lyon: IARC Press; 2004.
73. French CA, Alexander EK, Cibas ES, et al. Genetic and biological subgroups of low-stage follicular thyroid cancer. Am J Pathol 2003;162(4):1053–60.
74. Pu RT, Yang J, Wasserman PG, et al. Does Hurthle cell lesion/neoplasm predict malignancy more than follicular lesion/neoplasm on thyroid fine-needle aspiration? Diagn Cytopathol 2006;34(5):330–4.

75. Giorgadze T, Rossi ED, Fadda G, et al. Does the fine-needle aspiration diagnosis of "Hurthle-cell neoplasm/follicular neoplasm with oncocytic features" denote increased risk of malignancy? Diagn Cytopathol 2004;31(5):307–12.
76. Chung D, Ghossein RA, Lin O. Macrofollicular variant of papillary carcinoma: a potential thyroid FNA pitfall. Diagn Cytopathol 2007;35(9):560–4.
77. Renshaw AA. Focal features of papillary carcinoma of the thyroid in fine-needle aspiration material are strongly associated with papillary carcinoma at resection. Am J Clin Pathol 2002;118(2):208–10.
78. Logani S, Gupta PK, LiVolsi VA, et al. Thyroid nodules with FNA cytology suspicious for follicular variant of papillary thyroid carcinoma: follow-up and management. Diagn Cytopathol 2000;23(6):380–5.

Surgical Management of Thyroid Disease

Rizwan Aslam, DO[a],*, David Steward, MD[b]

KEYWORDS

- Thyroid management • Nodule • Goiter • Papillary
- Follicular • Thyroidectomy

Surgery of the thyroid gland has evolved in many ways since its modernization by Theodor Kocher in the late nineteenth century. Along with procedural modifications, the surgical indications for benign and malignant disease have also continued to evolve and have often been a source of controversy. Recently, the American Thyroid Association (ATA) and the National Comprehensive Cancer Network have developed task forces aimed at delineating the indications for surgery of both benign and malignant thyroid disease. The algorithms introduced in these guidelines were intended to simplify decisions on the surgical management of controversial issues. The authors at their institution use these guidelines, clinical experience, and informed patient preferences to perform appropriate surgical procedures. This article describes the indications, surgical management, and postoperative care for both benign and malignant processes of the thyroid gland.

PREOPERATIVE PLANNING

Before any surgical procedure, a detailed patient history, thyroid function testing, physical examination including laryngoscopy, and appropriate imaging studies should be performed. Patient history including family history, history of prior radiation exposure, and overall health should be solicited. If the patient or family history reveals findings suggestive of multiple endocrine neoplasia (MEN) IIA or IIB, a work-up for pheochromocytoma should be performed preoperatively.[1] To avoid unfavorable outcomes associated with a thyroid storm, preoperative screening thyroid functions tests should be performed. In addition, laryngoscopy should be performed routinely before surgery. Recurrent laryngeal nerve (RLN) compression or invasion may be

[a] Head and Neck Oncology, Microvascular Reconstruction, Department of Otolaryngology–Head and Neck Surgery, University of Cincinnati College of Medicine, 231 Albert B. Sabin Way, ML 0528, Cincinnati, OH 45267–0528, USA
[b] Division of Thyroid/Parathyroid Surgery, Department of Otolaryngology–Head and Neck Surgery, University of Cincinnati College of Medicine, 231 Albert B. Sabin Way, ML 0528, Cincinnati, OH 45267–0528, USA
* Corresponding author.
E-mail address: aslamrn@ucmail.uc.edu

Otolaryngol Clin N Am 43 (2010) 273–283
doi:10.1016/j.otc.2010.01.004
0030-6665/10/$ – see front matter © 2010 Elsevier Inc. All rights reserved.

oto.theclinics.com

asymptomatic or slow to progress necessitating visualization to determine vocal fold function.[1] The authors routinely use in-office ultrasound to evaluate lesions for their size and presence of any suspicious sonographic features. Suspicious radiographic findings include microcalcifications, hypoechoic solid nodules, hypervascularity, irregular borders, or a taller rather than wider nodule on transverse imaging. Preoperative awareness of contralateral nodules can also facilitate surgical planning. In cases of cytologically or sonographically suspicious nodules, the extent of disease including lymph node involvement in both the central and lateral neck can be demonstrated with ultrasound. The routine use of preoperative CT scan is not necessary in most cases; however, noncontrast CT scan is beneficial for determining the caudal extent and degree of tracheal compression secondary to large substernal goiters (SSG). Preoperative CT scans may also provide useful insight if there is a concern of laryngotracheal invasion associated with a malignant process. A careful synthesis of the aforementioned tools can help the surgeon optimize the extent of surgery and avoid potential shortcomings in their surgical interventions.

INDICATIONS FOR THYROIDECTOMY

Thyroidectomy can be performed for both benign and malignant disease. The first category includes hyperthyroidism, SSG, and nodular goiter. Hemithyroidectomy may also be of diagnostic use in the case of a suspicious nodule. In this discussion, the malignant category includes well-differentiated thyroid carcinoma (WDTC), medullary thyroid carcinoma (MTC), and anaplastic thyroid carcinoma.

Hyperthyroidism

Hyperthyroidism treatment is aimed at symptomatic relief with control of associated systemic morbidity. Optimal treatment of hyperthyroidism is dependent on the etiology. Hyperthyroidism associated with Hashimoto or de Quervain thyroiditis is self-limited. In general, medical management with the use of β-blockers and antithyroid medications (methimazole or propylthiouracil) achieves good control in most clinical scenarios. Antithyroid treatment may not be ideal long-term therapy in patients with toxic multinodular goiter or toxic adenoma because of the natural history of disease progression. Surgery and radioiodine therapy are definitive management options for toxic nodular disease or Graves disease.

Surgical options for those with hyperthyroidism include hemithyroidectomy for toxic adenoma or total thyroidectomy for toxic multinodular goiter or Graves disease. Patients who may benefit from surgery include those who cannot tolerate or are noncompliant with antithyroid medication, or have absolute or relative contraindications or aversion to radioactive iodine (RAI). Individuals desiring return to normal thyroid function sooner than can be achieved with RAI may also consider thyroidectomy. Shindo[2] recommended that before surgery hyperthyroid patients receive antithyroid medication, propanolol, and potassium iodide especially for patients with Graves disease. The patient should be rendered euthyroid and have a resting heart rate less than 80.[2] Potassium iodide or Lugol solution has the potential benefit of decreasing the thyroid gland vascularity, and minimizing glandular hemorrhage during surgery. This can be administered in 1 to 2 lingual drops 7 to 10 days before surgery.[2] Occasionally, corticosteroids may be necessary in medically refractory Graves disease patients.

SSG

SSG can be challenging for both the patient and surgeon. SSGs generally behave in an indolent manner, following a path of least resistance through the thoracic inlet. Most patients remain asymptomatic until the goiter impedes on adjacent structures of the thoracic cavity. Commonly associated symptoms include supine dyspnea, dysphagia, cough, and hoarseness.[3] Vascular compression of the superior vena cava and vertebral arteries have been reported. The reported malignant potential for SSG is approximately 3% to 21%.[4] Technically, obtaining a fine-needle aspirate for cytologic analysis can be limited by the intrathoracic or retrosternal position of SSGs. If there is not a significant cervical portion, obtaining tissue for diagnosis is contingent on removal of the SSG. Because the single most effective treatment for SSG is surgery, and because of the relative safety associated with this procedure, it is believed that the presence of SSG is an indication for surgery, irrespective of associated clinical manifestations especially in young or middle aged patients.[5] A CT scan can help the surgeon identify its inferior extent and location within the mediastinum (anterior vs posterior), degree of tracheal compression, malignancy, and caudal extent of SSG (**Fig. 1**).

It is generally accepted that most benign SSGs can be removed through a cervical incision. For the remaining lesions not amenable for removal through a cervical approach, the authors use a ministernotomy, which is performed in conjunction with thoracic surgery. They involve the thoracic surgery service preoperatively for possible sternotomy on patients with posterior mediastinal goiters, those goiters with extension below the level of the aortic arch, and known malignancy in the chest. In addition, Cohen[6] has recommended a sternotomy for the extraction of ectopic goiters. Anatomically, one must recognize the potential anterior displacement of the RLN by a posterior mediastinal goiter. Prior knowledge of this allows the surgeon to anticipate the location of the RLN during surgical dissection. Additional surgical exposure is gained by positioning the patients' head in neck extension allowing for a cephalad displacement of the SSG. This facilitates improved delivery and visualization of the goiter.

Nodular Goiter

Thyroid nodules are a common finding, and often a source of diagnostic and management dilemmas. The low cost and availability of ultrasound have made detection of thyroid nodules very easy and has led to the 10 times increased detection rates.[7] Coupled with the incidental detection of nodules during imaging for nonthyroid processes clinicians are seeing an epidemic. Although most of the nodules are benign, 5% to 10% of nodules are malignant. Surgeons should familiarize themselves with the sonographic characteristics of thyroid nodule pathology and their appropriate management.

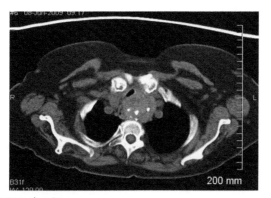

Fig. 1. CT scan substernal goiter.

Appropriate treatment of thyroid nodules relies on diagnostic cytology obtained through fine-needle aspiration biopsy (FNAB). The risk of malignancy is the same for patients with a solitary nodule or multiple nodules. Sonographically benign-appearing nodules larger than 1.5 cm or sonographically or clinically suspicious nodules should be considered for biopsy. The results of FNAB combined with ATA published treatment guidelines help direct the management of thyroid nodules. FNAB results are classified as benign (70%); indeterminate (10%, "suspicious for malignancy" or possible follicular neoplasm); malignant (5%); and nondiagnostic (15%).[8]

Ultrasound-guided FNAB greatly improves diagnostic accuracy over palpation with reduction in false-negative and nondiagnostic rates. Management of cytologically benign thyroid nodules includes observation with interval follow-up caused by the FNAB false-negative rates of up to 5%. A significant increase in nodule size greater than 20% to 50% or development of suspicious sonographic features warrants repeat ultrasound-guided FNAB or surgical excision.

Nodules with FNAB demonstrating indeterminate cells ("suspicious," "follicular," or Hurthle cell neoplasm) carry approximately a 10% to 20% risk of malignancy.[9–11] Solid or complex nodules yielding persistent nondiagnostic findings may demonstrate a 5% to 10% risk of malignancy.[12] For these patients with associated risk factors, the ATA suggests thyroid lobectomy as an initial treatment. Following lobectomy, intraoperative frozen histopathologic analysis positive for carcinoma requires a total thyroidectomy and possible central node dissection if gross nodal metastasis is identified. If the pathologist defers diagnosis until permanent sectioning, all patients with malignancy except those with a single focus or subcentimeter disease should undergo completion thyroidectomy. Completion thyroidectomy is usually performed in the first month following the initial procedure.[7] Scenarios that may benefit from a total thyroidectomy rather than lobectomy include (1) individuals with tumors greater than 4 cm and cytologic atypia, (2) FNAB "suspicious for papillary carcinoma," (3) patients with family history of thyroid carcinoma, and (4) childhood radiation exposure caused by increased risk of malignancy in these clinical settings.

Malignancy

Optimal surgical management of thyroid malignancy is dependent on the type and extent of malignancy: WDTC, papillary thyroid carcinoma (PTC), follicular thyroid carcinoma (FTC), Hurthle cell carcinoma (HCC), MTC, or anaplastic thyroid carcinoma.

Several variations of thyroidectomy exist but total or near total thyroidectomy is indicated for most thyroid malignancies. It is necessary to become familiar with the definitions, to communicate effectively with various members of the team. Partial lobectomy involves removing a portion of a single thyroid lobe and is not indicated in diagnosis or treatment of malignancy. Thyroid lobectomy or hemithyroidectomy involves resection of one thyroid lobe and may be sufficient for an isolated, subcentimeter FTC or PTC. Near total thyroidectomy is the resection of all grossly visible thyroid tissue, leaving a small fragment (1 g) of residual thyroid gland near the insertion of the RLN and ligament of Berry. A subtotal thyroidectomy involves leaving residual thyroid tissue greater than 1 g or with the ipsilateral posterior capsule intact. This is not an oncologically acceptable maneuver in the treatment of thyroid carcinoma.[8] Total thyroidectomy implies complete removal of the thyroid gland and is the procedure of choice for PTC, FTC, HCC, and MTC. Completion thyroidectomy refers to the removal of the contralateral residual thyroid lobe following a prior hemithyroidectomy when the diagnosis is made postoperatively.

PTC represents approximately 80% of thyroid malignancies. It may display multicentricity in the ipsilateral or contralateral lobe in a high proportion of cases. This multicentricity poses the predicament of hemithyroidectomy versus total thyroidectomy as definitive surgical therapy. At the Mayo Clinic, Hay and colleagues[13] compared patients treated with ipsilateral thyroid lobectomy plus isthmusectomy with bilateral resection (total thyroidectomy, bilateral subtotal, or near total thyroidectomy) for PTC. This study analyzed long-term 20-year results of these procedures. The data revealed local recurrence rates of 14% and 2% for thyroid lobectomy and bilateral resection, respectively. Also, rates for nodal metastasis were less with bilateral resection compared with thyroid lobectomy, 6% and 19%, respectively. Although near-total–total thyroidectomy is considered the definitive surgical modality for PTC, there are certain clinical circumstances in which hemithyroidectomy may be performed. The ATA states that hemithyroidectomy may be adequate for less than 10-mm, low-risk, isolated, intrathyroidal papillary carcinomas without evidence of cervical nodal disease.

PTC can manifest with cervical nodal metastasis in 20% to 90% of cases.[9] Some authors have demonstrated the presence of central and lateral neck metastases with rates of 62.2% and 25.6%, respectively.[14] Preoperative ultrasound is a sensitive tool in detecting the presence of cervical nodal disease, but may be more sensitive for the lateral rather than central compartment. The central compartment or level VI is defined by the carotid arteries laterally, hyoid bone superiorly, and suprasternal notch or brachiocephalic vessels inferiorly.[15] Therapeutic central compartment dissection should be considered in patients with PTC and nodal metastasis. For those with lateral nodal metastasis a functional level II to V neck dissection should be included.

FTC can be categorized as either minimally or widely invasive. Minimally invasive is the more common of the two and has no extension through the thyroid capsule with or without vascular invasion. Patients with lesions less than 1 to 1.5 cm may undergo hemithyroidectomy. For tumors described as minimally invasive with vascular invasion and widely invasive FTC near total or total thyroidectomy without central neck dissection is acceptable.[7,8] Unlike PTC and HCC that spread through lymphatics, FTC primarily spreads hematogenously or by direct extension. This behavior eliminates the need for elective or prophylactic neck dissections.

HCC is considered a variant of follicular carcinoma. This rare tumor comprises a small percentage of thyroid cancers, in the neighborhood of 2% to 3%. They tend to behave aggressively, and can readily demonstrate lymphatic spread. Near-total–total thyroidectomy is the recommended intervention. Like PTC, therapeutic central compartment node dissection should be performed in the presence of nodal metastasis. Evidence of lateral compartment nodal disease requires a functional neck dissection of levels II to V.

MTC is derived from parafollicular C cells of the thyroid gland and is embryologically distinct and differs in its behavior from WDTC. It is unresponsive to RAI, and surgery is the accepted basis of treatment. MTCs are multifocal and metastatic in most patients, and total thyroidectomy with elective or therapeutic central compartment neck dissection is the procedure of choice. This has been shown to achieve 80% biochemical cure rate, with a return to normocalcitonemia.[16,17] If there is evidence of levels II to V nodal disease, a therapeutic lateral neck dissection is suggested. Patients with MTC require genetic testing for somatic RET mutations associated with MEN IIA and IIB. Al-Rawi and Wheeler[16] suggest that despite total thyroidectomy and selective neck dissection 20% of patients recur or have residual disease. MTC association with MEN IIA and MEN IIB requires all first-degree relatives including children be tested for RET mutations.[18,19] It is generally accepted that children with MTC and those with MEN IIA should undergo a thyroidectomy by age 6 years. Those with the more aggressive

MEN IIB should have surgery within the first year of life. In addition, one can use micro-dissection effectively in this population.

SURGICAL TECHNIQUE

Contemporary thyroid surgery aims at eradicating disease while preserving parathyroid gland function, RLN integrity, and minimizing overall patient morbidity. In this discussion the authors' technique with conventional thyroidectomy is described and minimally invasive approaches are briefly discussed.

Preoperative Planning

Before surgery, the authors have an open discussion with the patient regarding benefits and potential postoperative complications of their procedure that include postoperative hypocalcemia, laryngeal nerve injury, bleeding, and infection. Informed consent is then obtained. High-resolution ultrasound is performed and CT scans obtained when indicated. Biochemical tests and imaging are reviewed with the patient and again the day of surgery.

Intraoperative Details

The patient is appropriately marked and transferred from the preoperative holding area to the operating room. After the patient and procedures have been confirmed using standard time-out technique, general anesthesia is induced and the patient is orotracheally intubated with a Nerve Integrity Monitoring (NIM) tube (NIM-Response, Medtronic USA, Jacksonville, FL, USA). Anesthesia is instructed to use only short-acting muscle relaxants and no topical laryngeal anesthetics with the use of NIM. NIM is useful as a training tool and to confirm accurate identification and preservation of the laryngeal nerves. The authors conducted a retrospective review of 165 patients who underwent thyroidectomy at their institution to assess if NIM is associated with a decreased risk of postoperative RLN injury. Primary outcome measures included postoperative RLN paralysis, paresis, and total injury rates. They found that there were no statistically significant differences in RLN paralysis, paresis, or total injury rates between control and NIM groups, even in subsets with advanced T stage and increased baseline risk.

The patient's neck is not extended but rather kept in a neutral position to minimize postoperative cervicalgia. A slight reverse Trendelenberg position prevents venous congestion. Superficial landmarks including cricoid cartilage and thyroid isthmus are identified. Ideal incision placement is in a natural skin crease at the level of the isthmus or cricoid. In most instances the authors are able to perform a thyroidectomy through a 3- to 5-cm incision. A 2- to 3-cm horizontal incision near the level of the cricoid for minimally invasive video assisted thyroidectomy (MIVATs) is preferred. Resection of larger inferior or mediastinal-based goiter requires a more traditional low cervical collar incision. When necessary a midline horizontal incision can be extended laterally for level V. The need for vertical cervical incisions is not required.

Next, the platysmal fascia (superficial cervical) is incised. The anterior jugular veins are identified and preserved. The midline linea alba is identified and dissected. The strap muscles are separated in the midline. The sternohyoid and sternothyroid muscles are grasped with Dabakey forceps on their medial surface. In so doing one does not inadvertently injure the anterior jugular veins. Next, dissection is carried laterally over the anterior and lateral surface of the thyroid glands with care to avoid disruption of the middle thyroid veins. Retraction of the straps laterally with an army navy is maintained while another retractor is placed under the superior aspect of the sternothyroid muscle, which is retracted superiorly to expose the superior vasculature pole and cricothyroid muscle. Anterolateral retraction of the superior pole allows visualization of the triangular space created by the medial border of the superior pole laterally and the cricothyroid muscle medially. Dissection is carried between the superior pole and cricothyroid muscle until the superior laryngeal nerve (SLN) is identified. Visual identification can be confirmed using electrical stimulation with a Prass probe (Medtronic USA, Jacksonville, FL, USA). Stimulation of the SLN at 0.5 to 1 mA results in diffuse movement of the cricothyroid muscle. Preservation of the SLN maintains pitch, which is important in patients whose careers rely on their voices and patients involved in recreational voice use, such as singing. Right angle clamps are used to dissect and retract the superior pole. The authors routinely use the Harmonic Focus (Ethicon Endo-Surgery, Cincinnati, OH, USA) to free the superior pole by coagulation and ligation of the superior thyroid vasculature. Cordon and colleagues[17] showed that operative time was decreased with the use of harmonic scalpel compared with electrocautery. Another similar study compared harmonic scalpel with conventional knot tying that showed harmonic scalpel shortened operative time by approximately 30 minutes.[20] Once the superior pole has been mobilized the middle thyroid veins are taken and the thyroid gland is isolated medially to expose the RLN near the inferior thyroid artery as it courses anterior to the superior parathyroid gland. Once identified the anterior motor RLN branches are neurophysiologically confirmed and preserved. The superior parathyroid gland is identified posterior to the RLN and the vascular supply maintained from the inferior thyroid artery. Remaining fibrous attachments are dissected from the lateral surface of the thyroid gland, and the procedure is directed toward the inferior lobe. The inferior parathyroid glands may be less consistent in their location. These glands are dissected from the inferior pole and the thyroid is mobilized medially. The inferior thyroid veins and thyrothymic ligament are released to expose the anterior trachea (**Fig. 2**). Antegrade dissection of the RLN is again carried toward the trachea following the RLN toward the ligament of Berry (**Fig. 3**). The RLN turns posterolaterally through the inferior pharyngeal constrictor and then the ligament of Berry is sharply transected (**Fig. 4**). If a pyramidal lobe is present it is taken with the dissection. If a nodule is present in the midline, the isthmus is resected with a margin. If a total thyroidectomy is being performed a similar dissection is undertaken on the contralateral side. Drains are then placed in patients with very large or SSGs; otherwise routinely the wound is closed in a layered fashion without a drain. A meta-analysis of 11 randomized trials comparing routine drain with no drains found no significant difference in respiratory distress or wound re-exploration but found an increased length of stay with drain usage. The skin is closed with subcuticular running 5-0 polysorb suture.

Recently, minimally invasive procedures have become increasingly popular among patients and surgeons. A desire for improved cosmesis and shorter recovery periods has led to the creation of video-assisted techniques. In 1998, Micolli and colleagues[21] described the first gasless endoscopic MIVAT. Studies suggest that this procedure does not carry an increased potential for complications including hypoparathyroidism and RLN palsy. A minority of patients are amenable to this procedure, making most surgeons reluctant to perform them. The current indications include nodules less than 3 cm in diameter in glands less than 25 mL in volume, Graves disease with volume less than 20 mL, no history of thyroiditis, no previous neck surgery or radiation, follicular or "low-risk" papillary carcinoma, and RET gene mutation carriers.[21] The patient is placed in a neutral supine position and a 2- to 3-cm incision is performed. A narrow flap is elevated in the midline playtsmal dehiscence. Elevation of lateral superior and inferior subplatysmal flaps is avoided because no benefit is gained with this

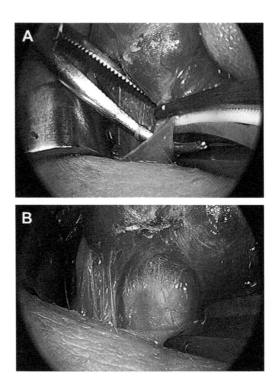

Fig. 2. (*A*) Release of the thyrothymic ligament. (*B*) Trachea exposed after release of thyro-thymic ligament.

maneuver. The strap muscles are divided as described in the conventional approach. A thirty-degree endoscope is introduced into the surgical field for visualizing critical structures during thyroidectomy, especially the SLN and RLN. The gland is delivered through the wound and the remainder of the thyroidectomy is performed as previously mentioned. Some institutions use skin adhesives for closure with rubber band drains; the authors use a subcuticular polysorb suture without drain. Ikeda and colleagues[22] have also developed a unique endoscopic approach through the axilla. Recently, the

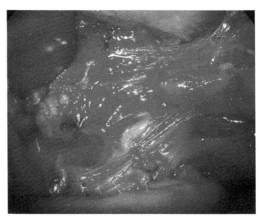

Fig. 3. RLN, superior parathyroid gland (SPG), and ligament of Berry (LB).

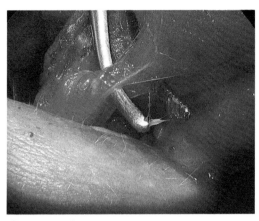

Fig. 4. Transection of ligament of Berry.

utilization of robotics has allowed to further minimize the need for an open cervical approach, by utilizing a transaxillary approach.

POSTOPERATIVE CARE

Postoperative care after thyroidectomy in the authors' institution is driven by the patient's need for a drain and postanesthesia care unit (PACU) parathyroid hormone (PTH) levels. In addition to risk from delayed hematoma formation, risk of hypocalcemia secondary to hypoparathyroidism has challenged ambulatory total or completion thyroidectomy. Patients are routinely discharge home following thyroidectomy if they meet the following criteria: no drain requirement and no evidence of hematoma with PACU PTH levels of at least 30 pg/mL or with PACU PTH levels of at least 20 pg/mL with oral calcium supplementation (Tums twice daily) and a calcium level at 1 week postoperatively. Routine calcium and vitamin D supplementation has been shown to reduce the risk of hypocalcemia. A meta-analysis of rapid postoperative PTH measurement confirmed a significantly increased risk of hypocalcemia for PTH less than 15 pg/mL.[23] If a patient has a PTH level less than 20 pg/mL in the PACU they are admitted for overnight observation and treatment. On postoperative day zero the patient is started on oral calcium, 500 mg four times daily, and oral calcitriol, 3 μg, as a bolus. This is followed on postoperative day 1 with 1 μg of calcitriol. On postoperative day 2 the patient is discharged on 0.5 μg calcitriol daily with Tums (calcium carbonate, 500 mg) four times a day or oral calcium equivalent with a renal panel on postoperative day 3 or 4. The patient's calcium supplementation is then reduced in a stepwise fashion over the next 3 to 4 weeks. Specifically, the next week the patient takes 500 mg of calcium by mouth three times daily, then the patient's dose is decreased to twice daily, and then the dose is further decreased to once daily. A repeat renal panel is performed along with a thyroid-stimulating hormone (TSH) level 1 month postoperatively. If the patient has no comorbid conditions requiring inpatient care, and they meet the aforementioned conditions, they can be safely discharged with instructions to call for neck swelling, bleeding, or circumoral paresthesias.

FOLLOW-UP CARE

Patients undergoing hemithyroidectomy require TSH testing 1 month postoperatively and levothyroxine should be instituted for hypothyroidism. Those undergoing total thyroidectomy are started on levothyroxine, 1.5 μg/kg, with a TSH level and dose titration at 1 month postoperatively. Patients requiring supplementation with levothyroxine after surgery for benign disease should have a target TSH of 1 to 3 mIU/L.

Patients with malignancy should have follow-up surveillance every 6 months for the first 2 years, and annually thereafter. Patients with WDTC should have thyroglobulin and antithyroglobulin antibody levels every 6 to 12 months. Stimulated or unstimulated elevated or rising serum thyroglublin levels of greater than 2 ng/mL may indicate recurrence. Antithyroglobulin antibodies may falsely raise the thyroglobulin level. Cervical ultrasound to evaluate the thyroid bed and central and lateral cervical nodal compartments is recommended at 6 and 12 months and then annually for a minimum of 3 to 5 years.[8] Studies have shown that TSH suppression may decrease adverse clinical events of thyroid cancer. We use levothyroxine to suppress TSH levels below 0.10 for high-risk patients and below 0.5 for low-risk patients. TSH levels should be checked semiannually and 6 weeks after the levothyroxine dose changes. Finally, patients are referred for RAI ablation if they have stage III or IV disease; less than 45 years old with stage II disease; most patients age greater than 45 years with stage II disease; and stage I patients demonstrating multifocal disease, nodal metastases, extrathyroidal or vascular invasion, or aggressive histologies.[8]

SUMMARY

The surgical management of thyroid disease can often be challenging. The authors' experience with both benign and malignant pathologies is described. To eliminate ambiguity, they use experience, guidelines, and patient interest to drive the decision-making process. Current advancements in thyroid surgery are making the process more efficient and desirable for patients and surgeons. When managed appropriately thyroid surgery can be safe and rewarding.

REFERENCES

1. Randolph G. Thyroid and parathyroid surgery. In: Bailey B, Johnson J, Newlands S, editors. Head and neck surgery: otolaryngology. 4th edition. Philadelphia: Lippincott Williams & Wilkins; 2006. p. 1637–45.
2. Shindo M. Surgery for hyperthyroidism [review]. ORL J Otorhinolaryngol Relat Spec 2008;70(5):298–304.
3. De Perrot M, Fadel M, Mercier O, et al. Surgical management of mediastinal goiters: when is a sternotomy required? Thorac Cardiovasc Surg 2007;55:39–43.
4. Sand ME, Laws HL, McElvein RB. Substernal and intrathoracic goiter. Am Surg 1983;49:196–202.
5. Cho HT, Cohen JP, Som ML. Management of substernal and intrathoracic goiters. Otolaryngol Head Neck Surg 1986;94:282–7.
6. Cohen JP. Substernal goiters and sternotomy. Laryngoscope 2009;119:683–8.
7. Yeung MJ, Serpell JW. Management of the solitary thyroid nodule. Oncologist 2008;13:105–12.
8. Cooper DS, Doherty GM, Haugen B, et al. Management guidelines for patients with thyroid nodules and differentiated thyroid cancer. Thyroid 2006;16:1–32.
9. Gharib H, Goellner JR, Zinsmeister AR, et al. Fine-needle aspiration biopsy of the thyroid: the problem of suspicious cytologic findings. Ann Intern Med 1984;101:25–8.
10. Baloch ZW, Fleisher S, LiVolsi VA, et al. Diagnosis of follicular neoplasm: a gray zone in thyroid fine-needle aspiration cytology. Diagn Cytopathol 2002;26:41–4.

11. Sclabas GM, Staerkel GA, Shapiro SE, et al. Fine-needle aspiration of the thyroid and correlation with histopathology in a contemporary series of 240 patients. Am J Surg 2003;186:702–9 [discussion: 709–10].

12. de los Santos ET, Keyhani-Rofagha S, Cunningham JJ. Cystic thyroid nodules: the dilemma of malignant lesions. Arch Intern Med 1990;150:1422–7.

13. Hay ID, Grant CS, Bergstralh EJ, et al. Unilateral total lobectomy: is it sufficient surgical treatment for patients with AMES low-risk papillary thyroid carcinoma? Surgery 1998;124:958–64 [discussion: 964–6].

14. Pai SI, Tufano RP. Central compartment neck dissection for thyroid cancer: technical considerations. ORL J Otorhinolaryngol Relat Spec 2008;70:292–7.

15. Shindo M, Wu JC, Park EE, et al. The importance of central compartment elective lymph node excision in the staging and treatment of papillary thyroid cancer. Arch Otolaryngol Head Neck Surg 2006;132:650–4.

16. Al-Rawi M, Wheeler MH. Medullary thyroid carcinoma: update and present management controversies. Ann R Coll Surg Engl 2006;88(5):433–8.

17. Cordon C, Fajardo R, Ramirez J, et al. A randomized, prospective, parallel group study comparing the harmonic scalpel to electrocautery in thyroidectomy. Surgery 2005;137:337–41.

18. Kloos RT, Eng C, Evans DB, et al. Medullary thyroid cancer: management guidelines of the American Thyroid Association. Thyroid. 2009;19(6):565–612.

19. Kang SW, Jeong JJ, Nam KH, et al. Robot-assisted endoscopic thyroidectomy for thyroid malignancies using a gasless transaxillary approach. J Am Coll Surg 2009;209(2):e1–7.

20. Siperstein AE, Berber E, Morkoyun E. The use of the harmonic scalpel vs conventional knot tying for vessel ligation in thyroid surgery. Arch Surg 2002;137:137–42.

21. Miccoli P, Berti P, Frustaci GL, et al. Video assisted thyroidectomy: indications and results. Langenbecks Arch Surg 2006;391:68–71.

22. Ikeda Y, Takami H, Sasaki Y, et al. Endoscopic neck surgery by the axillary approach. J Am Coll Surg 2000;191:336–40.

23. Hopkins B, Steward D. Outpatient thyroid surgery and the advances making it possible. Curr Opin Otolaryngol Head Neck Surg 2009;17(2):95–9.

Surgical Management of Cervical Lymph Nodes in Differentiated Thyroid Cancer

Danielle Fritze, MD[a], Gerard M. Doherty, MD[b],*

KEYWORDS

• Cervical lymph nodes • Differentiated thyroid cancer
• Prognosis • Nodal metastases • Dissection

Approximately 37,200 people are expected to be diagnosed with thyroid cancer in the United States this year.[1] Prognosis largely depends on the degree of tumor differentiation. In contrast to anaplastic tumors, well-differentiated thyroid cancer (DTC), including papillary and follicular carcinomas and their subtypes, has an excellent prognosis.[2] Although long-term survival can exceed 90%, regional lymph node metastases are common and contribute significantly to morbidity.[2] Surgical management of cervical lymph nodes is integral to the comprehensive treatment of DTC. Unfortunately, data from large randomized clinical trials do not exist to aid in defining optimal surgical treatment. The choice of surgical strategy is thus founded on a thorough understanding of the behavior and significance of lymphatic metastases in DTC and guided by observational data.

BACKGROUND
Differentiated Thyroid Cancer Growth and Spread

The malignant behavior of well-differentiated thyroid cancer is characterized by varying degrees of local invasion, lymphatic infiltration, and hematogenous dissemination. Papillary thyroid cancers (PTCs) compose 77% of thyroid malignancies and demonstrate a strong propensity for regional nodal involvement.[2] The most recent analysis of Surveillance, Epidemiology and End Results (SEER) data, including more than 33,000 patients with DTC, reports a 22% incidence of lymphatic involvement at initial operation in patients with PTC. Extrathyroidal extension was less common, involving 15% of patients, and distant metastases affected only 1% of patients at

[a] Department of Surgery, University of Michigan, 2207 Taubman Center, 1500 East Medical Center Drive, Ann Arbor, MI 48109, USA
[b] Department of Surgery, University of Michigan, 2920 Taubman Center, 1500 East Medical Center Drive, Ann Arbor, MI 48109, USA
* Corresponding author.
E-mail address: gerardd@umich.edu

Otolaryngol Clin N Am 43 (2010) 285–300
doi:10.1016/j.otc.2010.01.005
0030-6665/10/$ – see front matter © 2010 Elsevier Inc. All rights reserved.

oto.theclinics.com

diagnosis.[3] Other studies demonstrate lymphatic metastases in up to 50% of patients with DTC, depending on the timing of evaluation and diagnostic criteria.[4–12]

In contrast to PTCs, follicular thyroid cancers (FTCs) are less common, with a low rate of lymphatic involvement but more frequent distant metastasis. According to SEER data, 10% of patients with FTC present with extrathyroidal spread, 3% with distant metastases, and only 2% with lymphatic involvement.[3]

Anatomy of Cervical Lymphatics

The thyroid gland is seated amid a rich lymphatic network. The cervical lymph nodes are divided into levels I to VI and grouped into central and lateral compartments (**Fig. 1**).[13] Level I nodes are submental and submandibular. Levels II to IV consist of the upper, mid-, and lower jugular nodes, respectively, with level V nodes lateral to the jugular groups in the posterior triangle. The pretracheal, paratracheal, and prelaryngeal (delphian) nodes compose level VI. Level VII lymph nodes are located in the superior mediastinum inferior to the sternal notch. Although not technically included in the cervical lymphatic system, the superior mediastinal group is another common site of DTC metastasis.[14] Further subdivision of the levels I, II, and V nodes has been proposed based on significant anatomic landmarks. Ia refers to submental nodes whereas Ib nodes are submandibular. Level II is divided into superior (IIa) and inferior (IIb) nodes by the spinal accessory nerve, with IIb lateral to the nerve. Level Va is located superior to the level of the cricoid cartilage and Vb inferior. The spinal accessory nerve divides Va into inferior and superior sublevels.[14] Grouping adjacent nodal levels together has practical application. Levels II to V compose the lateral or posterolateral compartment, whereas level VI is synonymous with the central or anterior compartment.[14]

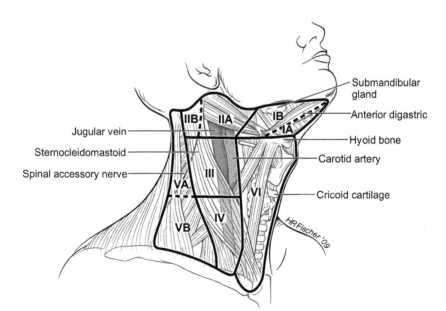

Fig. 1. The designation of lymph node levels in the neck. (*Reproduced from* American Thyroid Association Guidelines Taskforce on Thyroid Nodules and Differentiated Thyroid Cancer, et al. Revised American Thyroid Association management guidelines for patients with thyroid nodules and differentiated thyroid cancer [see comment]. Thyroid 2009;19[11]:1167–214; with permission.)

Patterns of Nodal Metastases

Several studies of cervical metastases in thyroid cancer suggest a general pattern of lymphatic spread from medial to lateral in the ipsilateral, then contralateral, neck. The incidence of nodal involvement is higher in the central compartment than the lateral compartment. Jugular lymph node metastases occur with greater frequency than do supraclavicular lymph node metastases, and involvement of submental or submandibular nodes is rare. Contralateral lymph node metastases greater than 1 cm have been described in 25% of patients with PTC. The majority of contralateral metastases are found in the central rather than lateral compartment.[8] Mediastinal lymph node involvement is rare, occurring in only 5% of node-positive patients with PTC.[15]

Incidence and location of nodal metastasis is ideally studied in a representative cohort of patients with thyroid cancer who undergo complete bilateral modified radical neck dissection (MRND) regardless of clinical node status. Mirallie and colleagues[8] examined 119 patients with PTC who underwent bilateral cervical neck dissection, excluding only node-negative patients with microcarcinomas less than 1 cm in diameter: 60.5% of patients were found to have cervical lymph node metastases. Of node-positive patients, 83% had central, 61% had midjugular, 36% had supraclavicular, and 28% had subdigastric involvement on the ipsilateral side. Contralateral involvement in the paratracheal nodes occurred in 35% of node-positive patients, with contralateral jugular metastases in less than 25%.[8] DTC metastases are thus most common within the central compartment; they are also frequent in the ipsilateral jugular groups. Contralateral involvement is less likely but nonetheless affects a significant proportion of patients.

Although central and jugular involvement is common, several studies have suggested infrequent involvement of levels I, IIb, and V. A series of 52 patients with lateral metastases at initial diagnosis who underwent MRND identified lymph node metastases by neck level. Levels IIa, III, and VI were each involved in more than 70% of patients. Involvement of other levels was significantly less common: only 16.7% of patients had positive nodes at level IIb, 13% at Vai, and 3.7% at Vb and Ib; there was no involvement of Vas. Level Ia was not dissected. Involvement of Level Ib, IIb, or V was associated with multilevel disease in all cases.[16] In contrast, another small series reported positive nodes above the spinal accessory nerve (level I or IIb) in 21% of 34 patients; nearly half of those had no involvement of level IIa.[17]

Many investigators have also described a relationship between the location of the cancer within the thyroid and the location of involved nodes. Quabain and coworkers[9] prospectively studied a population of patients with DTC who underwent prophylactic MRND and were staged as pN0 by standard histopathology. Micrometastatic disease was identified by immunohistochemistry in 53% of the 80 patients enrolled, primarily occurring in those with tumors larger than 1 cm. Examination of the location of micrometastases indicated a tendency for upper-pole lesions to metastasize to more superior nodes, with isthmus and lower-pole lesions metastasizing to inferior nodes. Within the central compartment, all micrometastases occurred ipsilateral to the tumor unless the tumor was within the isthmus.

Despite the general pattern of medial to lateral spread, skip metastases — lateral compartment metastases without central compartment involvement — occur in a significant proportion of patients (**Table 1**). In the study by Qubain and coworkers,[9] 7% of patients with DTC micrometastases had lateral compartment involvement without evidence of central disease. In a prospective series of 52 patients with DTC and clinically positive lateral nodes who underwent MRND, 5 patients (9.6%) had no evidence of central compartment disease.[11,16] Machens and colleagues[19] examined

Table 1
Location of lymph node metastases at MRND in patients with DTC and positive lateral nodes[a]

	I	Ia	Ib	II	IIa	IIb	III	IV	V	Vai	Vas	Vb	VI	Skip Mets[b]
Pingpank[17] (n = 44)	38	—	—	49	43	21	76	59	28	—	—	—		
Roh[16] (n = 52)	—	—	4		72	17	72	76		13	0	4	90	10
Yanir[18] (n = 27)	—	—	—	54	—	—	68	57	20	—	—	—	95	5
Mirallie[8] (n = 72)	—	—	—	28	—	—	61	61	36	—	—	—	83	17
Average	38	—	4	39	59	19	68	64	31	13	0	4	88	12

[a] Values indicate the % of patients with positive lymph nodes at each level.
[b] Metastases to lateral nodes without evidence of central compartment involvement.

215 patients with thyroid cancer and lateral or mediastinal metastases and found skip metastasis in 19.7% of patients with PTC and 0 of 8 patients with FTC. A statistically significant inverse correlation was observed between the incidence of skip metastases and the number of positive lymph nodes. The presence of skip metastases was not significantly associated with tumor size or patient demographic characteristics.

Risk Factors for Initial Nodal Metastases and Nodal Recurrence

Several risk factors have been defined for nodal involvement in DTC (**Table 2**). At the time of initial treatment, patients with PTC and those younger than 45 years old are more likely to have lymph node metastases than their older counterparts or those with FTC.[20,21] Patients with distant metastases are also more likely to harbor nodal metastases.[21] Correlation between tumor size and lymph node metastases has been variably reported.[10,20–22] Patients with tumors larger than 4 cm are 2 to 6 times more likely to have lymph node metastases present at operation than those with smaller tumors.[21,22] In smaller tumors, the presence of lymph node metastases at initial operation correlated more strongly with vascular and soft tissue invasion than primary tumor size (<1 cm vs 1–2 cm).[10] Locally invasive primary tumor and pronounced elevation in thyroglobulin levels have also been identified as possible risk factors.[23] Patient and tumor characteristics associated specifically with mediastinal lymph node involvement include older age at diagnosis, poor tumor differentiation, more positive lymph nodes, and distant metastases.[15]

Several risk factors are associated with regional lymph node recurrence in DTC. Male gender and extrathyroidal extension of the primary tumor have been implicated by several studies.[5,22] Older age, larger tumor, and macroscopically involved nodes at initial surgery also are cited.[5,22,24]

Table 2
Risk factors for lymph node metastases in DTC

At Presentation	Recurrence
PTC	Male > female
Distant metastases	Extrathyroidal extension
Age <45 years	Age >55 years
Large tumor	Large tumor
Extrathyroidal extension	Macroscopically positive
Vascular invasion	Lymph nodes at initial operation
Elevated thyroglobulin	

Ito and colleagues[22] proposed a scoring system to stratify patients in terms of risk for lymph node recurrence, assigning 1 point each for

- Age older than 55 years
- Male gender
- Massive extrathyroid extension
- Tumor greater than 3 cm.

Patients with 0 points had a 10-year, lymph node disease-free survival of 98.4%. This declined in a stepwise fashion to 64.7% for patients with all 4 criteria.

Detection and Diagnosis

Regional metastases are routinely detected by physical examination and imaging studies. In the setting of a negative preoperative evaluation, unanticipated lymphatic metastases are also frequently discovered at thyroidectomy. Initial assessment for lymphadenopathy is by physical examination of the neck. The accuracy of this method varies with clinician experience and patient body habitus, but false-positive and -negative rates of 20% to 30% are reported.[25] Clinician and patient factors also affect the accuracy of ultrasonography; however, ultrasound may detect cervical lymph node metastases in up to 34% of patients with a negative physical examination (**Fig. 2**).[26] Reported sensitivities for ultrasound in diagnosis of lymphatic metastases in DTC are widely variable, ranging from 10% to 92%.[26–31] Specificity, as confirmed by fine-needle aspiration (FNA), is high, with a reported range of 89% to 99%.[26–31] The sensitivity of ultrasound is particularly limited in the central compartment due to the presence of the trachea and thyroid gland. In patients whose thyroid gland remains in place, the false-negative rate for ultrasound detection of central compartment lymph node metastases is 36%. This rate drops to 18% for patients whose thyroid gland is surgically absent.[26] Positive or indeterminate findings on physical examination or imaging can be evaluated with FNA, particularly if the presence or absence of malignancy influences the choice of surgical procedure.[32]

SIGNIFICANCE OF LYMPH NODE METASTASES

The impact of lymph node metastases on survival in DTC has yet to be unequivocally defined. Nonetheless, lymphatic involvement is well established as a predictor of locoregional recurrence and implicated as a harbinger of distant metastases.

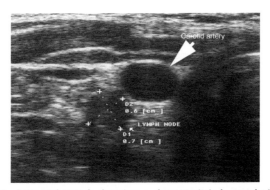

Fig. 2. Ultrasound of the right neck showing a characteristic hypoechoic rounded lymph node metastasis from PTC. The carotid artery is denoted by the large arrowhead.

Locoregional Recurrence

Lymph node metastasis is described as a risk factor for locoregional recurrence in several observational studies.[10,21,24,33–36] A retrospective review of 700 patients with DTC demonstrated a relative risk of recurrence of 4.2 in patients with lymph node metastases as compared with those without. This difference existed independent of treatment and other tumor and patient factors.[33] Similarly, McHenry and colleagues[24] reported recurrence of DTC in 19% of patients with initially positive nodes and 2% in node-negative patients after thyroidectomy and MRND.

Similar results are reported in series of patients with PTC only. According to a retrospective study by Salvesen and colleagues,[34] initial node-negative status in patients with PTC predicted recurrence-free survival with a hazard ratio (HR) of 3.6. Ninety percent of N0 patients were disease-free 10 years after resection compared with 65% of patients who presented with positive lymph nodes. Wada and colleagues[35] compared the rates of recurrence and mortality in 231 patients who had PTC with and without palpable lymphadenopathy. All patients underwent thyroidectomy and MRND; only a small minority received radioactive iodine postoperatively. The overall HR for disease-free survival in patients without palpable lymphadenopathy compared to those with nodal disease detectable on physical examination was 14.9 by multivariate analysis. The effect of lateral involvement was stronger than that of central compartment disease.

There are fewer studies exclusively concerned with nodal metastases in FTCs. Two retrospective reviews examined the effect of initial node-positive status on subsequent recurrence after total thyroidectomy with central lymph node dissection (CLND) and radioactive iodine therapy. Of patients who were initially node positive, 80% developed recurrence whereas only 34% of node-negative patients developed recurrence. This difference remained statistically significant on multivariate analysis.[36]

The effect of nodal involvement is more pronounced in certain subgroups of patients with DTC. A retrospective review of 342 patients with PTC revealed nodal status as a statistically significant predictor of recurrence and survival in patients with T1, T2, and T3 tumors but not in patients with T4 tumors.[21] In a study of patients with small DTC less than 2 cm, 20-year disease-free survival was 71% in N0 patients versus 56% in initially node-positive patients ($P = .02$).[10]

Distant Metastases

Nodal metastases have been identified as a predictor of systemic disease. In the series by McHenry and colleagues[24], 6% of patients with nodal involvement and 0.1% of patients without nodal involvement developed distant metastases. In another series stratified by tumor size, 0.7% of patients initially T1-T3N0 had distant metastases at diagnosis and 2.9% eventually developed distant spread. For T1-T3N1 patients, 8.5% had systemic involvement at diagnosis, and 15.1% later developed systemic disease.[21] Reflexively, patients with metastatic disease are more likely to have lymphatic involvement. Analysis of 231 patients with PTC who underwent MRND revealed a significantly higher burden of positive regional lymph nodes, particularly lateral nodes, in patients with systemic metastases.[35] These studies suggest that nodal involvement is reflective of more advanced or aggressive DTC.

Survival

Lymph node metastases have not traditionally been associated with mortality in DTC; however, recent evidence is accumulating to suggest decreased long-term survival in patients with lymphatic involvement. At least 6 case series have demonstrated no significant mortality risk associated with lymph node metastases in

DTC.[10,12,24,34,37,38] In contrast, a large, population-based, nested case-control study of all patients diagnosed with DTC in Sweden over 30 years suggests that lymph node metastases are associated with increased mortality. In a multivariate analysis controlling for TNM stage, the odds ratio for DTC-related death was 1.9 in patients with lymphatic involvement compared with those without.[39] Analysis of SEER data from more than 19,000 patients demonstrated a statistically significant survival difference in patients with DTC based on nodal status. The 14-year survival was 82% in node-negative patients versus 79% in node-positive patients.[40] A more recent review of SEER data from more than 33,000 patients demonstrated no significant difference in all-cause mortality between patients with PTC younger than age 45 with and without positive lymph nodes. For patients age 45 and older with PTC, however, mortality was 46% greater in patients with lymphatic metastases compared with those without.[3] Lymphatic metastases in patients with follicular cancers were significantly associated with increased mortality in patients older (HR 11.23) and younger (HR 2.86) than 45 years.[3] A single institution series of 700 patients with DTC analyzing disease-specific mortality also reports a statistically significant risk ratio of 2.6 for patients with nodal metastases compared with those without.[33] A study of papillary microcarcinomas <1 cm in size noted a statistically significant effect on survival for lateral but not central compartment lymph node metastases.[41] Although a mortality risk is not uniformly identified in every series, high-quality observational data strongly suggest lower long-term survival rates in DTC patients with lymphatic metastases.

Lymphatic Metastases and DTC Staging

Historically, nodal status has been conspicuously absent from staging systems for DTC, primarily because of lack of data implicating nodal status as a negative prognostic indicator. Several such systems, including AGES, AMES, MACIS, and the European Organization for Research and Treatment of Cancer (EORTC) system, do not include an assessment of lymph node status, yet are useful predictors of survival. In 1987, the American Joint Committee on Cancer and International Union Against Cancer adopted a TNM classification for DTC with separate staging criteria for patients younger and older than 45 years (**Table 3**).[42] For younger patients, stage is based entirely on the presence or absence of distant metastases. For older patients, nodal involvement equates to stage IIIb, with distant metastases stage IV. Several retrospective studies have demonstrated a correlation between TNM stage and mortality in thyroid cancer, with independent validation of the prognostic value of the regional lymph node or N classification.[12,33,34,39]

SURGICAL TREATMENT OF CERVICAL LYMPH NODES IN DTC

Surgical treatment of cervical lymph nodes in DTC remains a subject of debate. There is widespread consensus that clinically involved cervical nodes should be resected when detected, provided that distant metastases do not preclude curative operation. Resection of involved cervical nodes is also appropriate in patients with M1 disease to prevent or treat aerodigestive compression by nodal metastases. In these circumstances, neck dissection is therapeutic. Prophylactic neck dissection also is proposed and variably practiced for patients without clinically evident lymph node involvement, preoperatively or at thyroidectomy. The optimal role of prophylactic dissection and the appropriate extent of neck dissection for DTC remain controversial.

Techniques

The superiority of systematic lymphadenectomy with removal of all lymphatic tissue in a particular level or compartment to berry-picking procedures has been repeatedly

Table 3
Thyroid Cancer Staging

Primary Tumor (T)
Note: All categories may be subdivided: (a) solitary tumor, (b) multifocal tumor (the largest determines the classification).

TX	Primary T cannot be assessed
T0	No evidence of primary T
T1	T < 2 cm in greatest dimension limited to the thyroid
T2	T > 2 cm but not > 4 cm in greatest dimension limited to the thyroid
T3	T > 4 cm in greatest dimension limited to the thyroid or any T with minimal extrathyroid ext (e.g., ext. to sternothyroid muscle or perithyroid soft tissues)
T4a	T of any size extending beyond the thyroid capsule to invade subcutaneous soft tissues, larynx, trachea, esophagus, or recurrent laryngeal nerve
T4b	T invades prevertebral fascia or encases carotid artery or mediastinal vessels

All anaplastic carcinomas are considered T4 tumors.

T4a	Intrathyroidal anaplastic carcinoma – surgically resectable.
T4b	Extrathyroidal anaplastic carcinoma – surgically unresectable.

Regional Lymph Nodes (N)

Regional lymph nodes are the central compartment, lateral cervical, and upper mediastinal lymph nodes.

	NX	Regional lymph nodes cannot be assessed.
	N0	No regional lymph node metastasis
	N1	Regional lymph node metastasis
	N1a	Metastasis to Level VI (pretracheal, paratracheal, and prelaryngeal/Delphian lymph nodes)
	N1b	Metastasis to unilateral, bilateral, or contralateral cervical or superior mediastinal lymph nodes

Distant Metastasis (M)

MX	Distant metastasis cannot be assessed
M0	No distant metastasis
M1	Distant metastasis

STAGE GROUPING

Separate stage groupings are recommended for papillary or follicular, medullary, and anaplastic (undifferentiated) carcinoma.

Papillary or Follicular
UNDER 45 YEARS

Stage I	Any T	Any N	M0
Stage II	Any T	Any N	M1

Papillary or Folicular
45 YEARS AND OLDER

Stage I	T1	N0	M0
Stage II	T2	N0	M0
Stage III	T3	N0	M0
	T1	N1a	M0
	T2	N1a	M0
	T3	N1a	M0
Stage IVA	T4a	N0	M0
	T4a	N1a	M0

	T1	N1b	M0
	T2	N1b	M0
	T3	N1b	M0
	T4a	N1b	M0
Stage IVB	T4b	Any N	M0
Stage IVC	Any T	Any N	M1
Medullary Carcinoma			
Stage I	T1	N0	M0
Stage II	T2	N0	M0
Stage III	T3	N0	M0
	T1	N1a	M0
	T2	N1a	M0
	T3	N1a	M0
Stage IVA	T4a	N0	M0
	T4a	N1a	M0
	T1	N1b	M0
	T2	N1b	M0
	T3	N1b	M0
	T4a	N1b	M0
Stage IVB	T4b	Any N	M0
Stage IVC	Any T	Any N	M1
Anaplastic Carcinoma			
All anaplastic carcinomas are considered Stage IV			
Stage IVA	T4a	Any N	M0
Stage IVB	T4b	Any N	M0
Stage IVC	Any T	Any N	M1

demonstrated. Systematic lymphadenectomy is associated with lower rates of persistent and recurrent disease and possible survival benefit.[6,17,21,43] For example, a recent single institution series studied patients with DTC referred for MRND after a berry-picking procedure in the lateral neck demonstrated metastasis. The rate of additional metastases discovered at formal neck dissection was 81%, suggesting that resecting only macroscopically involved nodes is likely to result in persistent nodal disease.[17] Tisell and colleagues[43] described a technique of surgical microdissection with en bloc resection of all lymphatic tissue within a compartment. Central compartment dissection was performed in all patients and lateral compartment dissection in patients with macroscopically positive lateral nodes. Mortality from thyroid cancer was 1.6% in his series compared with 8.6% in a series of historical controls who underwent node-picking procedures, despite a higher rate of radioactive iodine therapy in the control series. The superiority of systematic dissection was confirmed in a study demonstrating increased survival and decreased recurrence rates in those undergoing systematic compartment-oriented lymphadenectomy as opposed to other techniques.[21]

Central Neck Dissection

Central compartment cervical lymph nodes metastases are common, with a reported incidence of up to 50% in patients with PTC.[44] Therapeutic central neck dissection prevents serious sequelae including compression or invasion of critical aerodigestive and neural structures. It also decreases the incidence of lymphatic recurrence, and may improve survival.[5,21,43,45] Because of its clear benefits, therapeutic neck dissection is widely accepted. The role of prophylactic central neck dissection, however, remains controversial. As this practice has gained acceptance only recently, studies comparing thyroidectomy alone to thyroidectomy with CLND in patients with clinically negative node status have had short follow-up and differ in their conclusions. A decision of whether or not to perform prophylactic CLND for patients with DTC must be based on the anticipated risks and benefits of operation.

Unfortunately, central compartment involvement is inconsistently identified pre- and intraoperatively. Studies involving prophylactic central neck dissection report unanticipated central metastases in 38% to 45% of patients with PTC.[44,46,47] Without prophylactic neck dissection, these metastases remain in situ as foci of persistent carcinoma. Prophylactic neck dissection thus results in more thorough clearance of disease in more than one-third of patients with PTC. As the frequency of lymphatic metastases in FTC is low, prophylactic dissection is not advocated for these patients.

Central neck dissection also is associated with lower thyroglobulin levels after thyroidectomy, neck dissection, and radioiodine ablation for PTC. Patients who underwent prophylactic central neck dissection were more likely to have undetectable thyroglobulin levels than those whose surgical treatment consisted of thyroidectomy alone.[44] This confirms a more complete removal of thyroid tissue from the central neck in patients who underwent lymphadenectomy. The significance of undetectable thyroglobulin levels for survival or recurrence is unclear; however, low levels of thyroglobulin do facilitate surveillance for recurrent disease.

As the practice of prophylactic central neck dissection is recent, few studies directly address recurrence after this operation. One study reports no central node metastases in 28 patients at 5 years' follow-up; however, this series is limited by small size and short duration.[46] A retrospective review of patients without macroscopically positive lymph nodes noted no difference in recurrence rates at 10 years whether or not central neck dissection was performed.[5] Therapeutic central neck dissection in patients with macroscopically positive central nodes is associated with decreased recurrence rates.[6,45] Preventing nodal recurrence leads to fewer operations to resect involved nodes, which represents a significant reduction in the morbidity of DTC.

Although clearance of thyroid tissue and lymphatic metastases is improved by prophylactic central neck dissection, and recurrence rates may be reduced, the implications for survival are not clear. Several studies have failed to demonstrate a survival advantage but may be underpowered to detect small differences in mortality. In a study of nearly 1000 patients with DTC, 20-year survival was not influenced by surgical treatment with lymph node dissection versus thyroidectomy alone.[48] Another retrospective analysis that identified nodal metastasis as a negative prognostic indicator failed to demonstrate a survival benefit to prophylactic neck dissection at 20-year follow-up.[49]

When evaluating the additional morbidity of prophylactic CLND compared to thyroidectomy alone, it is imperative to also consider the risk of reoperation in the central compartment should the patient develop recurrence. The most frequent complications of thyroidectomy and neck dissection include temporary or permanent hypocalcemia due to hypoparathyroidism, temporary or permanent recurrent laryngeal nerve (RLN) palsy, and injury to the superior branch of the external laryngeal nerve. Rare complications include bleeding requiring reoperation, infection, chyle leak, tracheal injury, and pneumothorax.

For experienced surgeons performing total thyroidectomy, the accepted incidence of permanent RLN injury and permanent hypoparathyroidism is 1% to 2%, with rates less than 1% reported in large series.[50,51] The reported incidence in case series ranges from 1% to 16% for permanent hypoparathyroidism and 1% to 9% for permanent RLN injury.[5,38,44,47] A similar range of complication rates is reported for thyroidectomy with CLND, including therapeutic and prophylactic dissections (**Table 4**). Select series by experienced endocrine surgeons report rates of permanent nerve injury and hypoparathyroidism of 1% to 2% in patients undergoing thyroidectomy with CLND, indicating that central node dissection may be added to total thyroidectomy with little additional morbidity.[38,44] One single-surgeon series of 300 patients with PTC undergoing total thyroidectomy alone, prophylactic unilateral CLND, or therapeutic bilateral CLND demonstrated a trend toward significantly increased rates of transient hypocalcemia with more extensive surgery. No difference in rates of permanent hypoparathyroidism or nerve injury were observed.[52] In contrast, reoperation within the central neck has been repeatedly shown to carry higher morbidity than initial operation, particularly with respect to RLN injury.[45,50,53,54] Prophylactic central neck dissection thus carries little additional morbidity compared with thyroidectomy alone but may decrease the rate of locally persistent or recurrent disease, thereby preventing the need for reoperation within the central compartment and its associated morbidity.

Bilateral and unilateral central compartment dissections have been proposed.[55] Within the central compartment, ipsilateral metastases are more common than contralateral; however, contralateral involvement still occurs in 10% to 20% of individuals.[8,56,57] Multifocal disease involving both thyroid lobes is often not discovered at the time of operation and is associated with increased incidence of bilateral central metastases.[9] For patients with macroscopically positive lymph nodes, bilateral lymphadenectomy should be performed; however, high rates of athyroglobulinemia may be achieved with unilateral central compartment dissection in patients with macroscopically negative lymph nodes.[44]

Lateral Neck Dissection

As with the central compartment, lateral compartment lymphadenectomy is indicated in the presence of clinically positive lymph nodes. Lateral lymphadenopathy detected on examination or imaging should be confirmed as metastatic thyroid cancer by FNA. For patients with DTC, MRND results in decreased local recurrence and fewer reoperative procedures than less extensive operations.[5] For patients with macroscopically

Table 4					
Frequency of complications after thyroidectomy with and without neck dissection (%)					
	Temporary Hypocalcemia	Permanent Hypoparathyroidism	Temporary RLN Palsy	Permanent RLN Palsy	Bleeding
Thyroidectomy without CLND	4–16	>1–15	1–4	>1–6	1.0–1.3
Thyroidectomy with CLND	18–60	0–14	1.8	0–9	1.8
Reoperative CLND		0–13		0–25	

Both prophylactic and therapeutic CLND are included.
Data from Refs.[4,5,22,44,50,51,61,62]

positive lateral nodes, MRND is associated with statistically significant improvement in disease-specific survival compared with thyroidectomy alone.[58]

Several investigators have examined potential indications for MRND in the absence of clinically positive lymph node disease. A series of 500 patients with DTC who underwent thyroidectomy with or without CND or MRND demonstrated no difference in lymphatic recurrence at 15 years in the absence of macroscopic nodal disease.[5] This was confirmed in a series consisting only of patients with FTC where no significant difference in recurrence or mortality was detected based on MRND, even in patients of more advanced stage.[36] Although not appropriate for all clinically node-negative patients, ipsilateral MRND is advocated for patients with significant risk factors for lateral metastasis. Confirmed risk factors include extrathyroidal extension, older age, male gender, larger primary tumor size, and large metastatic burden within the central compartment. For patients with these disease characteristics, MRND may be beneficial.[28,58,59]

Any potential benefits to MRND must be evaluated in the context of the procedure's morbidity. In one series of 1231 patients,[22] the overall complication rate for prophylactic MRND was 24.1%. This included RLN injury, transient hypocalcemia and permanent hypoparathyroidism, chlye leak, pneumothorax, Horner syndrome, and injury to the phrenic, facial, and spinal accessory nerves. The lateral compartment is not breached during thyroidectomy, so MRND performed at a separate operation does not involve a previously operated field. Given the risk of complication at initial operation and the lack of additional risk to MRND performed in a staged fashion after thyroidectomy, dissection of the lateral compartment is routinely limited to patients with FNA-proved lateral node metastases or obvious involvement at thyroidectomy.

The extent of lateral neck dissection necessary for regional control also is debated but not prospectively evaluated. Several studies have demonstrated the low incidence of metastases to levels IIb and V.[16] These observations suggest that dissection in these areas may be low yield but confer increased risk of complication and higher morbidity.

Suprahyoid and Superior Mediastinal Dissection

Metastatic involvement of levels I and VII (superior mediastinal) lymph nodes is rare. In a review of patients with lateral cervical metastases of PTC, less than 5% of patients had suprahyoid involvement.[16] Similarly, approximately 5% of patients with PTC were identified as having superior mediastinal metastases.[11,15] Suprahyoid dissection is not routinely included in lymph node dissections for DTC unless there is macroscopic involvement of this compartment. When nodal metastases are identified, suprahyoid dissection is associated with a low risk of complication and can be performed without additional morbidity.

As is recommended for the other nodal groups, dissection of the superior mediastinal lymph nodes should be performed in the presence of gross nodal involvement. This can often be accomplished via a standard cervical incision; however, sternotomy may result in more complete clearance of nodal tissue. Some investigators advocate for routine prophylactic superior mediastinal dissection in patients with PTC; however, data indicating a survival or recurrence advantage are lacking.

GUIDELINES AND SUMMARY

In 2006, the American Thyroid Association Guidelines Taskforce published management guidelines for patients with DTC. Recently revised guidelines recommend total thyroidectomy with level VI neck dissection for patients with clinically involved central or lateral lymph nodes.[60] For those patients with PTC who are clinically node negative, particularly with larger primary tumors, unilateral or bilateral prophylactic central compartment dissection was deemed worthy of consideration but not specifically recommended. Therapeutic lateral neck dissection was recommended for patients with biopsy-proved lateral node involvement. No recommendations were included regarding prophylactic lateral neck dissection or the optimal extent of lateral dissection.[32]

In the absence of definitive level 1 data from a prospective, randomized controlled trial, the surgical management of cervical lymph node metastasis in DTC is based on observational data and knowledge of disease behavior and relevant anatomy. The decisions for a specific patient must be made with a clear understanding of the natural history of the disease, the likelihood that therapy can change that natural history, and the morbidity of the therapeutic options.

REFERENCES

1. Society AC. Cancer facts and figures 2009. Atlanta (GA): American Cancer Society; 2009.
2. Hundahl SA, Fleming ID, Fremgen AM, et al. A National Cancer Data Base report on 53,856 cases of thyroid carcinoma treated in the U.S., 1985–1995 [comments]. Cancer 1998;83(12):2638–48.
3. Zaydfudim V, Feurer ID, Griffin MR, et al. The impact of lymph node involvement on survival in patients with papillary and follicular thyroid carcinoma. Surgery 2008;144(6):1070–7 [discussion: 1077–8].
4. Ahuja S, Ernst H, Lenz K. Papillary thyroid carcinoma: occurrence and types of lymph node metastases. J Endocrinol Invest 1991;14(7):543–9.
5. Bardet S, Malville E, Rame JP, et al. Macroscopic lymph-node involvement and neck dissection predict lymph-node recurrence in papillary thyroid carcinoma. Eur J Endocrinol 2008;158(4):551–60.
6. Davidson HC, Park BJ, Johnson JT. Papillary thyroid cancer: controversies in the management of neck metastasis. Laryngoscope 2008;118(12):2161–5.
7. Kupferman ME, Patterson M, Mandel SJ, et al. Patterns of lateral neck metastasis in papillary thyroid carcinoma. Arch Otolaryngol Head Neck Surg 2004;130(7): 857–60.
8. Mirallie E, Visset J, Sagan C, et al. Localization of cervical node metastasis of papillary thyroid carcinoma. World J Surg 1999;23(9):970–3 [discussion: 973–4].
9. Qubain SW, Nakano S, Baba M, et al. Distribution of lymph node micrometastasis in pN0 well-differentiated thyroid carcinoma. Surgery 2002;131(3):249–56.
10. Reddy RM, Grigsby PW, Moley JF, et al. Lymph node metastases in differentiated thyroid cancer under 2 cm. Surgery 2006;140(6):1050–4 [discussion: 1054–5].
11. Roh JL, Kim JM, Park CI. Central cervical nodal metastasis from papillary thyroid microcarcinoma: pattern and factors predictive of nodal metastasis. Ann Surg Oncol 2008;15(9):2482–6.
12. Sato N, Oyamatsu M, Koyama Y, et al. Do the level of nodal disease according to the TNM classification and the number of involved cervical nodes reflect prognosis in patients with differentiated carcinoma of the thyroid gland? J Surg Oncol 1998;69(3):151–5.
13. Hamoir M, Desuter G, Gregoire V, et al. A proposal for redefining the boundaries of level V in the neck: is dissection of the apex of level V necessary in mucosal squamous cell carcinoma of the head and neck? Arch Otolaryngol Head Neck Surg 2002;128(12):1381–3.

14. Robbins KT, Clayman G, Levine PA, et al. Neck dissection classification update: revisions proposed by the American Head and Neck Society and the American Academy of Otolaryngology-Head and Neck Surgery. Arch Otolaryngol Head Neck Surg 2002;128(7):751–8.
15. Machens A, Dralle H. Prediction of mediastinal lymph node metastasis in papillary thyroid cancer. Ann Surg Oncol 2009;16(1):171–6.
16. Roh JL, Kim JM, Park CI. Lateral cervical lymph node metastases from papillary thyroid carcinoma: pattern of nodal metastases and optimal strategy for neck dissection. Ann Surg Oncol 2008;15(4):1177–82.
17. Pingpank JF Jr, Sasson AR, Hanton AL, et al. Tumor above the spinal accessory nerve in papillary thyroid cancer that involves lateral neck nodes: a common occurrence. Arch Otolaryngol Head Neck Surg 2002;128(11):1275–8.
18. Yanir Y, Doweck I. Regional metastases in well-differentiated thyroid cancer: pattern of spread. Laryngoscope 2008;118:433–6.
19. Machens A, Holzhausen HJ, Dralle H. Skip metastases in thyroid cancer leaping the central lymph node compartment. Arch Surg 2004;139(1):43–5.
20. Wang TS, Dubner S, Sznyter LA, et al. Incidence of metastatic well-differentiated thyroid cancer in cervical lymph nodes. Arch Otolaryngol Head Neck Surg 2004; 130(1):110–3.
21. Scheumann GF, Gimm O, Wegener G, et al. Prognostic significance and surgical management of locoregional lymph node metastases in papillary thyroid cancer. World J Surg 1994;18(4):559–67 [discussion: 567–8].
22. Ito Y, Higashiyama T, Takamura Y, et al. Risk factors for recurrence to the lymph node in papillary thyroid carcinoma patients without preoperatively detectable lateral node metastasis: validity of prophylactic modified radical neck dissection. World J Surg 2007;31(11):2085–91.
23. Alzahrani AS, Al Mandil M, Chaudhary MA, et al. Frequency and predictive factors of malignancy in residual thyroid tissue and cervical lymph nodes after partial thyroidectomy for differentiated thyroid cancer. Surgery 2002;131(4):443–9.
24. McHenry CR, Rosen IB, Walfish PG. Prospective management of nodal metastases in differentiated thyroid cancer. Am J Surg 1991;162(4):353–6.
25. Ali S, Tiwari RM, Snow GB. False-positive and false-negative neck nodes. Head Neck Surg 1985;8(2):78–82.
26. Kouvaraki MA, Shapiro SE, Fornage BD, et al. Role of preoperative ultrasonography in the surgical management of patients with thyroid cancer. Surgery 2003;134(6):946–54 [discussion: 954–5].
27. Gonzalez HE, Cruz F, O'Brien A, et al. Impact of preoperative ultrasonographic staging of the neck in papillary thyroid carcinoma. Arch Otolaryngol Head Neck Surg 2007;133(12):1258–62.
28. Ito Y, Tomoda C, Uruno T, et al. Ultrasonographically and anatomopathologically detectable node metastases in the lateral compartment as indicators of worse relapse-free survival in patients with papillary thyroid carcinoma. World J Surg 2005;29(7):917–20.
29. Park JS, Son KR, Na DG, et al. Performance of preoperative sonographic staging of papillary thyroid carcinoma based on the sixth edition of the AJCC/UICC TNM classification system. AJR Am J Roentgenol 2009;192(1):66–72.
30. Shimamoto K, Satake H, Sawaki A, et al. Preoperative staging of thyroid papillary carcinoma with ultrasonography. Eur J Radiol 1998;29(1):4–10.
31. Stulak JM, Grant CS, Farley DR, et al. Value of preoperative ultrasonography in the surgical management of initial and reoperative papillary thyroid cancer. Arch Surg 2006;141(5):489–94 [discussion: 494–6].

32. Cooper DS, Doherty GM, Haugen BR, et al. Management guidelines for patients with thyroid nodules and differentiated thyroid cancer. Thyroid 2006;16(2): 109–42.
33. Loh KC, Greenspan FS, Gee L, et al. Pathological tumor-node-metastasis (pTNM) staging for papillary and follicular thyroid carcinomas: a retrospective analysis of 700 patients. J Clin Endocrinol Metab 1997;82(11):3553–62.
34. Salvesen H, Njolstad PR, Akslen LA, et al. Papillary thyroid carcinoma: a multivariate analysis of prognostic factors including an evaluation of the p-TNM staging system. Eur J Surg 1992;158(11–12):583–9.
35. Wada N, Masudo K, Nakayama H, et al. Clinical outcomes in older or younger patients with papillary thyroid carcinoma: impact of lymphadenopathy and patient age. Eur J Surg Oncol 2008;34(2):202–7.
36. Witte J, Goretzki PE, Dieken J, et al. Importance of lymph node metastases in follicular thyroid cancer. World J Surg 2002;26(8):1017–22.
37. Hughes CJ, Shaha AR, Shah JP, et al. Impact of lymph node metastasis in differentiated carcinoma of the thyroid: a matched-pair analysis. Head Neck 1996; 18(2):127–32.
38. Steinmuller T, Klupp J, Rayes N, et al. Prognostic factors in patients with differentiated thyroid carcinoma. Eur J Surg 2000;166(1):29–33.
39. Lundgren CI, Hall P, Dickman PW, et al. Clinically significant prognostic factors for differentiated thyroid carcinoma: a population-based, nested case-control study. Cancer 2006;106(3):524–31.
40. Podnos YD, Smith D, Wagman LD, et al. The implication of lymph node metastasis on survival in patients with well-differentiated thyroid cancer. Am Surg 2005;71(9):731–4.
41. Ito Y, Jikuzono T, Higashiyama T, et al. Clinical significance of metastasis to the central compartment from papillary microcarcinoma of the thyroid. World J Surg 2006;30(1):91–9.
42. Hay ID, Grant CS, Taylor WF, et al. Ipsilateral lobectomy versus bilateral lobar resection in papillary thyroid carcinoma: a retrospective analysis of surgical outcome using a novel prognostic scoring system. Surgery 1987;102(6):1088–95.
43. Tisell LE, Nilsson D, Molne J, et al. Improved survival of patients with papillary thyroid cancer after surgical microdissection. World J Surg 1996;20(7):854–9.
44. Sywak M, Cornford L, Roach P, et al. Routine ipsilateral level VI lymphadenectomy reduces postoperative thyroglobulin levels in papillary thyroid cancer. Surgery 2006;140(6):1000–5 [discussion: 1005–7].
45. Simon D, Goretzki PE, Witte J, et al. Incidence of regional recurrence guiding radicality in differentiated thyroid carcinoma. World J Surg 1996;20(7):860–6 [discussion: 866].
46. Pereira JA, Jimeno J, Miquel J, et al. Nodal yield, morbidity, and recurrence after central neck dissection for papillary thyroid carcinoma. Surgery 2005;138(6): 1095–100 [discussion: 1100–1].
47. Salvesen H, Njolstad PR, Akslen LA, et al. Thyroid carcinoma: results from surgical treatment in 211 consecutive patients. Eur J Surg 1991;157(9):521–6.
48. Cross S, Wei JP, Kim S, et al. Selective surgery and adjuvant therapy based on risk classifications of well-differentiated thyroid cancer. J Surg Oncol 2006; 94(8):678–82.
49. Eichhorn W, Tabler H, Lippold R, et al. Prognostic factors determining long-term survival in well-differentiated thyroid cancer: an analysis of four hundred eighty-four patients undergoing therapy and aftercare at the same institution. Thyroid 2003;13(10):949–58.

50. White ML, Gauger PG, Doherty GM. Central lymph node dissection in differenti-ated thyroid cancer. World J Surg 2007;31(5):895–904.
51. Bliss RD, Gauger PG, Delbridge LW. Surgeon's approach to the thyroid gland: surgical anatomy and the importance of technique. World J Surg 2000;24(8):891–7.
52. Palestini N, Borasi A, Cestino L, et al. Is central neck dissection a safe procedure in the treatment of papillary thyroid cancer? Our experience. Langenbecks Arch Surg 2008;393(5):693–8.
53. Kim MK, Mandel SH, Baloch Z, et al. Morbidity following central compartment re-operation for recurrent or persistent thyroid cancer. Arch Otolaryngol Head Neck Surg 2004;130(10):1214–6.
54. Monchik JM, DeLellis RA. Re-operative neck surgery for well-differentiated thyroid cancer of follicular origin. J Surg Oncol 2006;94(8):714–8.
55. American Thyroid Association Surgery Working Group, American Association of Endocrine Surgeons, American Academy of Otolaryngology-Head and Neck Surgery, et al. Consensus statement on the terminology and classification of central neck dissection for thyroid cancer. Thyroid 2009;19(11):1153–8.
56. Grodski S, Cornford L, Sywak M, et al. Routine level VI lymph node dissection for papillary thyroid cancer: surgical technique. ANZ J Surg 2007;77(4):203–8.
57. Gimm O, Rath FW, Dralle H. Pattern of lymph node metastases in papillary thyroid carcinoma. Br J Surg 1998;85(2):252–4.
58. Noguchi S, Murakami N, Yamashita H, et al. Papillary thyroid carcinoma: modified radical neck dissection improves prognosis. Arch Surg 1998;133(3):276–80.
59. Goropoulos A, Karamoshos K, Christodoulou A, et al. Value of the cervical compartments in the surgical treatment of papillary thyroid carcinoma. World J Surg 2004;28(12):1275–81.
60. American Thyroid Association Guidelines Taskforce on Thyroid Nodules and Differentiated Thyroid Cancer, Cooper DS, Doherty GM, et al. Revised American Thyroid Association management guidelines for patients with thyroid nodules and differentiated thyroid cancer [comment]. Thyroid 2009;19(11):1167–214.
61. Witt RL, McNamara AM. Prognostic factors in mortality and morbidity in patients with differentiated thyroid cancer. Ear Nose Throat J 2002;81(12):856–63.
62. Cheah WK, Arici C, Ituarte PH, et al. Complications of neck dissection for thyroid cancer. World J Surg 2002;26(8):1013–6.

Prognosis and Management of Invasive Well-differentiated Thyroid Cancer

Mark L. Urken, MD[a,b,c],*

KEYWORDS

- Invasive thyroid cancer • Tracheal resection
- Nerve anastomosis • Esophagus
- Extrathyroidal extension • Extracapsular spread

Gross involvement of the trachea or esophagus is almost a certain sign against curability, and yet one may be tempted into an extensive and dangerous operation to remove the diseased tissue....

D Balfour, Medical Record, 1918[1]

The rapid increase in well-differentiated thyroid cancer, in particular papillary thyroid cancer, has led to a proportionate increase in the volume of thyroid surgery performed in the United States and abroad.[2,3] The 3 primary disciplines involved in treating thyroid cancer are surgery, endocrinology, and nuclear medicine.

Surgery remains the initial form of treatment of virtually all patients who have well-differentiated thyroid malignancies. The surgeon performing that surgery is charged with the responsibility of removing all evidence of disease located in the central compartment of the neck, including the mediastinum, as well as nodal disease that is often present in the lateral compartments of the neck. That surgery is currently being performed by surgeons with a range of training experience in performing routine thyroidectomy, paratracheal node dissection, lateral compartment nodal dissection, and mediastinal dissection. Although most cases of well-differentiated thyroid cancer do not require the skill sets to manage aerodigestive tract involvement or nerve

[a] Department of Otorhinolaryngology-Head and Neck Surgery, Albert Einstein College of Medicine, New York, NY, USA
[b] Department of Otolaryngology, Beth Israel Medical Center, Continuum Cancer Centers of New York, New York, NY, USA
[c] Phillips Ambulatory Care Center, Institute for Head and Neck and Thyroid Cancer, Suite 5B, 10 Union Square East, New York, NY 10003, USA
* Phillips Ambulatory Care Center, Institute for Head and Neck and Thyroid Cancer, Suite 5B, 10 Union Square East, New York, NY 10003.
E-mail address: Murken@chpnet.org

Otolaryngol Clin N Am 43 (2010) 301–328
doi:10.1016/j.otc.2010.02.002
0030-6665/10/$ – see front matter © 2010 Elsevier Inc. All rights reserved.

involvement, when the disease requires that such intervention is essential for a complete resection, it is incumbent on the surgeon to be able to manage such cases of advanced disease in the primary setting. Closing the wound after performing a more limited resection and referring the patient to a surgeon who performs that type of surgery after the patient develops a recurrence has been shown to lead to a less favorable outcome.[4]

Specialties that are involved in the surgical management of thyroid cancer include otolaryngologists, endocrine surgeons, general surgeons, and surgeons with fellowship training in surgical oncology. Although statistics show that most of the incremental new cases of thyroid cancer that are treated each year are for early stage disease, there remains an ever-present danger that a patient presenting with thyroid cancer may have invasive disease that will complicate the surgical procedure and challenge the surgeon to perform a complete resection and render the patient functionally intact. It is imperative that all specialties performing thyroid cancer surgery are trained in all aspects of upper aerodigestive tract resection and reconstruction so that they are prepared to meet the demands that disease in these patients can present.

IDENTIFYING THE PATIENT WITH INVASIVE THYROID CANCER

One of the major challenges in treating patients with invasive thyroid cancer is that most patients with this form of the disease are asymptomatic and the disease takes the patient and the surgeon unawares. Four types of patients can be identified before surgery as having an increased likelihood of invasive disease:

1. Asymptomatic patients who present with an abnormal examination related to either vocal cord dysfunction or evidence of a subglottic or tracheal mass. The identification of vocal cord paralysis is 1 of the first clues that the surgeon is dealing with invasive disease that has extended outside the normal bounds of the thyroid gland to involve the recurrent laryngeal nerve (RLN).
2. Patients with recurrent thyroid cancer in the central compartment.
3. Symptomatic patients with biopsy-proven thyroid cancer who present with a change in voice, dyspnea, hemoptysis, or dysphagia.
4. Patients with documented invasive disease based on preoperative cross-sectional imaging of the central compartment showing invasion of the central viscera, or lateral compartment nodal metastases showing extracapsular extension.

All patients in the first 3 groups should undergo cross-sectional imaging before surgery to better anticipate the extent of the surgery that is required to achieve a complete resection. One additional category of patient is the one who presents with pulmonary or other systemic metastases that are found to be of thyroid origin. Such patients should undergo cross-sectional imaging of the neck and the mediastinum.

Despite the ominous appearance of an intraluminal tracheal mass in a patient with biopsy-proven thyroid cancer, the surgeon should be aware that all that is present in the trachea is not always invasive thyroid cancer. In 1 of my own memorable cases of thyroid cancer arising in an opera singer, preoperative imaging showed the presence of what was believed to be intraluminal extension of her disease, only to find out on the final pathologic review that the tracheal component was actually a benign thyroid rest that was not identified as benign disease until after the tracheal resection had been performed.[5] In another symptomatic patient with a biopsy suspicious for thyroid cancer, preoperative imaging identified an intraluminal mass that proved to be a chondrosarcoma arising from a tracheal ring. The fine-needle aspiration had traversed the thyroid and led to a false-positive cytologic report (**Fig. 1**). A patient with a large thyroid mass and a suspicious cytology was found to have intraluminal narrowing on preoperative imaging performed because of her symptomatic respiratory difficulty. The thyroidectomy proved to be benign, and the tracheal narrowing was caused by a benign tracheal stenosis of unknown cause (**Fig. 2**). Yet another patient developed severe airway compromise as a result of intraluminal extension of a paratracheal mass, which proved to be a schwannoma of the RLN (**Fig. 3**). Although most patients with an intraluminal mass and biopsy-proven thyroid cancer do indeed have invasive thyroid disease, it is not always the case.

There is a well-documented entity know as a collision tumor of the upper aerodigestive tract that results from 2 separate neoplastic processes arising in a contiguous manner to involve either the thyroid gland alone with 2 separate histologic subtypes, or the thyroid gland and the aerodigestive tract. The author recently reported such a case in which a papillary thyroid cancer was diagnosed preoperatively and a coexistent vocal cord paralysis led to cross-sectional imaging. The computed tomography (CT) scan showed findings that were interpreted as invasive thyroid cancer. Fiberoptic examination did not show any signs of a mucosal-based neoplastic process; however, because of destruction of the cricoid in this older male patient, the decision was made to proceed with a total thyroidectomy and a total laryngectomy. Final pathologic review identified a subglottic squamous cell cancer that had caused the cartilage destruction, and abutted against the intraglandular papillary thyroid cancer.[6]

INCIDENCE OF INVASIVE WELL-DIFFERENTIATED THYROID CANCER

It is difficult to know the true incidence of invasive thyroid cancer because it seems to be a moving target. With the increased incidence of small thyroid cancers detected as a result of more widespread use of ultrasonography, the percentage of cases of invasive disease has decreased accordingly.[2] However, there are several institutional case series that give a glimpse of the reported incidence of aerodigestive tract invasion in tertiary referral centers. The range of invasive well-differentiated thyroid cancer is 1% to 23%.[7] In the Mayo Clinic series reported by Djalilian and colleagues[8] 18 patients had thyroid cancer extending into the lumen of the larynx or trachea out of a total of 2000 patients treated for thyroid cancer at that institution from 1913 to 1973. The risk of upper aerodigestive tract involvement, nerve involvement, and muscle involvement is directly related to the presence of extrathyroidal extension (ETE) of the primary

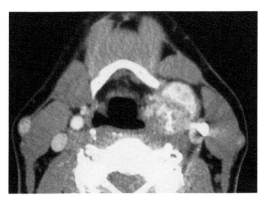

Fig. 1. Chondrosarcoma of the thyroid ala misdiagnosed as an invasive thyroid cancer.

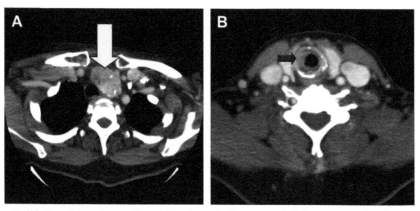

Fig. 2. (*A*) Thyroid nodule with calcifications (*yellow arrow*). (*B*) Benign tracheal stenosis (*blue arrow*).

tumor and extracapsular invasion in a metastatic lymph node. Numerous prognostic factors have been evaluated and adopted by the various staging systems for well-differentiated thyroid cancer; among them:

1. Size of the tumor
2. Age of the patient
3. Presence of ETE.

The incidence of extrathyroidal disease increases with increasing size of the primary malignancy[9]; however, even micropapillary cancers can extend outside the thyroid gland to place the RLN, the tracheal cartilage, the larynx, and esophagus at risk. The risk of ETE is related to the biology of the tumor as well as its geographic location within the thyroid lobe, whether it is in the middle or on the periphery of the gland. The incidence of ETE in micropapillary carcinomas has been reported to be as high as 31.9%.[10] The presence of ETE is associated with an increased incidence of recurrent disease and death caused by disease.[11] Breaux and Guillamondegui[12] reviewed the institutional experience with invasive thyroid cancer at MD Anderson Cancer Center and found that primary tumor size greater than 4 cm was associated with an increased incidence of mortality from disease. Involvement of more than 4 structures by the invasive disease was reported to be uniformly fatal. Similarly, primary tumor size greater

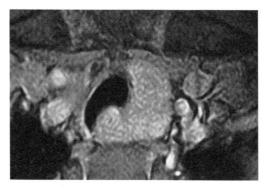

Fig. 3. Benign schwannoma of the RLN.

than 4 cm was identified as a significant adverse prognostic factor by Andersen and colleagues[13] in patients older than 45 years with invasive thyroid cancer.

The presence of disease extension outside the capsule of lymph nodes has been identified as a significant negative prognostic factor in patients with metastatic squamous cell cancer. Few studies have reported the incidence and prognostic significance of extracapsular extension in nodal metastases from papillary thyroid cancer. Yamashita and colleagues[14] reported the results of a multivariate analysis in 1997 in which they concluded that disease extension outside the capsule of a lymph node harboring metastatic papillary thyroid cancer had a significant effect on the risk of distant disease as well as the risk of dying from disease. In addition, these investigators identified the risk of extranodal extension as being higher in larger lymph nodes than smaller nodes, and also found that large nodal deposits and extrathyroidal invasion correlated with the development of distant disease and death. In the Yamashita study, 50% of the patients who died of disease succumbed within the first 10 years following treatment. Akslen and colleagues[15] reported that extracapsular extension of well-differentiated thyroid cancer was associated with a short recurrence-free survival interval, but not with increased 10-year mortality. It is unclear whether the lack of longer-term follow-up led to this discrepancy between these 2 studies.

STRUCTURES INVOLVED BY INVASIVE THYROID CANCER

A variety of different structures can be involved in invasive thyroid cancer. Central compartment disease can invade the viscera and nerves of the central compartment as well as to extend laterally or extend caudally to involve mediastinal structures. Those structures can be divided in several different ways: they might be classified based on visceral structures, muscles, nerves, and vessels; alternatively, dividing the structures at risk based geographically on central compartment and lateral compartment is the more common way to approach this topic.

The central compartment viscera include the larynx, trachea, and esophagus. In addition, the strap muscles are the structures most commonly involved by invasive thyroid cancer. The RLN is the nerve most commonly affected by invasive disease in the central compartment. The superior laryngeal nerve is rarely reported separately in large series of invasive thyroid disease. The caudal portion of the central compartment extends to the mediastinum, where the innominate artery and vein are at risk.

In the lateral compartment, the major vascular structures are the internal jugular vein and the common carotid artery. The neurologic structures include the vagus nerve, cervical sympathetic chain, phrenic nerve, and the spinal accessory nerve. Although theoretically possible, it is rare that the hypoglossal nerve is invaded by nodal disease in the upper jugular region. The sternocleidomastoid (SCM) muscle can also be invaded by extracapsular extension of metastatic nodes.

Some series have identified the incidence of involvement of various cervical structures by invasive thyroid cancer. In the series reported by Breaux and Guillamondegui,[9] 47 patients with invasive disease were analyzed. The RLN was involved in 22 (47%), the trachea was involved in 28 (60%), the larynx in 16 (34%), the esophagus in 8 (17%), and the strap muscles or platysma in 20 (43%) patients. In addition, the vagus nerve was involved in 2 (4%) patients, the jugular vein in 6 (13%), the carotid artery in 3 (6%), and the skin in 2 (4%) patients. In Nakao's series of 31 patients requiring tracheal resection, the following structures also required resection: RLN (61%), phrenic nerve (10%), vagus (13%), and spinal accessory nerve (6%), strap muscles or SCM (78%), jugular vein (45%), and esophageal muscle in 29%. Transmural extension to involve the esophageal mucosa was reported in only 6% of patients.[16] Nishida and colleagues[17] reported the following structures involved by invasive thyroid cancer in 117 patients: trachea (59%), esophagus (31%), internal jugular vein (38%), carotid artery (7%), strap muscles and SCM (77%), vagus nerve (8%), and RLN (61%). Kowalski and Filho[17] reported the following structures involved in 46 patients with invasive thyroid cancer: trachea (46%), muscle (41%), RLN (33%), larynx (24%), major vessel (13%), and esophagus (9%). From a review of these 4 series alone it is apparent that there is significant variability in the incidence of the various structures involved. The incidence of esophageal involvement ranges from 9% to 31%, the involvement of the RLN ranges from 33% to 61%, tracheal involvement ranges from 46% to 100%, and carotid artery involvement from 0% to 7%.

In the Mayo Clinic series reported by McCaffrey and colleagues, the invasion of different structures was found to have a different effect on survival. In that series, the involvement of muscle was found in 53%, the trachea in 37%, the RLN in 47%, esophagus in 21%, larynx in 12%, and a variety of other sites in 30%. Analysis of the different subsites identified the trachea and esophagus as having a statistically significant independent effect on survival, whereas completeness of resection approached statistical significance. Alternatively, invasion of muscle, the RLN, and larynx did not have a significant independent effect on survival.[18] It is unclear why involvement of different structures should lead to a different effect on survival. The biology of ETE and extracapsular invasion from a lymph node is seemingly the same and is a reflection of the aggressiveness of the tumor, although the actual structures involved are in part a product of the geographic location as well as the size of the tumor within the thyroid gland or the location of the lymph node within the central or lateral compartments of the neck or mediastinum.

DECISION MAKING IN MANAGEMENT OF INVASIVE THYROID CANCER

The central premise of managing patients with invasive thyroid cancer is to clear the central compartment of the neck to protect the patient's vital functions of being able to breathe comfortably, speak, and maintain nutrition through oral alimentation. Although a tracheostomy and a feeding gastrostomy tube can be placed, the unchecked growth of disease in the central neck challenges the patency of even a surgically created airway. The histology of the tumor, the degree of differentiation and the age of the patient are critical parameters in determining the opportunity and the likelihood of success of treating invasive thyroid cancer with adjuvant therapy once a resection has been performed. The likelihood of disease response to radioiodine (^{131}I) therapy has significant importance for the surgeon in terms of how complete a resection must be accomplished and what the implications are of leaving macro- or microscopic disease.

Recurrent thyroid cancer most often presents as nodal recurrence and often has a documented biology that is resistant to ^{131}I therapy. The decision to perform extensive central compartment resections in patients with metastatic disease involves a complex decision-making process. It raises the issue as to how extensive the work-up should be before performing surgery. The most commonly reported sites for metastatic thyroid cancer are the lung and bone. The liver and brain are less frequently involved.[19] In contemporary thyroid cancer management, the performance of a positron emission tomography CT scan can provide valuable information regarding the extent of disease as well as the likelihood of ^{131}I uptake. However, the luxury of obtaining that information is lost when the invasive nature of a thyroid cancer is unsuspected before the initiation of the surgery.

SITE-SPECIFIC MANAGEMENT OF INVASIVE THYROID CANCER
Strap Muscle and SCM Muscle Invasion

Involvement of the strap, platysma, and the SCM muscles rarely causes any specific symptoms (**Fig. 4**). The initial approach during thyroid surgery involves elevation of the sternothyroid muscle off the surface of the thyroid gland. Adherence of the strap muscles to the surface of the gland can be seen with thyroiditis but it is often the first indication for the surgeon of the biologic aggressiveness of the thyroid cancer. Resection of the strap muscles and the SCM muscles causes little functional effect on most patients, except for professional voice users, who may be negatively affected by loss of the accessory muscles of voice production. Resection of the SCM muscle has little functional effect but does lead to loss of volume in the lateral neck, producing a contour deformity. In most instances, a cuff of muscle should be resected to obtain clearance around a biologically aggressive thyroid cancer (**Fig. 5**).

Laryngotracheal Complex

Because most patients who die of thyroid cancer die of airway obstruction due to invasion of the structures in the midline visceral compartment with encroachment on the airway, surgeons probably should expend as much effort on the problem of what to do at the primary operation when there is invasion of the visceral compartment, superficial or otherwise, as they do on the problem of cervical lymph node metastasis.

Djalilian M, 1974[8]

Involvement of the larynx and trachea led to preoperative symptoms in 28% and 18% of patients, respectively with documented invasive thyroid cancer in Kowalski's series (**Fig. 6**).[18] In the series by McCarty and colleagues,[20] 40 patients with frank airway invasion were analyzed and 11% reported hemoptysis, dyspnea was reported in 5%, and only 22% were found to have hoarseness. The poor correlation between voice changes and the presence of vocal cord paralysis is discussed in the section on nerve involvement. However, the development of dyspnea is seen only when the cross-sectional airway of the trachea has been narrowed by at least 50%, either by intrinsic disease or extrinsic compression.[21] The rate of narrowing of the airway also

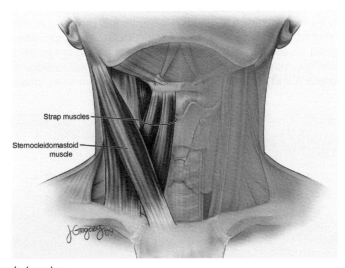

Strap muscles

Sternocleidomastoid muscle

Fig. 4. Muscle invasion.

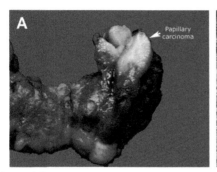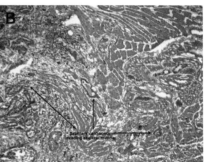

Fig. 5. (*A*) Papillary thyroid carcinoma arising in the superior pole of the thyroid with involvement of the sternothyroid muscle, which was resected. (*B*) Histology showed invasion of the muscle by papillary thyroid carcinoma.

affects the patient's awareness of dyspnea. When the process occurs slowly, patients often report that they accommodate in remarkable ways and often are incorrectly diagnosed with reactive airway disease or sleep apnea before the correct diagnosis is established.

Virtually all patients who are advised to undergo thyroid surgery have had an ultrasound examination as part of their preoperative evaluation. The performance of cross-sectional imaging is less common unless symptoms, the presence of recurrent disease, or physical findings warrant that intervention. Shimamoto and colleagues[22] reported the sensitivity for ultrasound detection of tracheal invasion was 42.9% and for esophageal invasion it was 28.6%. Yamamura and colleagues[23] reported a higher level of sensitivity, with 9 of 10 patients with intercartilaginous involvement predicted by ultrasound along with 9 of 10 patients with mucosal involvement. The experience of thyroid ultrasonographers varies greatly. In addition, the number of cases of invasive thyroid cancer that are seen regularly by most endocrinologists who are performing thyroid ultrasound and ultrasound-guided biopsies makes it unlikely that most patients with invasive disease are accurately diagnosed before surgery.

The mechanism for invasion of the upper aerodigestive tract by an invasive thyroid cancer has been delineated by McCaffrey and colleagues.[24] Disease may gain access to the airway by way of the primary tumor in the thyroid or via a paratracheal node involved by metastatic disease. **Fig. 7**A illustrates the routes of invasion around the posterior thyroid ala to gain access to the paraglottic space. In **Fig. 7**B the entry is from a paratracheal node, which can directly invade the tracheal cartilage or gain entry to the membranous wall of the trachea at the level of the tracheoesophageal groove.

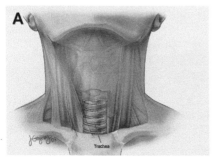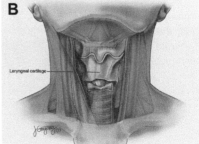

Fig. 6. (*A*) Invasion of the trachea. (*B*) Invasion of the larynx.

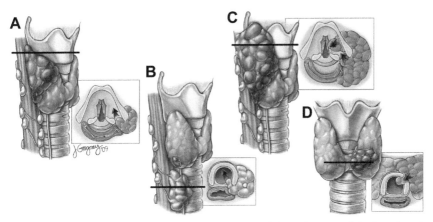

Fig. 7. Mechanisms of tracheal and laryngeal invasion of thyroid cancer. (*A*) Direct invasion around the posterior border of the thyroid ala to involve the paraglottic space. (*B*) Invasion of the trachea by a metastatic lymph node. (*C*) Direct invasion of the thyroid ala from a primary tumor in the superior pole of the gland. (*D*) Direct invasion of the anterior trachea from a primary tumor in the thyroid lobe or isthmus. (*Adapted from* McCafftrey T, Bergstralh E, Hay I. Locally invasive papillary thyroid carcinoma: 1940–1990. Head Neck 1994;16:168; with permission.)

Direct invasion of the thyroid cartilage may occur through larger primary thyroid malignancies (see **Fig. 7**C). Anterior airway invasion may occur through primary tumors involving the isthmus or from delphian or pretracheal lymph nodes involved by metastatic disease manifesting extracapular extension (see **Fig. 7**D). A delphian lymph node involved by metastatic papillary thyroid cancer is shown in **Fig. 8**.

Shin and colleagues[25] characterized 4 stages of airway invasion (**Fig. 9**):

- In stage 1 tracheal invasion, the tumor shows ETE and abuts the perichondrium, but does not invade through it.
- In stage 2 invasion, there is evidence of cartilage erosion but no evidence of transmural extension.
- In stage 3, the tumor extends through the cartilage along natural pathways that include vessels traversing the tracheal wall (**Fig. 10**). The disease is present within the trachea but not through the mucosa.

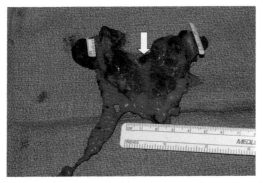

Fig. 8. Total thyroidectomy showing multifocal disease and a metastatic papillary thyroid cancer involving the paratracheal, pretracheal, and delphian lymph nodes (*yellow arrow*).

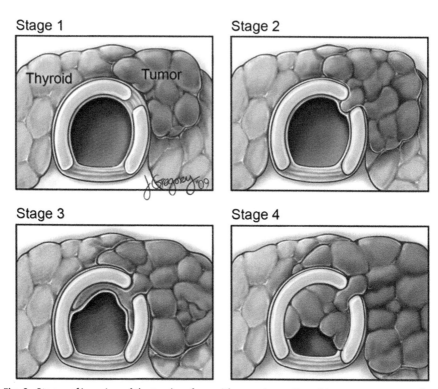

Fig. 9. Stages of invasion of the trachea from either a primary thyroid cancer or a paratracheal or pretracheal lymph node. (*Adapted from* Shin DH, Mark EJ, Suen HC, et al. Pathologic staging of papillary carcinoma of the thyroid with airway invasion based on the anatomic manner of extension to the trachea. Hum Pathol 1993;24:866; with permission.)

- Stage 4 disease extends through the mucosa and is present within the lumen of the trachea.

From a prognostic perspective, Shin and colleagues[25] reported that none of the patients with stage 1, 2, or 3 disease died within the first 5 years following initial therapy, but 1 patient did succumb to disease after 5 years. In the cohort of 11 patients with stage 4 disease, 5 of the patients succumbed within the first 5 years and 1 died of disease after that period.

In addition to these findings it is evident that preoperative tracheobronchoscopy in patients with stages 1, 2, and 3 disease would not show any abnormal tissue for biopsy unless a transmucosal biopsy is performed in stage 3 disease. Randolph and Kamani[26] reported a series of 21 patients with invasive thyroid cancer and found that tracheobronchoscopy was abnormal in 6 of the 7 patients in whom the procedure was performed. The exact abnormal findings were not described; however, these investigators reported that the prediction of tracheal invasion by preoperative imaging was achieved in only 3 of 15 patients in whom that disease was identified at the time of surgery. Although ETE is deemed to be important in virtually all staging systems, the depth of airway invasion is not accounted for in any of the current staging systems.

Nakao and colleagues[16] reported the depth of invasion of tumor involving the tracheal wall and found adventitial involvement in 6%, intercartilaginous extension

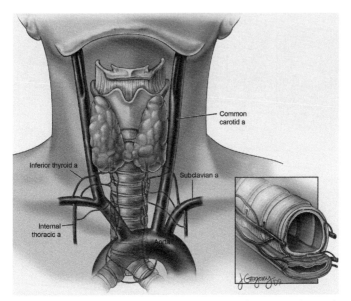

Fig. 10. Vascular supply to the cervical and mediastinal trachea. Inset shows the intercartilaginous pathway of vessels entering from a lateral direction and coursing through the wall of the trachea. (*Adapted from* Salassa J, Pearson B, Payne WS. Gross and microscopic blood supply of the trachea. Ann Thorac Surg 1977;24:103; with permission.)

of disease in 10%, submucosal involvement in 48%, and mucosal involvement in 35%. They did not report the effect of the depth of invasion on prognosis.

Dralle and colleagues[27] classified 6 types of laryngotracheal resections that are required based on the extent and location of the visceral invasion (**Fig. 11**):

- Type 1 was described as a limited area of invasion at the laryngotracheal junction, less than 2 cm in the longitudinal direction and less than or equal to one-third of the circumference. In type 1, the RLN is often invaded.
- Type 2 has a similar dimension but is located lower in the trachea away from the larynx.
- Type 3 tumor invasion is similar in location to type 1, at the laryngotracheal junction, but differs because of the larger dimension, greater than 2 cm longitudinally or more than one-third of the circumference.
- Type 4 invasion involves the trachea with dimensions that are greater than 2 cm longitudinally or more than one-third of the circumference.
- Type 5 invasion involves so much of the larynx that the only option for a complete resection is to perform a total laryngectomy. The minimum critical portion of the larynx that must be retained to reconstruct and restore function has been characterized in the extensive literature on laryngeal cancer surgery.[28] The critical structure needed to restore function is an intact cricoarytenoid joint with a functioning RLN. Sophisticated reconstructive techniques have been described to import lining and structure to restore an adequate caliber to the laryngotracheal lumen and a sphincter to allow protection of the airway during deglutition.[29]
- Type 6 resections involve the entire laryngopharynx and possibly the cervical esophagus requiring a total laryngopharngectomy with or without a cervical esophagectomy. There are numerous options for reconstruction of this type of defect,

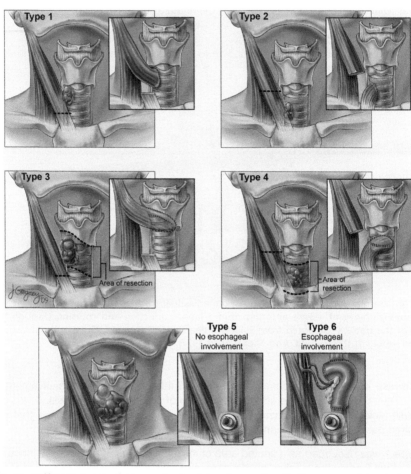

Fig. 11. Different types of laryngotracheal involvement with the appropriate design of resection and repair. (*Adapted from* Dralle H, Brauckhoff, M, Machens A, Gimm O. Surgical management of advanced thyroid cancer invading the aerodigestive tract. In: Clark OH, Duh QY, editors. Textbook of endocrine surgery. Philadelphia: WB Saunders; 2005. p. 325; with permission.)

which include a tubed cutaneous free flap or a free visceral flap such as jejunum or a gastro-omental flap.[30]

One of the important points for a surgeon is to estimate the amount of the laryngo-tracheal complex that must be resected to achieve clear margins around the tumor. One of the important challenges is encountered by the surgeon who is unaware of the invasive nature of a thyroid cancer that is found serendipitously to be extending outside the thyroid gland and involving the tracheal, cricoid, or thyroid cartilages. It is evident from the work of Shin and colleagues[25] that looking from the outside, the surgeon risks underestimating the full extent of the disease extent on the luminal aspect of the airway. Without imaging it is difficult to know whether the disease has reached the extent of stage 1 or stage 4. Ozaki and colleagues[31] evaluated the difference in the external extent of the disease and compared it with the internal extent of the disease (**Fig. 12**). The results of that pathologic assessment showed that the

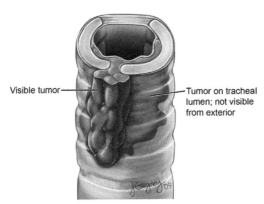

Visible tumor

Tumor on tracheal lumen; not visible from exterior

Fig. 12. Extent of invasion of the trachea, showing the greater risk of underestimating the circumferential extent rather than the longitudinal extent based on visible extent of tumor from the outside of the trachea.

extirpative surgeon runs the risk of underestimating the circumferential extent of the luminal portion of the tumor more than the longitudinal extent of the disease. As a result the surgeon can fairly accurately gage the longitudinal resection parameters based on the longitudinal extent of the external involvement of the tumor but may have to take a greater circumference than indicated based on what is seen on the external surface.

One of the significant challenges in performing surgery on the aerodigestive tract for patients with well-differentiated thyroid cancer is to decide how much of the structure of the airway to resect, with the goal of achieving clear margins. Complete surgical resection has been identified as a significant prognostic factor in well-differentiated thyroid cancer.[32] In high-risk patients with invasive disease, in particular, the surgeon should do everything possible to achieve a complete resection. Kowalski and Filho[18] identified incomplete resection, along with age greater than 45 years, and preoperative diagnosis of ETE as significant predictors of worse prognosis in patients with invasive thyroid cancer. The value of intraoperative frozen sections to achieve that goal has been questioned. Nakao and colleagues[16] reported 2 patients with negative margins on frozen section, but who were found to have positive margins in the adventitial layer on permanent histologic review of the tracheal resection. These 2 patients developed recurrence at the anastomotic site; however, 6 patients with similar false-negative frozen sections did not develop anastomotic recurrence.

Patients with invasive thyroid cancer are more often older and more often have less differentiated forms of the disease, which are less likely to be treated successfully with radioactive iodine therapy. As a result, the ability to effectively treat residual disease with adjuvant modalities is usually not known at the time of surgery, but should not be assumed by the surgeon. Rather than making the intraoperative decision that "I can leave some disease because I can always give radioactive iodine," complete extirpation of the disease should be sought in all cases.

A variety of surgical procedures are currently in use to manage invasive thyroid cancer that involves the larynx and trachea:

Shave resections are defined as the removal of macroscopic disease from the surface of the trachea without a full thickness resection of the airway.

Window resections are defined as full thickness resection of a portion of the airway and closure of that window using a variety of techniques (Dralle types 1 and 2, see **Fig. 11**). It is usually considered that a maximum of one-third of the

circumference of the trachea can be resected without compromising the structure of the airway.
Sleeve resections of the trachea are defined as circumferential resections that
require repair using end-to-end anastomoses, with or without laryngeal release
procedures (Dralle types 3 and 4, see **Fig. 11**).

Shave excisions of the laryngotracheal complex do not require reconstruction
because the structural integrity and the lining of the airway are not disrupted. In window
resections, 3 common techniques can be used to reconstruct the airway defect:

1. The first is a sliding tracheoplasty or the excision of added portions of the airway to
   allow primary repair to be performed free of tension (**Fig. 13**).
2. The second is to patch the defect with either an inferiorly based or a superiorly
   based SCM flap to seal the defect. This technique results in remucosalization of
   the exposed muscle in the lumen of the airway.[33]

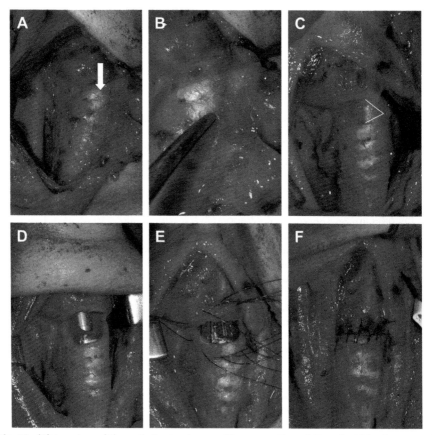

Fig. 13. (A) Invasion of the anterior trachea and lower portion of the cricoid (*yellow arrow*)
from a papillary thyroid carcinoma arising in the isthmus. (B) Disease on the surface of the
first tracheal ring is readily apparent. (C) Following a window resection, the opening in the
trachea is extended bilaterally (*white lines*) to facilitate primary repair. (D) The resulting
defect can be closed primarily with direct suturing. (E, F) Sutures are placed and then
secured, completing the repair.

3. The final technique is a staged repair of the airway with the initial creation of a formalized tracheal trough by suturing the skin to the mucosa. Following a 2-week period of healing, the second stage is performed by placement of a titanium mesh deep to the skin adjacent to the trough. In the final stage the composite flap composed of skin and mesh is turned inward to reline the airway with skin and provide structural integrity with the alloplast, which at that point has become incorporated through ingrowth of native tissue between and around the mesh (**Fig. 14**). Although this technique works well and allows for greater than one-third of the circumference to be resected, it does require a staged repair and is not favorable when the cervical skin is hair bearing, as is often the case in men. Planned postoperative external beam radiotherapy eliminates the problem of growth of hair on skin transposed into the airway.

Sleeve resection and end-to-end repair is a useful and reliable technique to achieve wide margins around the disease and primary reconstitution of the airway. The key to success in this technique is to achieve a tension-free repair to avoid the short-term risk of an anastomotic breakdown with the risk of fistula formation resulting in cervical or mediastinal infection, or the complete disruption of the airway repair with catastrophic

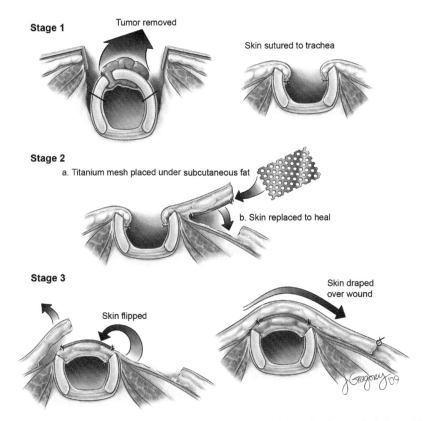

Fig. 14. Staged repair of a window resection by creation of a tracheal trough, followed by placement of titanium mesh in the subcutaneous tissue in stage 2. The final stage involves the transposition of the fabricated composite flap with placement of the skin into the lumen and then coverage of the neck with regional skin.

consequences. The surgeon must remember that the blood supply to the trachea enters laterally (see **Fig. 10**) and must be preserved to avoid ischemia of the mobilized tracheal segment. Therefore mobilization of the cervical and mediastinal portions of the trachea is best accomplished with blunt dissection along the anterior wall with minimal lateral dissection. When a tension-free repair cannot be achieved with blunt dissection and flexion of the neck, then a suprahyoid or infrahyoid release of the larynx should be performed to allow several additional centimeters of mobilization of the larynx to be achieved (**Fig. 15**). Monofilament sutures are placed in the airway with the knots placed outside the lumen to create as little intraluminal reaction as possible and the attendant risk of forming a tracheal stenosis (**Fig. 16**).

A growing body of literature is centered around the controversy regarding how radical the resection of the laryngotracheal complex needs to be to achieve long-term control.[7] This literature is flawed for several reasons because of the lack of a prospective randomized trial that appropriately stratifies patients according to the extent of the local disease based on the depth of invasion across the wall of the trachea, distinguishing between primary and recurrent disease, limiting the series to well-differentiated cancers, reporting the iodine-trapping ability of the tumor, the use of adjuvant external beam radiotherapy, the presence of distant metastases, the presence of regional adenopathy, and the adequacy of the margins around the resection. In addition, the appropriate length of follow-up is critical to determine the efficacy of the type of resection in controlling local disease. Control of local disease is a critical parameter in the successful management of thyroid cancer, because viable central compartment disease has been reported in half of the patients who die of thyroid cancer.[34] A review of this literature shows proponents of the more limited shave resection, as well as others who believe that all patients should have a sleeve resection to ensure clearance of transmural disease. A prospective, randomized, and appropriately stratified study of that nature cannot be performed at any single institution.

When the surgeon elects to perform a shave excision of a thyroid carcinoma that is adherent to the trachea it is difficult, if not impossible, to obtain an accurate assessment of the margins of resection. A shave excision is performed by sharply separating

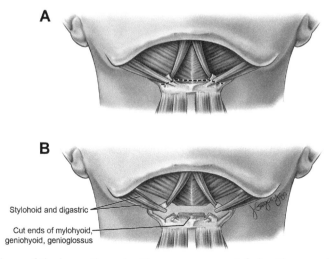

A

B

Stylohoid and digastric

Cut ends of mylohyoid,
geniohyoid, genioglossus

Fig. 15. Release of the larynx through either a supra- or an infrahyoid approach can facilitate the tension-free repair of the trachea.

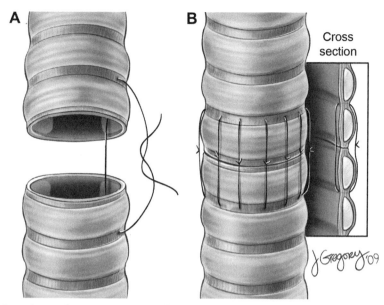

Fig. 16. End-to-end anastomosis is performed with sequential placement of sutures and tying of the knots on the outside of the lumen.

the thyroid gland from the wall of the trachea and is usually coupled with removal of an additional layer of cartilage. Using this technique, it is impossible to comprehensively address disease extension through the incartilaginous spaces where lymphatic and vascular channels penetrate to the luminal aspect of the trachea and provide access for unrecognized disease extension (see **Figs. 9** and **17**).[25] McCarty and colleagues[20] reported that residual microscopic disease was left on the wall of the trachea in all 35 patients in whom they performed a shave excision; however, only 17% of these patients developed local recurrence at a mean follow-up of 82 months. Alternatively, Park and colleagues[35] reported that 10 of 16 patients who underwent a shave procedure developed central compartment recurrence and 7 died of disease. The obvious advantage of performing a sleeve resection of the airway is that it provides an opportunity to assess the depth of invasion while also providing the most complete resection of the circumferential extent of the disease. This technique may be performed in the primary setting or, less optimally, in patients who are referred to a tertiary center after identifying invasive disease inadvertently. However, this technique should be part of the armamentarium of head and neck surgeons entrusted with providing surgical care of patients with thyroid cancer. Sleeve resections and primary end-to-end anastomoses can be performed successfully with acceptable risk and a low rate of operative mortality. There is a risk of tracheal stenosis as well as permanent tracheostomy, depending on the function of the RLNs.[7]

Although uncommon, a total laryngectomy may be required in patients with extensive laryngeal involvement in whom a functional cricoarytenoid joint cannot be preserved safely without compromising the oncologic soundness of the procedure. Although sophisticated reconstructive techniques can be used to restore a patent laryngeal airway and a functional laryngeal sphincter, such extensive surgery may be warranted in younger patients with well-differentiated thyroid cancer, whereas it is not appropriate in older patients.

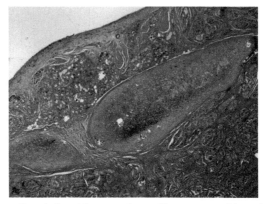

Fig. 17. Well-differentiated thyroid cancer is readily seen on either side of the tracheal cartilage.

ESOPHAGUS

Because of its malleable nature, the esophagus is rarely involved transmurally. None of the patients with esophageal invasion in Kowalski's series had symptoms before surgery (**Fig. 18**).[18] More often than not, the extent of involvement is limited to the muscular layer, and with the help of a bougie placed into the lumen, the muscle layer can be removed without creating a mucosal defect in the esophagus (**Fig. 19**). In the absence of mucosal involvement, the muscular layer can be safely removed with seemingly little effect on the swallowing mechanism. However, as with many such statements, no true objective studies have evaluated the effect of removing varying degrees of the esophageal musculature so we do not know the exact effect on the swallowing mechanism. It is rare that the necessity to remove the esophageal musculature is performed in isolation, without removal of the RLN or other associated central

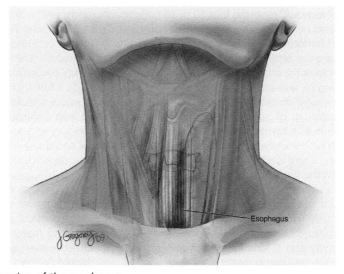

Fig. 18. Invasion of the esophagus.

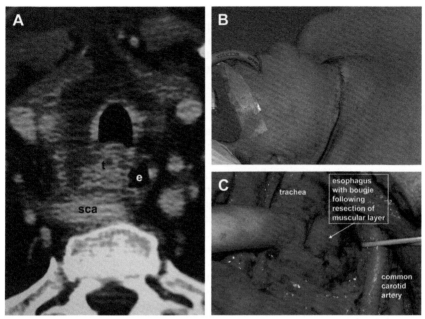

Fig. 19. (*A*) This patient was referred for definitive surgery when tumor (t) was found to be adherent to the wall of the esophagus (e) during the initial surgery. Of note is the aberrant course of the subclavian artery that was traversing the space behind the esophagus and this anomaly led to the development of a nonrecurrent laryngeal nerve. (*B*) Placement of a bougie helps in the dissection of the residual disease. (*C*) Following resection of the persistent tumor the muscular layer was stripped from the mucosa. The esophagus is stented by a bougie placed transorally.

compartment structures. As a result, the functional effect on the patient is often multifactorial.

If there is transmural invasion by biologically aggressive thyroid cancer, then the extent of the circumference involved determines whether primary repair can be accomplished or alternatively whether there is a need to import epithelial tissue to reconstitute the normal caliber of the esophagus. Skin represents the most readily available replacement tissue for esophageal mucosa and can be transferred to the neck as a regional flap or as a free flap. For long segments of circumferential involvement, options for management include the transfer of skin that is sutured to form a tube that provides an epithelial lined conduit. Alternatively, there is considerable experience with the transfer of segments of jejunum that can be used to replace segmental esophageal defects. The greater curvature of the stomach can also serve as a source of vascularized mucosa that can be transferred with the greater omentum to create a mucosal conduit. The added benefit of this donor site is that the greater omentum provides a unique flap of well-vascularized tissue that is extremely useful for severely compromised wounds with anticipated impaired wound healing, most commonly following external beam radiation therapy. When the disease extends to the thoracic esophagus then the time-honored approach to reconstruction is to perform a gastric pull-up procedure that allows the pharyngogastric anastomosis to be placed in the neck and to avoid placement of the anastomosis in the mediastinum, where a leak can have serious, life-threatening consequences.

The techniques described earlier can also be readily used in patients who require resection of the larynx and esophagus with the creation of a permanent tracheostome. In rare situations in which extensive disease requires resection of the laryngopharynx and portions of the thoracic trachea, a tracheal lengthening procedure can be performed with the use of a funnel-shaped tubed radial forearm flap.[30]

VASCULAR INVASION

It is rare that the major vessels in the neck and mediastinum are involved by disease that is deemed to be resectable (**Fig. 20**). In the 6 patients with major vessel involvement in Kowalski's series, only 1 had symptoms before surgery.[18] The exception to vascular invasion is the internal jugular vein, which can readily be removed without any morbidity to the patient. The clinical scenario that most often presents with jugular vein involvement is a metastatic node with extracapsular extension. Alternatively, venous involvement by disease extending along intraluminal pathways from the draining veins of the thyroid has been described (**Fig. 21**).[36–38] Resection of the internal jugular vein can be performed with little effect on the patient provided that the disease does not involve both internal jugular veins. In the event of bilateral involvement, a staged resection of the jugular veins should be performed, with a minimum of 2 weeks' delay to allow collateral venous circulation to develop.

The necessity for carotid artery resection is uncommon in invasive thyroid cancer. In most instances a carotid peel procedure can be performed, provided that there is a plane of resection that does not compromise the integrity of the wall of the carotid artery. In instances in which the artery is circumferentially involved or in which no surgical plane can be established, then a segmental resection of the artery can be considered. The usual guideline for such an undertaking in other malignancies arising in the head and neck is predicated on identifying that the disease that is adherent to the carotid artery is the only portion of the disease that stands in the way of achieving a complete resection. The inherent morbidity of interrupting the flow of the carotid

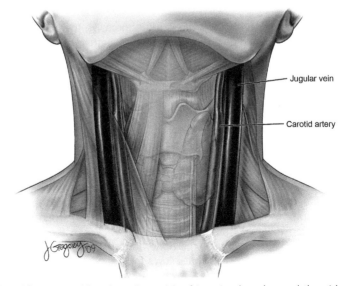

Fig. 20. Carotid artery and jugular vein at risk of invasion by advanced thyroid cancer.

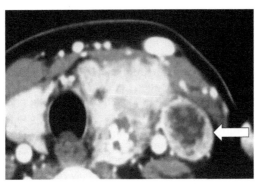

Fig. 21. Direct invasion of the internal jugular vein (*arrow*).

artery involves the risk of neurologic sequelae. In theory, carotid involvement by primary thyroid cancer represents a safer area to perform a carotid resection and replacement than what is usually encountered in squamous cell carcinoma involvement of the carotid artery. In the latter situation, the carotid bulb is most commonly involved, necessitating resection of the common carotid and a portion of the internal carotid arteries. Successful bypass requires temporary cross-clamping and interruption of flow to the brain. In thyroid cancer that involves direct extension from the gland to the lower portion of the common carotid artery, there is usually an opportunity to preserve the circulation through the region of the carotid bifurcation that permits cerebral protection through reverse flow from the external carotid artery (**Fig. 22**). It is therefore less likely that such a surgical undertaking of replacing the common carotid artery for an invasive thyroid cancer will result in as high a risk of neurologic sequelae

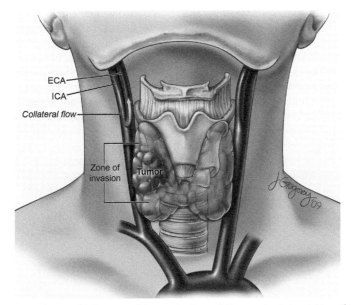

Fig. 22. Retrograde carotid flow provides protection of the cerebral circulation if the tumor involves the lower portion of the common carotid artery.

as has come to be associated with resection of the carotid artery for squamous cell cancer, in particular when the carotid bifurcation is involved. One final note of caution is related to the increased surgical risk of replacing the carotid artery in patients following entry into the upper aerodigestive tract, where the potential for postoperative fistulae can lead to catastrophic vascular complications.[39]

There are no data to provide information regarding the oncologic value of extending the resection to include the internal jugular vein or the carotid artery. The age of the patient, the degree of differentiation of the tumor, the presence of metastatic disease, the extent of prior therapy and the opportunity to treat with radioactive iodine are all important parameters that affect that decision. As noted earlier, the decision to replace the carotid artery should be made only after the surgeon is convinced that the disease adherent to the carotid artery is the only remaining gross disease that stands in the way of a complete resection of the tumor.

NERVE INVOLVEMENT

The range of nerves involved by invasive thyroid cancer includes virtually the entire spectrum of central and lateral compartment nerves (**Fig. 23**). The RLN is undoubtedly the most common nerve to be reported as being affected by invasive disease. In Nakao's series on invasive cancer,[16] the RLN was affected in 61%, whereas the vagus was involved in 13%, the phrenic nerve in 10%, and the spinal accessory nerve in 6% of 31 patients. As noted earlier, it is rare that the superior laryngeal nerve is reported as a separate nerve in the large series on invasive thyroid cancer.

Randolph and Kamani[26] reported a series of 21 patients with invasive thyroid cancer and compared the preoperative laryngeal examination with a group of 344 patients with either noninvasive thyroid cancer or benign thyroid disease who required surgery. RLN paralysis was identified in 70% of patients with invasive disease compared with only 0.3% of patients with benign or noninvasive disease. Voice change was identified in only 40% of patients with documented vocal cord paralysis.

The appropriate management of the RLN that is involved by a thyroid cancer within the gland or metastatic to a paratracheal node depends on several factors: the presence or absence of preoperative vocal cord paralysis, the involvement of the opposite RLN, and the histology of the tumor. If the vocal cord is functional, then the decision to sacrifice the nerve is more difficult. In these cases the nerve should be preserved as long as all gross disease can be removed. In the case of tumor involving the only functioning RLN, then that nerve should rarely be sacrificed in light of the need to perform a tracheostomy and subsequent lateralization procedures. Disease left in proximity to

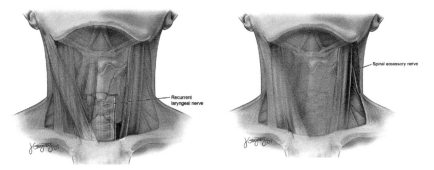

Fig. 23. Nerve invasion by thyroid cancer in the central or lateral compartments.

a functioning RLN leads to the necessity to treat postoperatively with radioactive iodine and possibly external beam radiotherapy. The decision to leave microscopic disease attached to the RLN does not seem to affect the survival or the risk of recurrence compared with the decision to perform a resection of the nerve.[40]

If an RLN has to be sacrificed there are 3 options for management of the resulting deficit:

1. The first is to perform a medialization procedure postoperatively.
2. The second is to perform an immediate nerve graft to bridge the gap between the 2 ends of the nerve.
3. A third alternative approach is to perform an anastomosis between the distal RLN and a motor branch of the ansa cervicalis (**Figs. 24** and **25**).

In either of the last 2 procedures, the patient may benefit from a temporary medialization procedure to achieve a functional improvement while the nerve is regenerating.

Involvement of other lateral compartment nerves is most often secondary to metastatic disease to cervical nodes. The vagus nerve is most often at risk and the surgeon should be aware of the lymphatic pathways that exit the central compartment of the neck along the inferior thyroid artery that courses deep to the carotid artery (**Fig. 26**). Lymph node involvement deep to the carotid artery is a common scenario and the surgeon should have a high index of suspicion to search for nodes along that lymphatic pathway in the primary and recurrent setting. In such situations, the structures within the carotid sheath are placed at risk from disease extending outside the capsule of the node (**Fig. 27**).

PROGNOSIS OF PATIENTS WITH INVASIVE THYROID CANCER

Although radioactive iodine is routinely administered to patients with advanced thyroid cancer, invasive thyroid cancers in patients with locally invasive disease, especially

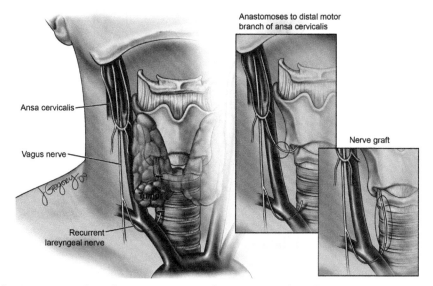

Fig. 24. Two options for management of an RLN involved by tumor that requires a segmental resection. Reinnervation of the cord can be achieved through an ansa to distal RLN anastomosis or a nerve graft.

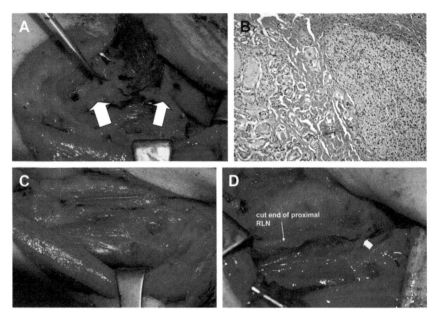

Fig. 25. (*A*) RLN encased by an invasive papillary thyroid cancer (*white arrows*). (*B*) Histologic section shows nerve invasion. (*C*) The distal branches of the ansa cervicalis are exposed. (*D*) The anastomosis of the distal ansa cervicalis to the distal RLN is shown (*yellow arrow*).

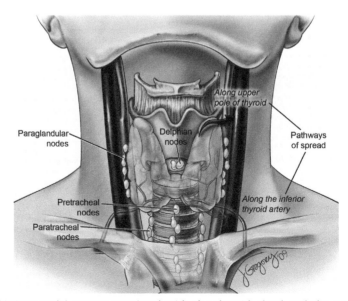

Fig. 26. Various nodal groups associated with the thyroid gland and the pathway for lymphatic spread outside the central compartment. The route along the inferior thyroid artery deep to the common carotid artery is shown.

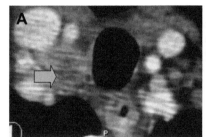
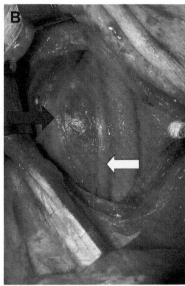

Fig. 27. (*A*) Recurrent thyroid cancer presenting with a lymph node (*green arrow*) deep to the common carotid artery. (*B*) At the time of the resection the vagus nerve (*yellow arrow*) was adherent to the capsule of the lymph node (*blue arrow*).

those in an older age group, have often lost the ability to trap iodine and therefore the ability to be effectively treated with this adjuvant modality. There is an increasing use of external beam radiotherapy in patients with this clinical profile; however, it has not been evaluated in a prospective fashion. In the contemporary series published by Chow and colleagues,[41] external beam radiotherapy was found to reduce the risk of locoregional failure in the particular subgroup of patients with gross residual disease following surgery. In that series of 842 patients with papillary thyroid cancer treated between 1960 and 1997, the 4 factors that were identified on multivariate analysis as leading to a poor prognosis were distant metastases at presentation, age greater than 45 years, gross residual locoregional disease following surgery, and lack of radioactive iodine treatment. The investigators used the following parameters to recommend external beam radiation: presence of gross locoregional disease, extensive ETE, and extensive lymph node metasases. Chow and colleagues[41] reported that the presence of postoperative residual disease was more important than other prognostic factors such as ETE, tumor size, lymph node involvement, and type of surgery.

Numerous survival statistics and local control rates have been reported for patients with invasive thyroid cancer. However, the heterogeneous nature of the patients in these series makes it difficult to draw meaningful conclusions. After complete resection of thyroid cancer invading the trachea, the 3-, 5-, and 10-year survival rates have been reported to be 87%, 78%, and 78%.[42] In the Mayo Clinic series reported by McCaffrey and colleagues,[24] the overall survival at 5 years was 79%, 63% at 10 years, and 54% at 15 years.

One of the more challenging clinical scenarios occurs in the patients who present with advanced local disease in conjunction with metastatic disease. The surgeon must decide how aggressive the treatment of the primary tumor should be in light of the adverse prognostic finding. Sugitani and colleagues[43] reported 86 patients with distant metastases, of which 42 were discovered at the time of presentation and 44 were identified from 1 to 25 years following initial thyroidectomy. Disease-specific survival in the group of 86 patients was 65% at 5 years and 45% at 10 years. The factors that appeared to be associated with a worse prognosis were metastatic disease to sites other than the lung, distant metastases greater than 2 cm, cervical nodal metastases greater than 3 cm, and less well-differentiated histologic features. All but 1 patient in that series underwent curative resection of the primary tumor and only 5 patients were identified as dying as a result of local disease progression or recurrence. The development of recurrent local disease was a poor prognostic feature: 60% of the patients who developed recurrent local disease in the face of distant metastases succumbed to thyroid cancer. The investigators concluded that the presence of distant metastases at the time of diagnosis of invasive local disease, whether primary or recurrent, should not preclude an aggressive approach to the resection of that local disease. They cautioned that a specific subset of patients with distant metastases at nonpulmonary sites and poorly differentiated papillary thyroid cancer were at highest risk of early demise as a result of distant disease and should not be treated with aggressive surgery.[43]

SUMMARY

The successful management of well-differentiated thyroid cancer requires a preparedness on the part of the surgeon for whatever circumstance the disease may present. Identification of the patient at risk and performing appropriate imaging studies to determine the full extent of the disease are critical to educating the patient and preparing for what is necessary for complete resection of the disease. Prevention of disease progression and disease recurrence in the central compartment is vital to the overall strategy for successful oncologic management. Various structures are at risk from invasive thyroid cancer or disease extending beyond the capsule of a metastatic lymph node. Effective management of those structures is critical to achieving a complete resection of the disease and a restoration or preservation of an optimal level of function for the patient.

ACKNOWLEDGMENTS

The author would like to acknowledge Jill Gregory for her extraordinary talents and dedication as a medical illustrator.

REFERENCES

1. Balfour D. Cancer of the thyroid gland, Medical Record, 1918.
2. Davies L, Welch HG. Increasing incidence of thyroid cancer in the United States 1973–2002. JAMA 2006;295(18):2164–7.
3. Mitchell I, Livingston E, Chang A, et al. Trends in thyroid cancer demographics and surgical therapy in the United States. Surgery 2007;142:823–8.
4. Gaissert H, Honings M, Grillo H, et al. Segmental laryngotracheal and tracheal resection for invasive thyroid carcinoma. Ann Thorac Surg 2007; 83(6):1952–9.
5. Brandwein M, Som P, Urken ML. Benign intratracheal thyroid tissue, a possible cause for preoperative overstaging. Arch Otolaryngol 1998;124:1266–9.
6. Jacobson AS, Wenig BM, Urken ML. Collision tumor of the thyroid and larynx: a patient with papillary thyroid carcinoma colliding with laryngeal squamous cell carcinoma. Thyroid 2008;18(12):1325–8.

7. Kim A, Maxhimer J, Quiros R, et al. Surgical management of well-differentiated thyroid cancer locally invasive to the respiratory tract. J Am Coll Surg 2005; 201(4):619–27.

8. Djalilian M, Beahrs O, Devine K, et al. Intraluminal involvement of the larynx and trachea by thyroid cancer. Am J Surg 1974;128:500–4.

9. Machens A, Holzhausen HJ, Dralle H. The prognostic value of primary tumor size in papillary and follicular thyroid carcinoma; a comparative analysis. Cancer 2005;103:2269–73.

10. Lim D, Baek K, Lee Y, et al. Clinical, histopathological, and molecular characteristics of papillary thyroid microcarcinoma. Thyroid 2007;17:883–8.

11. Kebebew E, Clark O. Differentiated thyroid cancer: "complete" rational approach. World J Surg 2000;24(8):942–51.

12. Breaux E, Guillamondegui O. Treatment of locally invasive carcinoma of the thyroid: how radical? Am J Surg 1980;140:514–7.

13. Andersen P, Kinsella J, Loree J, et al. Differentiated carcinoma of the thyroid with extrathyroidal extension. Am J Surg 1995;170:467–70.

14. Yamashita H, Noguchi S, Murakami N, et al. Extracapsular invasion of lymph node metastasis is an indicator of distant metastasis and poor prognosis in patients with thyroid papillary carcinoma. Cancer 1997;80:2268–72.

15. Akslen L, Myking A, Salvesen H, et al. Prognostic importance of various clinicopathological features in papillary thyroid carcinoma. Eur J Cancer 1993;29A: 44–51.

16. Nakao K, Kurozumi K, Fukushima S, et al. Merits and demerits of operative procedure to the trachea in patients with differentiated thyroid cancer. World J Surg 2001;25:723–7.

17. Nishida T, Nakao K, Hamaji M. Differentiated thyroid carcinoma with airway invasions: indication for tracheal resection based on the extent of cancer invasion. J Thorac Cardiovasc Surg 1997;114:84–92.

18. Kowalski LP, Filho JG. Results of the treatment of locally invasive thyroid carcinoma. Head Neck 2002;24:340–4.

19. Schlumberger M, Tubiana M, De Vathaire F, et al. Long-term results of treatment of 283 patients with lung and bone metastases from differentiated thyroid carcinoma. J Clin Endocrinol Metab 1986;63:960–7.

20. McCarty T, Kuhn J, Williams W, et al. Surgical management of thyroid cancer invading the airway. Ann Surg Oncol 1997;4:403–8.

21. Maassen W, Greschuchna D, Vogt-Moykopf I, et al. Tracheal resection state of the art. Thorac Cardiovasc Surg 1985;33:2–7.

22. Shimamoto K, Satake H, Sawaki A, et al. Preoperative staging of thyroid papillary carcinoma with ultrasonography. Eur J Radiol 1998;29:4–10.

23. Yamamura N, Fukushima S, Nakao K. Relation between ultrasonographic and histologic findings of tracheal invasion by differentiated thyroid cancer. World J Surg 2002;26:1071–3.

24. McCaffrey T, Bergstralh E, Hay I. Locally invasive papillary thyroid carcinoma: 1940–1990. Head Neck 1994;16:165–72.

25. Shin DH, Mark EJ, Suen HC, et al. Pathologic staging of papillary carcinoma of the thyroid with airway invasion based on the anatomic manner of extension to the trachea. Hum Pathol 1993;24:866.

26. Randolph G, Kamani D. The importance of preoperative laryngoscopy in patients undergoing thyroidectomy: voice, vocal cord function, and the preoperative detection of invasive thyroid malignancy. Surgery 2006;139: 357–62.

27. Dralle H, Brauckhoff M, Machens A, et al. Surgical management of advanced thyroid cancer invading the aerodigestive tract. In: Clark OH, Duh QY, editors. Textbook of endocrine surgery. Philadelphia: WB Saunders; p. 318–33.

28. Urken ML, Biller HF. Management of early vocal cord carcinoma. Oncology 1988; 2:48–59.

29. Urken ML, Blackwell K, Biller HF. Reconstruction of the laryngopharynx after hemicricoid/hemithyroid cartilage resection: preliminary functional results. Arch Otolaryngol Head Neck Surg 1997;123(11):1213–22.

30. Blackwell K, Urken ML. Laryngopharyngeal and pharyngoesophageal reconstruction. In: Urken ML, editor. Multidisciplinary head and neck reconstruction: a defect oriented approach. Philadelphia: Lippincott Williams and Wilkins; 2010. p. 689–778.

31. Ozaki O, Sugino K, Mimura T, et al. Surgery for patients with thyroid carcinoma invading the trachea: circumferential sleeve resection followed by end to end anastomosis. Surgery 1995;117:268.

32. Lundgren C, Hall P, Dickman P, et al. Clinically significant prognostic factors for differentiated thyroid carcinoma, a population-based, nested case-control study. Cancer 2006;106:524–31.

33. Friedman M, Toriumi D, Owens R, et al. Experience with the sternocleidomastoid myoperiosteal flap for reconstruction of subglottic and tracheal defects: modification of technique and report of long-term results. Laryngoscope 1988;98: 1003–11.

34. Ishahara T, Yamazaki S, Kobayashi K, et al. Resection of the trachea infiltrated by thyroid cancer. Ann Surg 1982;201:496–500.

35. Park C, Suh K, Min J. Cartilage-shaving procedure for the control of tracheal cartilage invasion by thyroid carcinoma. Head Neck 1993;15:289–91.

36. Onaran Y, Terzioglu T, Oguz H, et al. Great cervical vein invasion of thyroid carcinoma. Thyroid 1998;8:59–61.

37. Thompson NW, Brown J, Orringer M, et al. Follicular carcinoma of the thyroid with massive angioinvasion: extension of tumor thrombus to the heart. Surgery 1978; 83:451–7.

38. Perez D, Brown L. Follicular carcinoma of the thyroid appearing as an intraluminal superior vena cava tumor. Arch Surg 1984;119:323–6.

39. Biller HF, Urken ML, Lawson W, et al. Carotid artery resection and bypass for neck carcinoma. Laryngoscope 1988;98:181–3.

40. Samaan NA, Maheshwari Y, Nader S, et al. Impact of therapy for differentiated carcinoma of the thyroid: an analysis of 706 cases. J Clin Endocrinol Metab 1983;56:1131–8.

41. Chow S, Law S, Mendenhall W, et al. Papillary thyroid carcinoma: prognostic factors and the role of radioiodine and external radiotherapy. Int J Radiat Oncol Biol Phys 2002;52:784–95.

42. Ishahara T, Kobahashi K, Kikuchi K, et al. Surgical treatment of advanced thyroid carcinoma invading the trachea. J Thorac Cardiovasc Surg 1991;102:717–20.

43. Sugitani I, Fujimoto Y, Yamamoto N. Papillary thyroid carcinoma with distant metastases: survival predictors and the importance of local control. Surgery 2008;143:35–42.

Postoperative Management of Differentiated Thyroid Cancer

Amin Sabet, MD[a], Matthew Kim, MD[b],*

KEYWORDS

- Thyroid cancer • Radioactive iodine • Thyroglobulin
- Recombinant human thyroid-stimulating hormone

POSTOPERATIVE STAGING

In patients with differentiated thyroid cancer, postoperative staging helps to determine prognosis. Staging also has a role in guiding decisions regarding postoperative radioactive iodine treatment and thyroid hormone suppression therapy, in addition to aiding specific decisions regarding follow-up.[1]

The UICC (Union Internationale Contre le Cancer) and the American Joint Committee on Cancer (AJCC) have adopted a staging system for differentiated thyroid cancer based on the pathologic tumor-node metastasis (pTNM) system. The sixth edition of the AJCC staging manual presented a revised definition of stages T3 and T4 to reflect the extent of extrathyroidal extension which, along with age, is a major prognostic factor for survival and risk of local recurrence.[2–5] Stage T3 represents any primary tumor with minimal extrathyroidal extension or size greater than 4 cm limited to the thyroid. Stage T4a includes a tumor of any size extending beyond the thyroid capsule to invade subcutaneous soft tissues, the larynx, trachea, esophagus, or recurrent laryngeal nerve. Stage T4b refers to any tumor that invades prevertebral fascia or encases a carotid artery or mediastinal vessels.[2]

Patient age at the time of initial diagnosis and therapy is a major determinant of stage in the AJCC/UICC TNM classification. In the absence of distant metastases (M0), all patients younger than 45 years are classified as stage I. In the presence of distant metastases (M1), all patients younger than 45 years are classified as stage II.

[a] Division of Endocrinology, Diabetes & Metabolism, Harvard Medical School, Beth Israel Deaconess Medical Center, 330 Brookline Avenue, Gryzmish 6, Boston, MA 02215, USA
[b] Thyroid Section, Harvard Medical School, Brigham and Women's Hospital, 77 Avenue Louis Pasteur, HIM-645, Boston, MA 02115, USA
* Corresponding author.
E-mail address: mikim@partners.org

Otolaryngol Clin N Am 43 (2010) 329–351
doi:10.1016/j.otc.2010.02.003
oto.theclinics.com

Patients 45 years or older with a primary tumor smaller than 2 cm and limited to the thyroid (T1), in the absence of node or distant metastases (N0, M0) are classified as stage I, whereas those 45 years or older with a primary tumor larger than 2 cm but not larger than 4 cm and limited to the thyroid (T2), in the absence of node or distant metastases (N0, M0), are classified as stage II. Patients 45 years or older with T3 disease and/or metastases limited to level VI lymph nodes (N1a, M0) are stage III, whereas those 45 years or older with a more locally invasive primary tumor (T4a or T4b) and/or metastases to any location other than level VI lymph nodes (N1b and/or M1) are classified as stage IV.

The American Thyroid Association (ATA) management guidelines recommend application of the AJCC/UICC TNM classification, based on the premise that the system provides a useful method to describe tumor extent and is also used in cancer registries and epidemiologic studies.[1,6] Several other classification systems have been proposed, each differentially weighing prognostic values such as age, primary tumor size, presence of direct local invasion, multifocality, lymph node involvement, and distant metastases.[7] Each system identifies the majority of patients at low risk of disease-specific mortality, although none have established clear superiority.[8]

AJCC/UICC thyroid cancer staging fails to take into account some known prognostic factors such as histologic subtype, positron emission tomography (PET) positivity, presence or absence of multifocality, vascular invasion, and molecular characteristics.[9–12] In particular, activating mutations of *BRAF* have been associated with lymph node metastases, lack of response to radioactive iodine, and increased likelihood of clinically recurrent disease in low-risk patients.[13–15]

Although thyroid cancer staging systems are well suited to predicting cancer-associated mortality, they are relatively insensitive for predicting risk of clinical tumor recurrence. Furthermore, current staging systems rely primarily on data obtained during the initial evaluation, and are not well suited to modification as further studies obtained during follow-up provide key data regarding tumor aggressiveness and response to treatment. With regard to the risk of persistent or recurrent disease, the ATA guidelines designate as low risk those patients with the following characteristics after initial surgery and remnant ablation[1]:

1. Lack of local or distant metastases
2. No evidence of residual macroscopic tumor
3. Absence of tumor invasion of locoregional tissues or structures
4. Lack of vascular invasion or aggressive histologic features (such as tall cell, insular, or columnar cell carcinoma)
5. Lack of radioactive iodine uptake outside of the thyroid bed on the first posttreatment whole body scan (if the patient has been treated with radioactive iodine).

TREATMENT WITH RADIOACTIVE IODINE

Following thyroidectomy in patients with differentiated thyroid cancer, radioactive iodine treatment may be indicated for remnant ablation or for treatment of known residual or metastatic disease.

Postoperative Remnant Ablation

Postoperative remnant ablation with radioactive iodine has two main potential benefits.

First, by destroying remaining normal thyroid tissue, remnant ablation increases the sensitivity of subsequent surveillance using serum thyroglobulin levels and radioactive iodine whole body scanning to detect persistent or recurrent disease.

Second, remnant ablation may serve to destroy microscopic thyroid cancer foci remaining in the thyroid bed after surgery. In patients who are at high risk of developing de novo thyroid cancer due to prior radiation exposure or genetic predisposition, remnant ablation has the possible additional benefit of destroying remnant normal thyroid tissue that may harbor the potential to develop into de novo cancer.

Several large retrospective studies and a meta-analysis have shown significant reductions in thyroid cancer recurrence and disease-specific mortality in thyroid cancer patients treated with radioactive iodine for remnant ablation.[11,16–20] In these studies, the benefit has appeared to be restricted to those patients with tumors larger than 1.5 cm, multicentric disease, locally invasive cancer, or residual disease after surgery.[11,16,21,22]

Other studies have shown no such benefits, particularly with regard to low-risk differentiated thyroid cancer.[19,21,23–26] An updated systematic review did not confirm a benefit of remnant ablation in early-stage well-differentiated thyroid cancer with regard to either cause-specific mortality or recurrence, although a statistically significant decreased risk of distant metastasis was noted with remnant ablation.[27]

In the absence of data from a randomized controlled trial, significant controversy remains regarding the use of postoperative radioactive iodine treatment in patients with low-risk differentiated thyroid carcinoma. The ATA guidelines recommend radioactive iodine treatment for all patients who have distant metastatic disease, primary tumor greater than 4 cm, or evidence of gross extrathyroidal extension. In addition, the guidelines recommend radioactive iodine treatment for selected patients with primary tumor size of 1 to 4 cm limited to the thyroid who, based on tumor size, age, lymph node status, and histology, are predicted to be at intermediate or high risk of thyroid cancer recurrence or death. In the absence of other higher risk features, the ATA guidelines recommend against radioactive iodine treatment of patients with unifocal primary tumor smaller than 1 cm or multifocal cancer when all foci are smaller than 1 cm.[1]

Treatment of Known Residual Locoregional or Metastatic Disease

Residual local, regional, or metastatic disease may respond to radioactive iodine treatment. In general, radioactive iodine treatment appears to be most effective in patients younger than age 40 years with well-differentiated primary tumors and small-volume metastases.[28]

In patients with known residual local or metastatic thyroid cancer after initial surgery, the benefits of postsurgical radioactive iodine treatment are clear. Mazzaferri and Jhiang[11] found that thyroid cancer patients with residual local or regional disease after thyroidectomy who were treated with radioactive iodine had an approximately 50% decrease in 30-year recurrence and disease-specific mortality. A subsequent prospective multicenter study in 385 patients with high-risk thyroid cancer found that radioactive iodine treatment improved disease-specific mortality and rates of progression in patients with differentiated thyroid cancer.[20]

Iodine-avid pulmonary metastases, particularly micronodular disease, may respond to radioactive iodine treatment, whereas skeletal metastases typically do not show a good response.[29–34] FDG-avid metastatic lesions that are detected on PET scanning are generally refractory to radioactive iodine treatment.[35]

PREPARATION FOR RADIOACTIVE IODINE TREATMENT
Methods to Increase Thyroid-Stimulating Hormone

Iodine is taken up and concentrated in normal thyroid follicular cells and, to a lesser extent, differentiated thyroid cancer cells via a membrane sodium-iodide symporter.[36]

Iodine uptake is stimulated by thyroid-stimulating hormone (TSH). Postthyroidectomy patients are prepared for radioactive iodine treatment either via withdrawal from thyroid hormone, with an accompanying increase in endogenous TSH levels, or via injection of recombinant human TSH (rhTSH; Thyrogen). The optimal level of TSH elevation is not known. However, data from uncontrolled studies suggest a minimum TSH level of 30 mU/L.[37,38]

Withdrawal from thyroid hormone
Withdrawal from thyroid hormone is the traditional means of preparation for post-surgical remnant ablation and is typically accomplished by withholding levothyroxine (T4; Synthroid) therapy for 6 weeks after total or near total thyroidectomy, although 2 studies have demonstrated a satisfactory TSH elevation after an average duration of less than 3 weeks of T4 withdrawal.[39,40] To minimize the symptoms of hypothyroidism during T4 withdrawal, patients are commonly treated with the shorter acting hormone liothyronine (T3; Cytomel) during the first 2 to 3 weeks after surgery (or after stopping T4). Typical doses of T3 are 25 µg twice daily in most patients, or 12.5 µg twice daily in elderly patients or those with coronary artery disease. However, data from a recent small randomized controlled trial suggest that the administration of T3 makes no difference in hypothyroid symptom scores while significantly delaying the onset of hypothyroidism (32 ± 4 days vs 17 ± 9 days needed to reach a TSH level of >30 mU/L in the T3 and control groups, respectively).[41] Based on these data, it has been suggested that withdrawal preparation for remnant ablation can be simply and effectively accomplished via 2 to 3 weeks of T4 withdrawal without increasing morbidity associated with hypothyroidism. Regardless of the approach used, patients undergoing withdrawal before remnant ablation should undergo testing to confirm TSH elevation before therapy.

Recombinant human TSH
rhTSH was approved by the United States Food and Drug Administration (FDA) in 2007 for initial remnant ablation, and is being offered as the method of choice for routine remnant ablation in some centers. The major advantage of using rhTSH is that patients do not need to discontinue T4 therapy and go through a period of overt hypothyroidism in conjunction with radioactive iodine treatment. This agent is given as a 0.9-mg intramuscular injection on 2 consecutive days with a therapeutic dose of I-131 administered 24 hours after the second dose.[42]

Prospective studies using 30, 50, and 100 mCi of I-131 have shown similar ablation success rates using rhTSH compared with withdrawal, while one prospective study using 30 mCi reported a lower ablation success rate with rhTSH versus hormone withdrawal.[42–45] One retrospective study found that short-term clinical recurrence rates assessed at a median of 2.5 years after radioactive iodine remnant ablation (median I-131 dose of 108 mCi) were similar for patients prepared with rhTSH and those prepared with thyroid hormone withdrawal.[46] However, to date there are no published data comparing long-term outcomes of patients treated with radioactive iodine ablation after preparation using rhTSH versus thyroid hormone withdrawal. As such, many providers continue to primarily use thyroid hormone withdrawal for radioactive iodine treatment of intermediate- and high-risk thyroid cancer patients except in cases where iatrogenic hypothyroidism may be particularly high risk (eg, congestive heart failure) or ineffective (eg, pituitary disease).

The economic implications of using rhTSH as preparation for remnant ablation are unclear. While the cost of therapy is much higher when using rhTSH versus hormone withdrawal, several studies have shown that the use of rhTSH may be associated with substantial productivity benefits due to shorter hospital stays and reduced sick leave.[47-50]

Low Iodine Diet and Avoidance of Iodine-Containing Medications

High levels of iodine reduce uptake of radioactive iodine by normal thyroid cells as well as differentiated thyroid cancer cells. Before administering radioactive iodine, patients should take care to avoid iodine-containing drugs such as amiodarone as well as avoid computed tomography with iodinated intravenous contrast, which can impair the response to I-131 for up to 6 months.[51,52] To enhance the effectiveness of radioactive iodine treatment, it is recommended that patients adhere to a low iodine diet for 1 to 2 weeks before treatment.[51,53]

Pretherapy Radioactive Iodine Scanning

Using small amounts of radioactive iodine, a diagnostic scan may be performed to determine the amount of thyroid remnant and presence of metastatic disease before administration of the treatment dose of radioactive iodine. Diagnostic I-131 doses as low as 3 mCi may result in diminished uptake of the subsequent therapeutic dose, an effect referred to as "stunning," while lower doses are less sensitive for the detection of remaining thyroid tissue and metastases.[54-56] The use of low-dose I-123 has been demonstrated to produce high-quality images without stunning. However, widespread I-123 use has been limited by its availability and higher cost.[57]

DOSE OF I-131 ADMINISTERED FOR RADIOACTIVE IODINE TREATMENT

The dose of radioactive iodine may be determined by:

1. Empirical fixed dosing based on tumor stage
2. Upper bound limits defined by whole blood dosimetry
3. Quantitative lesional dosimetry.

There are no data from controlled, prospective trials to suggest superiority of one particular method of dosing radioactive iodine, and current guidelines do not endorse a specific approach.[1]

Empirical fixed dosing is the simplest and most commonly used form of radioactive iodine dose determination. The optimal dose of I-131 depends on whether treatment is intended solely for remnant ablation or to treat known locoregional or metastatic disease. Patients with low-risk disease, if treated with radioactive iodine for remnant ablation, are typically given a dose of 30 to 100 mCi. Those with larger remnants with higher fractional uptake are paradoxically treated with a lower dose of I-131 in order to decrease the incidence of painful radiation thyroiditis. The ATA guidelines recommend that the minimum activity necessary to achieve successful ablation be used, particularly in low-risk patients.[1] A systematic review of retrospective and prospective data comparing the use of low-dose (30 mCi) and high-dose (100 mCi) radioactive iodine concluded that based on available published data, it is not possible to reliably determine whether rates of successful ablation are similar using 30 mCi and 100 mCi.[58]

Patients with intermediate- or high-risk differentiated thyroid cancer are typically treated with higher activities (100–200 mCi) according to risk, although there is evidence to suggest that this empirical method of radioactive iodine dosing may result in unsafe levels of radiation exposure to bone marrow in the elderly as well as those with diffuse pulmonary metastases.[59-62]

Posttherapy Radioactive Iodine Scanning

Posttherapy whole body iodine scanning is typically performed 5 to 8 days after radioactive iodine dosing for initial remnant ablation, and represents an import component of staging for differentiated thyroid cancer. When compared with the pretreatment diagnostic scan, posttreatment scanning has been reported to demonstrate additional metastatic foci, most commonly in the neck, lungs, and mediastinum, in 10% to 26% of patients.[63,64] Disease identified on posttreatment scan may alter cancer staging in approximately 10% of patients and may change plans for therapy in up to 15% of patients.[63–65]

COMPLICATIONS OF RADIOACTIVE IODINE TREATMENT

At the typical dosages used for postoperative remnant ablation, radioactive iodine treatment is associated with a low risk of adverse events and long-term complications. The most common complications are due to radiation sialadenitis, characterized by pain and swelling in the parotid region, as well as hypogeusia and xerostomia. The incidence of sialadenitis is dose related, occurring in 5% to 40% of patients treated with radioactive iodine.[66,67] A related complication is nasolacrimal duct obstruction.[68] Mild, self-limited leukopenia and thrombocytopenia may be seen 6 weeks after treatment.[69] An increased risk of pneumonitis and pulmonary fibrosis may also be seen in some patients with diffuse pulmonary involvement. In patients with diffuse pulmonary radioactive iodine uptake, dosimetry studies with a limit of 80 mCi whole body retention at 48 hours should be considered.[70]

Acute complications of radioactive iodine treatment are uncommon. Hemorrhage and edema involving metastatic disease, which can occur 12 hours to 2 weeks after I-131 treatment, is of greatest concern in patients with intracranial and spinal cord metastases.[71] Bone pain may occur following radioactive iodine treatment in patients with skeletal metastases. Patients with a large thyroid remnant can develop radiation thyroiditis, characterized by pain and swelling. Airway compromise rarely may occur.[69] Patients with radiation thyroiditis are treated with prednisone and supportive airway maintenance. In up to two-thirds of patients treated with 200 mCi of I-131, radiation sickness characterized by headache and nausea may occur, typically resolving within 24 hours.[72]

Radioactive iodine treatment may also be associated with an increased risk of secondary malignancies. A multicenter cohort study demonstrated a small, dose-dependent increase in the risk of second primary malignancies in thyroid cancer patients treated with radioactive iodine. Extrapolating data from higher cumulative doses of I-131, the investigators calculated that 100 mCi of I-131 would be associated with an additional 53 solid nonthyroidal malignancies and 3 leukemias during a 10-year period of follow-up of 10,000 patients.[73] In contrast, a large cohort study using the Surveillance, Epidemiology, and End Results (SEER) database compared 10,000 patients administered I-131 for thyroid cancer with 19,000 control cases and found that use of radioactive iodine was not associated with an increased incidence of second primary malignancy during a 5-year follow-up period.[74]

Menstrual irregularities including amenorrhea and oligomenorrhea with a duration of 4 to 10 months may be seen in up to 27% of women treated with radioactive iodine for thyroid cancer. Data from a large retrospective study suggest that pregnancy should be postponed for 1 year following radioactive iodine treatment, because of a higher rate of miscarriage.[1,75] In men, radioactive iodine treatment may be accompanied by a transient reduction in sperm count and elevation of follicle-stimulating hormone (FSH) levels.[76,77]

THYROID HORMONE SUPPRESSION

Circulating TSH has a trophic effect on differentiated thyroid cancer cells that express the TSH receptor. Thyroid hormone administered in doses targeted to suppress TSH levels is an important component of the postoperative management of thyroid cancer. Suppression of endogenous TSH using supraphysiologic thyroid hormone levels has been associated with a 27% reduction in adverse clinical events in thyroid cancer patients, although this benefit has not been demonstrated in low-risk patients.[78–80] Subclinical hyperthyroidism is associated with an increased risk of atrial fibrillation, ventricular hypertrophy, and increased bone turnover; therefore, the appropriate extent of thyroid hormone suppression is determined based on thyroid cancer risk, which in turn is dependent on patient staging and clinical status.[81–83]

In the absence of specific contraindications, current heuristics target suppression of TSH to less than 0.1 mU/L for initial therapy for patients with stage III and IV disease as well as for all patients with persistent disease. For patients without evidence of persistent disease but at high risk of recurrence, it may be reasonable to adjust TSH suppressive therapy to achieve a TSH level of 0.1 to 0.5 mU/L for 5 to 10 years. Patients without evidence of persistent disease and at low risk of recurrence may be treated to maintain a TSH in the low normal range (0.5–2.0 mU/L).

EXTERNAL BEAM RADIATION

Adjuvant external beam radiation therapy has not been prospectively evaluated in randomized, controlled trials involving patients with thyroid cancer. Several retrospective studies have shown a decreased local recurrence rate after adjuvant external radiation therapy for high-risk disease, whereas others have shown either no benefit or an adverse effect.[17,84,85] A single-institution retrospective study including 154 patients older than 45 years with differentiated thyroid cancer and microscopic residual cancer after surgery found that among patients older than 60 years who had extrathyroidal extension but no gross residual disease, external beam radiation therapy was associated with improved 10-year cause-specific survival (81% vs 65%).[86] In one study of 137 patients older than 40 years with extrathyroidal tumor extension, all of whom were treated with thyroidectomy, radioactive iodine, and thyroid hormone suppression, those patients treated with adjuvant external beam radiation therapy had fewer local and regional recurrences.[87]

At present, there are no prospective data to suggest that adjuvant external beam radiation improves locoregional control or disease-specific survival in patients who receive conventional surgery and treatment with radioactive iodine. The ATA guidelines suggest that adjuvant external beam radiation therapy be considered for patients older than 45 years who have grossly visible extrathyroidal extension (T4 disease) and a high likelihood of residual microscopic disease, as well as for patients with gross residual disease that cannot effectively be addressed with further surgery or radioactive iodine treatment.[1] In addition, external beam radiation therapy has an important role in the management of painful bone metastases as well as other unresectable metastatic disease likely to result in fracture, compressive, or neurologic symptoms.[1,88,89]

CHEMOTHERAPY

There are no data to support a role for adjuvant chemotherapy in patients with differentiated thyroid cancer. Chemotherapy may be useful in the management of patients with progressive, advanced disease that is nonradioactive iodine avid and cannot be addressed through surgery or external beam radiation.

Studies of cytotoxic systemic chemotherapy for advanced thyroid cancer have historically been limited and generally disappointing, with typical response rates of 25% or less.[90,91] Early reports of partial responses to doxorubicin led to FDA approval for treatment of metastatic thyroid cancer, but durable responses are not common.[92,93] Results from studies using combination cytotoxic chemotherapy have demonstrated increased toxicity without improved response rates.[90]

Current understanding of cancer biology has led to interest in small molecule chemotherapy agents that target activating mutations of *BRAF*, *RAS*, and translocations producing *RET/PTC* oncogenes, all of which lead to activation of the MAPK pathway. Other treatments are directed at inhibition of proangiogenic growth factor receptors, in particular vascular endothelial growth factor receptor (VEGFR). Numerous recent and ongoing clinical trials have been performed to evaluate these and other novel therapies (for a recent review see Sherman[91]). Overall, partial responses have been infrequent and complete responses not seen in recent monotherapy trials. To date, no novel agent has been shown to prolong survival in patients with advanced thyroid cancer.

Selected patients with advanced, progressive, metastatic thyroid cancer who are appropriate candidates for chemotherapy but unable to participate in a clinical trial may be treated with sorafenib, an oral tyrosine kinase inhibitor targeting VEGFR, *RET*, and *BRAF*. Sorafenib has been approved by the FDA as treatment for advanced renal cell carcinoma and unresectable hepatocellular carcinoma, and is therefore available for off-label use in patients with metastatic thyroid carcinoma. In phase 2 clinical trials, partial responses were seen in 15% to 23% of metastatic thyroid cancer patients treated with sorafenib.[94,95] In up to 56% of patients, stable disease was observed for at least 6 months. Common toxicities with sorafenib include hand-foot rash, oral mucositis, fatigue, diarrhea, and hypertension. Sorafenib has also been associated with the uncommon development of skin cancers, including squamous cell carcinoma and keratoacanthoma.[96]

MONITORING

Detection of persistent or recurrent well-differentiated thyroid cancer relies on monitoring protocols that incorporate a range of testing modalities including measurement of serum thyroglobulin, functional imaging, anatomic imaging, and direct sampling of suspected sites of involvement. Approaches adopted in clinical practice may vary based on a range of factors including the stage of disease at the time of initial treatment, the availability of different imaging and sampling technologies, and the level of institutional experience with the management of advanced cases.

Thyroglobulin

Measurement of serum thyroglobulin levels in both suppressed and stimulated states has emerged as a principal modality used to track patients with well-differentiated thyroid cancer. Thyroglobulin is a 660-kDa storage protein that is directly involved in the synthesis and storage of thyroid hormone in normally functioning thyroid tissue. Thyroglobulin may be secreted in detectable levels by remnant normal thyroid tissue that persists after thyroid surgery, or by foci of well-differentiated thyroid cancer that persists after treatment with radioactive iodine. Secretion of thyroglobulin is known to vary in direct relation to changes in TSH levels.

Given the high likelihood that remnants of normal thyroid tissue will be present after initial thyroid surgery, thyroglobulin levels are usually not held to be meaningfully interpretable until an interval of up to 6 months after completion of radioactive iodine treatment. Although measurement in the immediate postoperative period may not provide a reliable index for long-term comparison, it has been shown that thyroglobulin levels that are greater than 2.3 ng/mL 3 weeks after total thyroidectomy are correlated with the presence of cervical lymph node or distant metastases.[97]

Static thyroglobulin levels checked while patients are maintained on doses of levothyroxine targeted to suppress TSH levels have proven to be a sensitive index of recurrent disease. A thyroglobulin level that is less than 1.0 ng/mL 2 years after thyroid surgery is associated with a low 5-year risk of recurrence.[98] By the same token, a previously undetectable or low thyroglobulin level that becomes detectable or demonstrates a relative increase in the setting of adequate TSH suppression usually signifies recurrence.

Accurate measurement of serum thyroglobulin levels may be confounded by the presence of circulating antithyroglobulin antibodies. These antibodies, which are often measured as markers of underlying thyroid autoimmunity, have been shown to be more prevalent in the setting of well-differentiated thyroid cancer. The antibodies may be detected in up to 25% of patients diagnosed with papillary or follicular thyroid cancer in comparison with 10% of general population controls.[99] When appreciable titers of antithyroglobulin antibodies are present, a fraction may form complexes with circulating thyroglobulin, precluding accurate measurement of free levels.[100] In relative terms, the accuracy of measurement in the presence of antithyroglobulin antibodies may vary depending on the method used to perform the assays. When elevated titers of antithyroglobulin antibodies are present in serum, agglutination assays may not be able to reliably measure thyroglobulin levels less than 10 ng/mL that are readily detected with chemiluminescent assays.[101] Discordance has also been noted between thyroglobulin levels measured by radioimmunoassay and immunometric assay in antithyroglobulin antibody-positive sera.[99] The degree of discordance noted between these 2 methods has been shown to correlate with the concentration of antibodies present in tested samples. Radioimmunoassays that have been purposefully constructed with a high-affinity first antibody and a species-specific second antibody may be less prone to interference.[99]

When elevated antithyroglobulin antibody titers have been detected during the course of monitoring, their longevity and variance may serve as a secondary marker of persistent or recurrent disease. A study involving the serial measurement of antithyroglobulin antibodies in patients with undetectable thyroglobulin levels measured by immunometric assay showed that 49% of patients with detectable antibodies (vs 3.4% of patients without antibodies) had evidence of recurrent disease demonstrated through combinations of anatomic imaging, functional imaging, and surgical exploration.[102] After treatment of accessible disease, 71% of patients with initially detectable antibodies demonstrated an appreciable decline in titers.

Measurement of thyroglobulin mRNA has been proposed as an alternative method of detecting persistent or recurrent well-differentiated thyroid cancer that may circumvent discrepancies related to the presence of antithyroglobulin antibodies.[103,104] A study evaluating revere transcription-polymerase chain reaction (RT-PCR) measurement of circulating thyroglobulin mRNA in patients with varying degrees of recurrence based on radioactive iodine scanning showed that there were higher rates of positive threshold mRNA levels detectable in cases of more advanced disease.[105] When positive threshold mRNA levels were compared with simultaneously measured thyroglobulin levels, they demonstrated greater sensitivity and equivalent specificity for detection of recurrent disease. Proportionate increases were noted when mRNA levels measured on suppressive doses of levothyroxine were compared with levels measured after TSH stimulation. A study that used RT-PCR to measure circulating thyroglobulin mRNA in patients with treated thyroid cancer over a 12-month period demonstrated a higher degree of correlation with the detection of recurrent disease on radioactive iodine scanning when compared with suppressed thyroglobulin levels.[106] No interference from antithyroglobulin antibodies was noted in the measurement of serial mRNA levels. Despite its seeming promise, use of thyroglobulin mRNA measurement in clinical practice has been precluded by its current expense and by the low specificity of methods tested to date. An efficacy study that used a similar approach to evaluate patients determined to be disease free after a mean interval of 9.5 years of follow-up showed a high false-positive rate, with detection of high-threshold thyroglobulin mRNA levels in 76% of disease-free patients.[103] Technical factors related to the nonspecific expression and illegitimate transcription of thyroglobulin mRNA have been cited as potential explanations for this low specificity rate.[107]

Monitoring Protocols

Current approaches to monitoring that involve combinations of different imaging and sampling modalities can be loosely stratified based on:

1. Estimated risk of recurrence extrapolated from the stage of disease at the time of initial treatment
2. Use of radioactive iodine treatment after thyroid surgery
3. Degree of correlation between functional imaging results and suppressed and stimulated thyroglobulin measurements.

Low-Risk Patients Not Treated with Radioactive Iodine

Analysis of data collected in tracking thyroid cancer patients treated at the Mayo Clinic over the course of decades has shown that radioactive iodine treatment may be deferred in patients determined to be at low risk for recurrence, without any significant adverse effects.[108] Those patients determined to have MACIS scores (distant Metastasis, patient Age, Completeness of resection, local Invasion, tumor Size) less than 6 (MACIS score = 3.1 (if aged 39 years) or 0.08 × age (if aged 40 years) + 0.3 × tumor size in cm + 1 (if not completely resected) + 1 (if locally invasive) + 3 (if distant metastases)) on the day of their initial surgery who elected to defer subsequent treatment with radioactive iodine were eventually shown to have a 30-year cause-specific mortality rate of 1% with a 15% cumulative rate of recurrence at any site. This finding, which came under great scrutiny in light of the prior long-standing practice of treating all thyroid cancer patients with radioactive iodine, has had a bearing on the modification of published guidelines related to the management of well-differentiated thyroid cancer. Current ATA guideline recommendations stipulate that the beneficial effects of radioactive iodine may be limited to patients who present with tumors greater than 1.5 cm in maximal diameter or have evidence of residual disease after their initial surgery.[1] At present, it is unclear as to what extent this shift in outlook has had on the impact on the practice of clinicians who oversee the treatment of low-risk thyroid cancer patients.

In cases where a decision has been made to defer treatment with radioactive iodine after thyroid surgery, monitoring for possible persistent or recurrent disease necessarily relies on anatomic imaging with ultrasonography. Dedicated cervical ultrasonography has proven to be a sensitive and reproducible mode of imaging that allows for clear visualization of the thyroid bed, paratracheal regions, and lymph node chains, which are the most common sites of local recurrence.[109–111] Findings noted on ultrasonography can be localized within surgically defined anatomic regions within the neck (Levels I–VI) to allow for precise tracking of changes in appearance or dimension of any suspicious or indeterminate lymph nodes.[112] The accuracy of reported findings may vary to a significant extent in relation to institutional experience and operator expertise in recognizing and characterizing suspicious masses or lymph nodes.

To date, there does not seem to be any consensus regarding the utility of measuring suppressed and stimulated thyroglobulin levels in low-risk patients who have not undergone treatment with radioactive iodine. While it might be anticipated that an undetectable thyroglobulin level would indicate a better prognosis in this situation, it is unclear whether the significance of detectable or increasing levels can be determined in patients who are likely to have varying residual amounts of remnant thyroid tissue after thyroid surgery.

Low-risk Patients Treated with Radioactive Iodine

Stimulated whole body radioactive iodine scanning with measurement of a concomitant serum thyroglobulin level is the traditional modality used to monitor the status of patients treated with radioactive iodine after thyroid surgery.[64] Negative whole body scans checked at an appropriate interval after initial treatment are used to demonstrate clearance of remnant thyroid tissue that clarifies interpretation of suppressed and stimulated thyroglobulin levels. Positive whole body scans can be used to localize sites of persistent or recurrent disease to[113]:

1. Determine the need for possible further radioactive iodine treatment
2. Guide further imaging and sampling to confirm suspected sites of metastatic spread.

When stimulated whole body scanning is performed in the setting of possible further administration of therapeutic doses of radioactive iodine, the use of I-123 as a tracer in place of I-131 may offer the benefit of minimizing stunning of tissue that may limit the efficacy of treatment.[114]

Whole body scanning

The utility of ongoing monitoring with stimulated whole body scanning in low-risk patients has been questioned with the emergence and refinement of alternative approaches that may increase the detection sensitivity of recurrent disease.[115] A study that compared whole body scanning to measurement of stimulated thyroglobulin levels obtained at 6 to 12 months after treatment with radioactive iodine showed that an undetectable thyroglobulin level during this interval was highly predictive of disease-free status.[116] Stimulated thyroglobulin levels measured after radioactive iodine treatment have been shown to be more predictive of persistent or recurrent disease than levels measured immediately after surgery.[117,118] The relative magnitude of any change in thyroglobulin levels noted after stimulation may reflect the level of differentiation of responsive tissue. Normal thyroid tissue and well-differentiated thyroid cancer usually demonstrate greater than 10-fold increase in thyroglobulin levels in response to stimulation, whereas less differentiated thyroid cancer is usually marked by a less than 3-fold increase after exposure to elevated TSH levels.[98]

Recombinant human TSH

rhTSH administered in a sequence of intramuscular injections has been shown to provide an adequate level of stimulation for the acquisition of whole body scans used to monitor the status of low- to moderate-risk patients.[115,119] Use of rhTSH allows patients treated with replacement or suppressive doses of levothyroxine to avoid the unpleasant effects of hypothyroidism precipitated by gradual withdrawal of thyroid hormone to boost levels of TSH secreted by the pituitary gland. Whole body scans acquired after rhTSH stimulation followed by I-123 have been shown to be comparable to those acquired after administration of tracer doses of I-131.[120]

Studies evaluating low-risk patients have shown that serum thyroglobulin levels measured after administration of rhTSH may be a more sensitive index of persistent or recurrent disease than whole body scanning.[121,122] One of the larger mixed modality studies evaluating this approach showed that a threshold rhTSH-stimulated thyroglobulin level greater than 1 ng/mL detected active disease in 85% of cases, whereas whole body scanning was only able to detect active disease in 21% of cases.[123] The sensitivity of detection was further enhanced to a level of 96% when high-resolution ultrasonography was combined with rhTSH-stimulated thyroglobulin measurement. Thresholds of positivity demarcated in guidelines for the management of well-differentiated thyroid cancer tend to be slightly more conservative.[124] Current ATA guidelines stipulate that rhTSH-stimulated thyroglobulin levels less than 2 ng/mL should be considered to be less significant. Low-risk patients with levels in this range may benefit from continued monitoring with neck ultrasonography and measurement of suppressed thyroglobulin levels. Levels that range between 2 and 5 ng/mL are considered to be significant enough to warrant continued monitoring with neck ultrasonography and repeated measurement of rhTSH-stimulated thyroglobulin levels to track trends.[115] Levels that rise to greater than 5 ng/mL after rhTSH stimulation are considered to be significant enough to prompt further evaluation with functional or anatomic imaging to search for sites of local recurrence or distant metastasis.[125,126]

High-risk Patients

As most patients determined to be at high risk for persistent or recurrent disease at the time of initial surgery proceed to radioactive iodine treatment, assessments of response usually focus on stimulated whole body scanning and serum thyroglobulin measurement at intervals of 6 to 12 months after administration of therapeutic doses of radioactive iodine. Standard protocols based on withdrawal of thyroid hormone to promote increased secretion of TSH are usually employed as preparatory methods of stimulation. Administration of rhTSH may be considered in cases where comorbidities might be complicated by extended periods of hypothyroidism, but this approach has not been validated as an equivalent method of preparing high-risk patients for whole body scanning. To be effective, thyroid hormone withdrawal protocols aim to boost TSH to levels beyond 30 mU/L immediately before the administration of tracer doses of radioactive iodine.[39] Trials have shown that withdrawal involving direct cessation of levothyroxine is comparable to more traditional approaches that involve a brief period of transition to liothyronine before complete withdrawal of thyroid hormone.[40,127] Although most providers have adopted the practice of extending thyroid hormone withdrawal over periods of 3 to 6 weeks, at least one study has shown that the degree of TSH elevation reached after 1 week of thyroid hormone withdrawal is comparable with the degree reached after 3 weeks, with similar responses noted in patients withdrawn immediately after surgery and patients transitioning from suppressive doses of levothyroxine.[128]

Withdrawal-stimulated thyroglobulin levels measured before initial treatment with radioactive iodine have been shown to have low predictive values.[129] Levels measured at appropriate intervals after prior radioactive treatment are more likely to reflect the presence and extent of persistent or recurrent disease.[129,130] Current ATA guidelines stipulate that withdrawal-stimulated thyroglobulin levels greater than 10 ng/mL after rhTSH stimulation should be considered significant enough to prompt further evaluation with functional or anatomic imaging to search for sites of local recurrence or distant metastasis.[1]

Scan-negative/Thyroglobulin-positive Cases

The increasing sensitivity of refined thyroglobulin assays has led to the identification of many cases where patients who have negative whole body scans after radioactive iodine treatment that appear to be consistent with disease-free states also have detectable thyroglobulin levels that signal the presence of persistent or recurrent disease. This finding, which may be noted in up to 20% of all cases of well-differentiated thyroid cancer, suggests that the thyroid cancer cells that are present have dedifferentiated to a state whereby they have lost the ability to take up and concentrate radioactive iodine but retain the ability to produce thyroglobulin in response to TSH stimulation.[131] Detection of persistent or recurrent disease that may be amenable to further treatment in scan-negative/thyroglobulin-positive cases usually relies on a combination of anatomic imaging and direct sampling. Dedicated ultrasonography performed by experienced operators has proven to be the most reliable modality for the identification of suspicious cervical lymphadenopathy.[123] When ultrasonography has successfully identified an accessible mass or suspicious lymph node, fine-needle aspiration biopsy may be employed to obtain samples for cytopathologic analysis. Samples aspirated from small or cystic lymph nodes often prove to be nondiagnostic due to a lack of sampling of distinct thyroid carcinoma cells.[132] Detection of elevated thyroglobulin levels in aspirate washouts may be useful in identifying metastatic thyroid carcinoma in situations where fine-needle aspiration biopsy samples have been classified as negative or nondiagnostic.[132] A study evaluating aspirate washout samples taken from 168 ultrasonographically detected lymph nodes showed that when standardized preparations diluted in 1 mL normal saline (or undiluted cystic fluid) were assayed for thyroglobulin, a cutoff level of 10 ng/mL had a positive predictive value of 93% for the detection of metastatic well-differentiated thyroid cancer.[133]

When cervical ultrasonography fails to detect any suspicious masses or lymphadenopathy, and thyroglobulin levels increase to markedly elevated ranges that appear to be consistent with a larger burden of persistent or recurrent disease, it may be prudent to focus on imaging of the lung fields to check for evidence of pulmonary metastases. In this circumstance, chest computed tomography (CT) scans have proven to be more sensitive than standard plain film chest radiographs for the detection micronodules representing pulmonary metastases.[134] Interpreting radiologists should be aware of the fact that the presence of micronodules does not always signify active disease. Fibrotic changes that assume the same shape may persist after successful eradication of functional pulmonary metastases with radioactive iodine treatment.[135] Decisions regarding the use of iodinated intravenous contrast in performing chest CT scans should be based on the anticipated likelihood of possible empirical treatment with radioactive iodine. When iodinated intravenous contrast has been used to enhance imaging, it may be necessary to confirm adequate clearance of iodine before proceeding with empirical radioactive iodine treatment. Measurement of spot urine iodine with a threshold level of less than 200 µg/L may help to determine whether there has been adequate clearance of iodine after contrast administration.

Metastatic thyroid cancer that has dedifferentiated to the point of losing iodine avidity may demonstrate avid uptake of ^{18}F-fluorodeoxyglucose (FDG).[136] Studies evaluating FDG-PET scanning in scan-negative/thyroglobulin-positive cases have shown that static imaging has a positive predictive value of 92% to 100% and a negative predictive value of 27% to 93% for the detection of persistent or recurrent disease.[131,137,138] False-negative results have been shown to be more common in patients presenting with minimal cervical lymphadenopathy. Positive detection of disease that has a direct impact on plans for management has been shown to be more common in patients presenting with stage IV disease with suppressed thyroglobulin levels of greater than 10 ng/mL. The generalizability of these studies may be limited because they were not blinded and reference standards were inadequately defined for positive findings.[136] A small study that compared static FDG-PET scanning to rhTSH-stimulated FDG-PET scanning in 7 patients suggested that stimulation may augment the sensitivity of detecting disease.[139] A larger series that compared preparation modalities in 63 patients showed that while administration of rhTSH increased the total number of foci identified in patients with positive findings, it did not significantly change the overall number of patients with positive findings, and had little to no impact on plans for management in cases where additional foci were identified.[140]

POSTSURGICAL HYPOPARATHYROIDISM

While transient mild hypocalcemia is commonly noted to develop immediately after surgical resection for thyroid cancer, severe hypocalcemia that persists over the course of days to weeks should raise suspicion that devitalization or inadvertent removal of tissue may have led to postsurgical hypoparathyroidism. Low intact parathyroid hormone (PTH) levels checked 1 hour after surgery may predict the development of postoperative hypocalcemia requiring treatment.[141] Confirmation of a suspected diagnosis of postoperative hypoparathyroidism relies on detection of low or inappropriately normal PTH levels in tandem with low serum or ionized calcium levels.

Standard treatment of postsurgical hypoparathyroidism involves the administration of calcium carbonate or calcium citrate supplements in combination with vitamin D analogues that act to promote effective absorption.[142] Calcitriol (Rocaltrol), a synthetic form of 1,25-dihydroxyvitamin D3, is the most commonly prescribed analogue currently used in treatment of this disorder. Calcitriol is of high potency and demonstrates a relatively short half-life that reduces the likelihood of sustained vitamin D toxicity. Its principal disadvantages stem from its expense and that it usually has to be administered twice daily to provide effective absorption of dietary and supplemental calcium. Ergocalciferol is an inexpensive synthetic form of vitamin D2 that demonstrates a markedly lower level of affinity for the vitamin D receptor. Ergocalciferol can be administered once daily in high doses to treat postsurgical hypoparathyroidism, and may serve as an acceptable alternative in cases where extreme sensitivity to the effects of calcitriol limits its use. Doses of vitamin D analogues and calcium supplements are adjusted over time to target serum or ionized calcium levels that are at or just below the lower limits of reference ranges. In some patients, adequate relief of peiroral numbness and digital paresthesias may require treatment with doses that maintain slightly higher serum calcium levels. Loss of PTH-mediated regulation of renal calcium absorption and excretion is known to be associated with an increased risk of progressive renal dysfunction. Twenty-four–hour urine samples can be collected and tracked to guide adjustment of doses of vitamin D analogues and calcium supplements targeted to minimize urine calcium excretion.

Teriparatide (Forteo), a recombinant form of the 1-34 sequence of human PTH used to treat refractory osteoporosis, has been evaluated as a potential hormonal agent for use in the treatment of postsurgical hypoparathyroidism. An early trial that studied use of teriparatide showed that daily subcutaneous injections effectively maintained serum calcium levels within normal ranges while reducing urine calcium excretion.[143] The effect was noted to diminish after 12 hours, leading to periods of symptomatic hypocalcemia. Trials that studied twice daily subcutaneous injections showed that more frequent administration allowed for use of lower total daily doses with maintenance of higher average serum calcium levels.[144,145] Despite its seeming promise, teriparatide has not been adopted for general use in the treatment of postsurgical hypoparathyroidism, principally due to questions and concerns about its efficacy, expense, side effect profile, and potential impact on bone turnover with long-term administration.

REFERENCES

1. Cooper DS, Doherty GM, Haugen BR, et al. Revised American Thyroid Association management guidelines for patients with thyroid nodules and differentiated thyroid cancer. Thyroid 2009;19(11):1167–214.
2. Greene FL, Page DL, Fleming ID, editors. AJCC (American Joint Committee on Cancer) cancer staging manual. 6th edition. New York: Springer-Verlag; 2002. p. 77–87.
3. Brierley JD, Asa SL. Thyroid cancer. In: Gospodarowicz MK, O'Sullivan B, Sobin LH, editors. Prognostic factors in cancer. Hoboken (NJ): John Wiley and Sons, Inc; 2006. p. 119–22.
4. Baloch ZW, LiVolsi VA. Prognostic factors in well-differentiated follicular-derived carcinoma and medullary thyroid carcinoma. Thyroid 2001;11(7):637–45.
5. Vassilopoulou-Sellin R, Schultz PN, Haynie TP. Clinical outcome of patients with papillary thyroid carcinoma who have recurrence after initial radioactive iodine therapy. Cancer 1996;78(3):493–501.
6. Wada N, Nakayama H, Suganuma N, et al. Prognostic value of the sixth edition AJCC/UICC TNM classification for differentiated thyroid carcinoma with extrathyroid extension. J Clin Endocrinol Metab 2007;92(1):215–8.
7. Sherman SI. Toward a standard clinicopathologic staging approach for differentiated thyroid carcinoma. Semin Surg Oncol 1999;16(1):12–5.
8. Sherman SI, Brierley JD, Sperling M, et al. Prospective multicenter study of thyroid carcinoma treatment: initial analysis of staging and outcome. National Thyroid Cancer Treatment Cooperative Study Registry Group. Cancer 1998; 83(5):1012–21.
9. Ghossein RA, Leboeuf R, Patel KN, et al. Tall cell variant of papillary thyroid carcinoma without extrathyroid extension: biologic behavior and clinical implications. Thyroid 2007;17(7):655–61.
10. Are C, Hsu JF, Ghossein RA, et al. Histological aggressiveness of fluorodeoxyglucose positron-emission tomogram (FDG-PET)-detected incidental thyroid carcinomas. Ann Surg Oncol 2007;14(11):3210–5.
11. Mazzaferri EL, Jhiang SM. Long-term impact of initial surgical and medical therapy on papillary and follicular thyroid cancer. Am J Med 1994;97(5):418–28.
12. Grebe SK, Hay ID. Follicular thyroid cancer. Endocrinol Metab Clin North Am 1995;24(4):761–801.
13. Nikiforova MN, Kimura ET, Gandhi M, et al. BRAF mutations in thyroid tumors are restricted to papillary carcinomas and anaplastic or poorly differentiated carcinomas arising from papillary carcinomas. J Clin Endocrinol Metab 2003;88(11): 5399–404.

14. Xing M, Westra WH, Tufano RP, et al. BRAF mutation predicts a poorer clinical prognosis for papillary thyroid cancer. J Clin Endocrinol Metab 2005;90(12): 6373–9.

15. Kim TY, Kim WB, Rhee YS, et al. The BRAF mutation is useful for prediction of clinical recurrence in low-risk patients with conventional papillary thyroid carcinoma. Clin Endocrinol (Oxf) 2006;65(3):364–8.

16. DeGroot LJ, Kaplan EL, McCormick M, et al. Natural history, treatment, and course of papillary thyroid carcinoma. J Clin Endocrinol Metab 1990;71(2):414–24.

17. Samaan NA, Schultz PN, Hickey RC, et al. The results of various modalities of treatment of well differentiated thyroid carcinomas: a retrospective review of 1599 patients. J Clin Endocrinol Metab 1992;75(3):714–20.

18. Wong JB, Kaplan MM, Meyer KB, et al. Ablative radioactive iodine therapy for apparently localized thyroid carcinoma. A decision analytic perspective. Endocrinol Metab Clin North Am 1990;19(3):741–60.

19. Sawka AM, Thephamongkhol K, Brouwers M, et al. Clinical review 170: a systematic review and metaanalysis of the effectiveness of radioactive iodine remnant ablation for well-differentiated thyroid cancer. J Clin Endocrinol Metab 2004; 89(8):3668–76.

20. Taylor T, Specker B, Robbins J, et al. Outcome after treatment of high-risk papillary and non-Hurthle-cell follicular thyroid carcinoma. Ann Intern Med 1998; 129(8):622–7.

21. Hay ID, Thompson GB, Grant CS, et al. Papillary thyroid carcinoma managed at the Mayo Clinic during six decades (1940-1999): temporal trends in initial therapy and long-term outcome in 2444 consecutively treated patients. World J Surg 2002;26(8):879–85.

22. Mazzaferri EL. Thyroid remnant 131I ablation for papillary and follicular thyroid carcinoma. Thyroid 1997;7(2):265–71.

23. Hay ID. Selective use of radioactive iodine in the postoperative management of patients with papillary and follicular thyroid carcinoma. J Surg Oncol 2006;94(8): 692–700.

24. Simpson WJ, Panzarella T, Carruthers JS, et al. Papillary and follicular thyroid cancer: impact of treatment in 1578 patients. Int J Radiat Oncol Biol Phys 1988;14(6):1063–75.

25. Tubiana M, Schlumberger M, Rougier P, et al. Long-term results and prognostic factors in patients with differentiated thyroid carcinoma. Cancer 1985;55(4): 794–804.

26. Sanders LE, Cady B. Differentiated thyroid cancer: reexamination of risk groups and outcome of treatment. Arch Surg 1998;133(4):419–25.

27. Sawka AM, Brierley JD, Tsang RW, et al. An updated systematic review and commentary examining the effectiveness of radioactive iodine remnant ablation in well-differentiated thyroid cancer. Endocrinol Metab Clin North Am 2008; 37(2):457–80, x.

28. Durante C, Haddy N, Baudin E, et al. Long-term outcome of 444 patients with distant metastases from papillary and follicular thyroid carcinoma: benefits and limits of radioiodine therapy. J Clin Endocrinol Metab 2006;91(8):2892–9.

29. Sisson JC, Giordano TJ, Jamadar DA, et al. 131-I treatment of micronodular pulmonary metastases from papillary thyroid carcinoma. Cancer 1996;78(10): 2184–92.

30. Schlumberger M, Tubiana M, De Vathaire F, et al. Long-term results of treatment of 283 patients with lung and bone metastases from differentiated thyroid carcinoma. J Clin Endocrinol Metab 1986;63(4):960–7.

31. Samaan NA, Schultz PN, Haynie TP, et al. Pulmonary metastasis of differentiated thyroid carcinoma: treatment results in 101 patients. J Clin Endocrinol Metab 1985;60(2):376–80.
32. Hindie E, Melliere D, Lange F, et al. Functioning pulmonary metastases of thyroid cancer: does radioiodine influence the prognosis? Eur J Nucl Med Mol Imaging 2003;30(7):974–81.
33. Bal CS, Kumar A, Chandra P, et al. Is chest x-ray or high-resolution computed tomography scan of the chest sufficient investigation to detect pulmonary metastasis in pediatric differentiated thyroid cancer? Thyroid 2004;14(3): 217–25.
34. Schlumberger M, Challeton C, De Vathaire F, et al. Radioactive iodine treatment and external radiotherapy for lung and bone metastases from thyroid carcinoma. J Nucl Med 1996;37(4):598–605.
35. Wang W, Larson SM, Tuttle RM, et al. Resistance of [^{18}F]-fluorodeoxyglucose-avid metastatic thyroid cancer lesions to treatment with high-dose radioactive iodine. Thyroid 2001;11(12):1169–75.
36. Spitzweg C, Harrington KJ, Pinke LA, et al. Clinical review 132: The sodium iodide symporter and its potential role in cancer therapy. J Clin Endocrinol Metab 2001;86(7):3327–35.
37. Samaan NA, Maheshwari YK, Nader S, et al. Impact of therapy for differentiated carcinoma of the thyroid: an analysis of 706 cases. J Clin Endocrinol Metab 1983;56(6):1131–8.
38. Edmonds CJ, Hayes S, Kermode JC, et al. Measurement of serum TSH and thyroid hormones in the management of treatment of thyroid carcinoma with radioiodine. Br J Radiol 1977;50(599):799–807.
39. Liel Y. Preparation for radioactive iodine administration in differentiated thyroid cancer patients. Clin Endocrinol (Oxf) 2002;57(4):523–7.
40. Serhal DI, Nasrallah MP, Arafah BM. Rapid rise in serum thyrotropin concentrations after thyroidectomy or withdrawal of suppressive thyroxine therapy in preparation for radioactive iodine administration to patients with differentiated thyroid cancer. J Clin Endocrinol Metab 2004;89(7):3285–9.
41. Leboeuf R, Perron P, Carpentier AC, et al. L-T3 preparation for whole-body scintigraphy: a randomized-controlled trial. Clin Endocrinol (Oxf) 2007;67(6): 839–44.
42. Pacini F, Ladenson PW, Schlumberger M, et al. Radioiodine ablation of thyroid remnants after preparation with recombinant human thyrotropin in differentiated thyroid carcinoma: results of an international, randomized, controlled study. J Clin Endocrinol Metab 2006;91(3):926–32.
43. Barbaro D, Boni G, Meucci G, et al. Radioiodine treatment with 30 mCi after recombinant human thyrotropin stimulation in thyroid cancer: effectiveness for postsurgical remnants ablation and possible role of iodine content in L-thyroxine in the outcome of ablation. J Clin Endocrinol Metab 2003;88(9): 4110–5.
44. Pilli T, Brianzoni E, Capoccetti F, et al. A comparison of 1850 (50 mCi) and 3700 MBq (100 mCi) 131-iodine administered doses for recombinant thyrotropin-stimulated postoperative thyroid remnant ablation in differentiated thyroid cancer. J Clin Endocrinol Metab 2007;92(9):3542–6.
45. Pacini F, Molinaro E, Castagna MG, et al. Ablation of thyroid residues with 30 mCi (131)I: a comparison in thyroid cancer patients prepared with recombinant human TSH or thyroid hormone withdrawal. J Clin Endocrinol Metab 2002;87(9): 4063–8.

46. Tuttle RM, Brokhin M, Omry G, et al. Recombinant human TSH-assisted radioactive iodine remnant ablation achieves short-term clinical recurrence rates similar to those of traditional thyroid hormone withdrawal. J Nucl Med 2008;49(5): 764–70.

47. Borget I, Corone C, Nocaudie M, et al. Sick leave for follow-up control in thyroid cancer patients: comparison between stimulation with Thyrogen and thyroid hormone withdrawal. Eur J Endocrinol 2007;156(5):531–8.

48. Borget I, Remy H, Chevalier J, et al. Length and cost of hospital stay of radioiodine ablation in thyroid cancer patients: comparison between preparation with thyroid hormone withdrawal and thyrogen. Eur J Nucl Med Mol Imaging 2008;35(8):1457–63.

49. Mernagh P, Campbell S, Dietlein M, et al. Cost-effectiveness of using recombinant human TSH prior to radioiodine ablation for thyroid cancer, compared with treating patients in a hypothyroid state: the German perspective. Eur J Endocrinol 2006;155(3):405–14.

50. Luster M, Felbinger R, Dietlein M, et al. Thyroid hormone withdrawal in patients with differentiated thyroid carcinoma: a one hundred thirty-patient pilot survey on consequences of hypothyroidism and a pharmacoeconomic comparison to recombinant thyrotropin administration. Thyroid 2005;15(10):1147–55.

51. Maxon HR, Thomas SR, Boehringer A, et al. Low iodine diet in I-131 ablation of thyroid remnants. Clin Nucl Med 1983;8(3):123–6.

52. Costa A, Testori OB, Cenderelli C, et al. Iodine content of human tissues after administration of iodine containing drugs or contrast media. J Endocrinol Invest 1978;1(3):221–5.

53. Pluijmen MJ, Eustatia-Rutten C, Goslings BM, et al. Effects of low-iodide diet on postsurgical radioiodide ablation therapy in patients with differentiated thyroid carcinoma. Clin Endocrinol (Oxf) 2003;58(4):428–35.

54. Medvedec M. Thyroid stunning in vivo and in vitro. Nucl Med Commun 2005; 26(8):731–5.

55. Morris LF, Waxman AD, Braunstein GD. Thyroid stunning. Thyroid 2003;13(4): 333–40.

56. Muratet JP, Giraud P, Daver A, et al. Predicting the efficacy of first iodine-131 treatment in differentiated thyroid carcinoma. J Nucl Med 1997;38(9):1362–8.

57. Urhan M, Dadparvar S, Mavi A, et al. Iodine-123 as a diagnostic imaging agent in differentiated thyroid carcinoma: a comparison with iodine-131 post-treatment scanning and serum thyroglobulin measurement. Eur J Nucl Med Mol Imaging 2007;34(7):1012–7.

58. Hackshaw A, Harmer C, Mallick U, et al. [131]I activity for remnant ablation in patients with differentiated thyroid cancer: a systematic review. J Clin Endocrinol Metab 2007;92(1):28–38.

59. Bal C, Padhy AK, Jana S, et al. Prospective randomized clinical trial to evaluate the optimal dose of ^{131}I for remnant ablation in patients with differentiated thyroid carcinoma. Cancer 1996;77(12):2574–80.

60. Doi SA, Woodhouse NJ. Ablation of the thyroid remnant and ^{131}I dose in differentiated thyroid cancer. Clin Endocrinol (Oxf) 2000;52(6):765–73.

61. Tuttle RM, Leboeuf R, Robbins RJ, et al. Empiric radioactive iodine dosing regimens frequently exceed maximum tolerated activity levels in elderly patients with thyroid cancer. J Nucl Med 2006;47(10):1587–91.

62. Van Nostrand D, Atkins F, Yeganeh F, et al. Dosimetrically determined doses of radioiodine for the treatment of metastatic thyroid carcinoma. Thyroid 2002; 12(2):121–34.

63. Fatourechi V, Hay ID, Mullan BP, et al. Are posttherapy radioiodine scans informative and do they influence subsequent therapy of patients with differentiated thyroid cancer? Thyroid 2000;10(7):573–7.
64. Sherman SI, Tielens ET, Sostre S, et al. Clinical utility of posttreatment radioiodine scans in the management of patients with thyroid carcinoma. J Clin Endocrinol Metab 1994;78(3):629–34.
65. Souza Rosario PW, Barroso AL, Rezende LL, et al. Post I-131 therapy scanning in patients with thyroid carcinoma metastases: an unnecessary cost or a relevant contribution? Clin Nucl Med 2004;29(12):795–8.
66. Van Nostrand D, Neutze J, Atkins F. Side effects of "rational dose" iodine-131 therapy for metastatic well-differentiated thyroid carcinoma. J Nucl Med 1986; 27(10):1519–27.
67. Wartofsky L, Sherman SI, Gopal J, et al. The use of radioactive iodine in patients with papillary and follicular thyroid cancer. J Clin Endocrinol Metab 1998;83(12): 4195–203.
68. Kloos RT, Duvuuri V, Jhiang SM, et al. Nasolacrimal drainage system obstruction from radioactive iodine therapy for thyroid carcinoma. J Clin Endocrinol Metab 2002;87(12):5817–20.
69. DiRusso G, Kern KA. Comparative analysis of complications from I-131 radioablation for well-differentiated thyroid cancer. Surgery 1994;116(6): 1024–30.
70. Benua RS, Cicale NR, Sonenberg M, et al. The relation of radioiodine dosimetry to results and complications in the treatment of metastatic thyroid cancer. Am J Roentgenol Radium Ther Nucl Med 1962;87:171–82.
71. Datz FL. Cerebral edema following iodine-131 therapy for thyroid carcinoma metastatic to the brain. J Nucl Med 1986;27(5):637–40.
72. Brierly J, Maxon HR. Radioiodine and external radiation therapy. Boston/Dordrecht. In: Fagin JA, editor. Thyroid cancer. London: Kluwer Academic Publishers; 1998. p. 285–317.
73. Adjadj E, Rubino C, Shamsaldim A, et al. The risk of multiple primary breast and thyroid carcinomas. Cancer 2003;98(6):1309–17.
74. Bhattacharyya N, Chien W. Risk of second primary malignancy after radioactive iodine treatment for differentiated thyroid carcinoma. Ann Otol Rhinol Laryngol 2006;115(8):607–10.
75. Schlumberger M, De Vathaire F, Ceccarelli C, et al. Exposure to radioactive iodine-131 for scintigraphy or therapy does not preclude pregnancy in thyroid cancer patients. J Nucl Med 1996;37(4):606–12.
76. Wichers M, Benz E, Palmedo H, et al. Testicular function after radioiodine therapy for thyroid carcinoma. Eur J Nucl Med 2000;27(5):503–7.
77. Hyer S, Vini L, O'Connell M, et al. Testicular dose and fertility in men following I(131) therapy for thyroid cancer. Clin Endocrinol (Oxf) 2002; 56(6):755–8.
78. McGriff NJ, Csako G, Gourgiotis L, et al. Effects of thyroid hormone suppression therapy on adverse clinical outcomes in thyroid cancer. Annu Mediaev 2002; 34(7-8):554–64.
79. Jonklaas J, Sarlis NJ, Litofsky D, et al. Outcomes of patients with differentiated thyroid carcinoma following initial therapy. Thyroid 2006;16(12):1229–42.
80. Cooper DS, Specker B, Ho M, et al. Thyrotropin suppression and disease progression in patients with differentiated thyroid cancer: results from the National Thyroid Cancer Treatment Cooperative Registry. Thyroid 1998;8(9): 737–44.

81. Merola B, Cittadini A, Colao A, et al. Chronic treatment with the somatostatin analog octreotide improves cardiac abnormalities in acromegaly. J Clin Endocrinol Metab 1993;77(3):790–3.
82. Sawin CT, Geller A, Wolf PA, et al. Low serum thyrotropin concentrations as a risk factor for atrial fibrillation in older persons. N Engl J Med 1994;331(19): 1249–52.
83. Toivonen J, Tahtela R, Laitinen K, et al. Markers of bone turnover in patients with differentiated thyroid cancer with and following withdrawal of thyroxine suppressive therapy. Eur J Endocrinol 1998;138(6):667–73.
84. Brierley JD, Tsang RW. External beam radiation therapy for thyroid cancer. Endocrinol Metab Clin North Am 2008;37(2):497–509, xi.
85. Lin JD, Tsang NM, Huang MJ, et al. Results of external beam radiotherapy in patients with well differentiated thyroid carcinoma. Jpn J Clin Oncol 1997; 27(4):244–7.
86. Brierley J, Tsang R, Panzarella T, et al. Prognostic factors and the effect of treatment with radioactive iodine and external beam radiation on patients with differentiated thyroid cancer seen at a single institution over 40 years. Clin Endocrinol (Oxf) 2005;63(4):418–27.
87. Farahati J, Reiners C, Stuschke M, et al. Differentiated thyroid cancer. Impact of adjuvant external radiotherapy in patients with perithyroidal tumor infiltration (stage pT4). Cancer 1996;77(1):172–80.
88. Tsang RW, Brierley JD, Simpson WJ, et al. The effects of surgery, radioiodine, and external radiation therapy on the clinical outcome of patients with differentiated thyroid carcinoma. Cancer 1998;82(2):375–88.
89. Brierley JD, Tsang RW. External-beam radiation therapy in the treatment of differentiated thyroid cancer. Semin Surg Oncol 1999;16(1):42–9.
90. Haugen BR. Management of the patient with progressive radioiodine nonresponsive disease. Semin Surg Oncol 1999;16(1):34–41.
91. Sherman SI. Advances in chemotherapy of differentiated epithelial and medullary thyroid cancers. J Clin Endocrinol Metab 2009;94(5):1493–9.
92. Gottlieb JA, Hill CS Jr. Chemotherapy of thyroid cancer with adriamycin. Experience with 30 patients. N Engl J Med 1974;290(4):193–7.
93. O'Bryan RM, Baker LH, Gottlieb JE, et al. Dose response evaluation of adriamycin in human neoplasia. Cancer 1977;39(5):1940–8.
94. Kloos RT, Ringel MD, Knopp MV, et al. Phase II trial of sorafenib in metastatic thyroid cancer. J Clin Oncol 2009;27(10):1675–84.
95. Gupta-Abramson V, Troxel AB, Nellore A, et al. Phase II trial of sorafenib in advanced thyroid cancer. J Clin Oncol 2008;26(29):4714–9.
96. Arnault JP, Wechsler J, Escudier B, et al. Keratoacanthomas and squamous cell carcinomas in patients receiving sorafenib. J Clin Oncol 2009;27(23): e59–61.
97. Lima N, Cavaliere H, Tomimori E, et al. Prognostic value of serial serum thyroglobulin determinations after total thyroidectomy for differentiated thyroid cancer. J Endocrinol Invest 2002;25(2):110–5.
98. Spencer CA, LoPresti JS, Fatemi S, et al. Detection of residual and recurrent differentiated thyroid carcinoma by serum thyroglobulin measurement. Thyroid 1999;9(5):435–41.
99. Spencer CA, Takeuchi M, Kazarosyan M, et al. Serum thyroglobulin autoantibodies: prevalence, influence on serum thyroglobulin measurement, and prognostic significance in patients with differentiated thyroid carcinoma. J Clin Endocrinol Metab 1998;83(4):1121–7.

100. Spencer CA. Challenges of serum thyroglobulin (Tg) measurement in the presence of Tg autoantibodies. J Clin Endocrinol Metab 2004;89(8):3702–4.
101. Rosario PW, Maia FF, Fagundes TA, et al. Antithyroglobulin antibodies in patients with differentiated thyroid carcinoma: methods of detection, interference with serum thyroglobulin measurement and clinical significance. Arq Bras Endocrinol Metabol 2004;48(4):487–92.
102. Chung JK, Park YJ, Kim TY, et al. Clinical significance of elevated level of serum antithyroglobulin antibody in patients with differentiated thyroid cancer after thyroid ablation. Clin Endocrinol (Oxf) 2002;57(2):215–21.
103. Elisei R, Vivaldi A, Agate L, et al. Low specificity of blood thyroglobulin messenger ribonucleic acid assay prevents its use in the follow-up of differentiated thyroid cancer patients. J Clin Endocrinol Metab 2004;89(1):33–9.
104. Wingo ST, Ringel MD, Anderson JS, et al. Quantitative reverse transcription-PCR measurement of thyroglobulin mRNA in peripheral blood of healthy subjects. Clin Chem 1999;45(6 Pt 1):785–9.
105. Ringel MD, Balducci-Silano PL, Anderson JS, et al. Quantitative reverse transcription-polymerase chain reaction of circulating thyroglobulin messenger ribonucleic acid for monitoring patients with thyroid carcinoma. J Clin Endocrinol Metab 1999;84(11):4037–42.
106. Grammatopoulos D, Elliott Y, Smith SC, et al. Measurement of thyroglobulin mRNA in peripheral blood as an adjunctive test for monitoring thyroid cancer. Mol Pathol 2003;56(3):162–6.
107. Eszlinger M, Neumann S, Otto L, et al. Thyroglobulin mRNA quantification in the peripheral blood is not a reliable marker for the follow-up of patients with differentiated thyroid cancer. Eur J Endocrinol 2002;147(5):575–82.
108. Hay ID. Management of patients with low-risk papillary thyroid carcinoma. Endocr Pract 2007;13(5):521–33.
109. Machens A, Hinze R, Thomusch O, et al. Pattern of nodal metastasis for primary and reoperative thyroid cancer. World J Surg 2002;26(1):22–8.
110. Qubain SW, Nakano S, Baba M, et al. Distribution of lymph node micrometastasis in pN0 well-differentiated thyroid carcinoma. Surgery 2002;131(3): 249–56.
111. Wang TS, Dubner S, Sznyter LA, et al. Incidence of metastatic well-differentiated thyroid cancer in cervical lymph nodes. Arch Otolaryngol Head Neck Surg 2004;130(1):110–3.
112. Robbins KT, Clayman G, Levine PA, et al. Neck dissection classification update: revisions proposed by the American Head and Neck Society and the American Academy of Otolaryngology-Head and Neck Surgery. Arch Otolaryngol Head Neck Surg 2002;128(7):751–8.
113. van Tol KM, Jager PL, de Vries EG, et al. Outcome in patients with differentiated thyroid cancer with negative diagnostic whole-body scanning and detectable stimulated thyroglobulin. Eur J Endocrinol 2003;148(6):589–96.
114. Gerard SK, Cavalieri RR. I-123 diagnostic thyroid tumor whole-body scanning with imaging at 6, 24, and 48 hours. Clin Nucl Med 2002;27(1):1–8.
115. Mazzaferri EL, Kloos RT. Is diagnostic iodine-131 scanning with recombinant human TSH useful in the follow-up of differentiated thyroid cancer after thyroid ablation? J Clin Endocrinol Metab 2002;87(4):1490–8.
116. Pacini F, Capezzone M, Elisei R, et al. Diagnostic 131-iodine whole-body scan may be avoided in thyroid cancer patients who have undetectable stimulated serum Tg levels after initial treatment. J Clin Endocrinol Metab 2002;87(4): 1499–501.

117. Eustatia-Rutten CF, Smit JW, Romijn JA, et al. Diagnostic value of serum thyroglobulin measurements in the follow-up of differentiated thyroid carcinoma, a structured meta-analysis. Clin Endocrinol (Oxf) 2004;61(1):61–74.
118. Toubeau M, Touzery C, Arveux P, et al. Predictive value for disease progression of serum thyroglobulin levels measured in the postoperative period and after (131)I ablation therapy in patients with differentiated thyroid cancer. J Nucl Med 2004;45(6):988–94.
119. Haugen BR, Pacini F, Reiners C, et al. A comparison of recombinant human thyrotropin and thyroid hormone withdrawal for the detection of thyroid remnant or cancer. J Clin Endocrinol Metab 1999;84(11):3877–85.
120. Anderson GS, Fish S, Nakhoda K, et al. Comparison of I-123 and I-131 for whole-body imaging after stimulation by recombinant human thyrotropin: a preliminary report. Clin Nucl Med 2003;28(2):93–6.
121. Pacini F, Molinaro E, Lippi F, et al. Prediction of disease status by recombinant human TSH-stimulated serum Tg in the postsurgical follow-up of differentiated thyroid carcinoma. J Clin Endocrinol Metab 2001;86(12):5686–90.
122. Haugen BR, Ridgway EC, McLaughlin BA, et al. Clinical comparison of whole-body radioiodine scan and serum thyroglobulin after stimulation with recombinant human thyrotropin. Thyroid 2002;12(1):37–43.
123. Pacini F, Molinaro E, Castagna MG, et al. Recombinant human thyrotropin-stimulated serum thyroglobulin combined with neck ultrasonography has the highest sensitivity in monitoring differentiated thyroid carcinoma. J Clin Endocrinol Metab 2003;88(8):3668–73.
124. Wartofsky L. Management of low-risk well-differentiated thyroid cancer based only on thyroglobulin measurement after recombinant human thyrotropin. Thyroid 2002;12(7):583–90.
125. David A, Blotta A, Rossi R, et al. Clinical value of different responses of serum thyroglobulin to recombinant human thyrotropin in the follow-up of patients with differentiated thyroid carcinoma. Thyroid 2005;15(3):267–73.
126. Kloos RT, Mazzaferri EL. A single recombinant human thyrotropin-stimulated serum thyroglobulin measurement predicts differentiated thyroid carcinoma metastases three to five years later. J Clin Endocrinol Metab 2005;90(9): 5047–57.
127. Sanchez R, Espinosa-de-los-Monteros AL, Mendoza V, et al. Adequate thyroid-stimulating hormone levels after levothyroxine discontinuation in the follow-up of patients with well-differentiated thyroid carcinoma. Arch Med Res 2002;33(5): 478–81.
128. Grigsby PW, Siegel BA, Bekker S, et al. Preparation of patients with thyroid cancer for 131I scintigraphy or therapy by 1-3 weeks of thyroxine discontinuation. J Nucl Med 2004;45(4):567–70.
129. Baudin E, Do Cao C, Cailleux AF, et al. Positive predictive value of serum thyroglobulin levels, measured during the first year of follow-up after thyroid hormone withdrawal, in thyroid cancer patients. J Clin Endocrinol Metab 2003;88(3): 1107–11.
130. Bachelot A, Cailleux AF, Klain M, et al. Relationship between tumor burden and serum thyroglobulin level in patients with papillary and follicular thyroid carcinoma. Thyroid 2002;12(8):707–11.
131. Wang W, Macapinlac H, Larson SM, et al. [^{18}F]-2-fluoro-2-deoxy-D-glucose positron emission tomography localizes residual thyroid cancer in patients with negative diagnostic (131)I whole body scans and elevated serum thyroglobulin levels. J Clin Endocrinol Metab 1999;84(7):2291–302.

132. Baloch ZW, Barroeta JE, Walsh J, et al. Utility of Thyroglobulin measurement in fine-needle aspiration biopsy specimens of lymph nodes in the diagnosis of recurrent thyroid carcinoma. Cytojournal 2008;5:1.
133. Kim MJ, Kim EK, Kim BM, et al. Thyroglobulin measurement in fine-needle aspirate washouts: the criteria for neck node dissection for patients with thyroid cancer. Clin Endocrinol (Oxf) 2009;70(1):145–51.
134. Ilgan S, Karacalioglu AO, Pabuscu Y, et al. Iodine-131 treatment and high-resolution CT: results in patients with lung metastases from differentiated thyroid carcinoma. Eur J Nucl Med Mol Imaging 2004;31(6):825–30.
135. Piekarski JD, Schlumberger M, Leclere J, et al. Chest computed tomography (CT) in patients with micronodular lung metastases of differentiated thyroid carcinoma. Int J Radiat Oncol Biol Phys 1985;11(5):1023–7.
136. Hooft L, Hoekstra OS, Deville W, et al. Diagnostic accuracy of ^{18}F-fluorodeoxyglucose positron emission tomography in the follow-up of papillary or follicular thyroid cancer. J Clin Endocrinol Metab 2001;86(8):3779–86.
137. Nahas Z, Goldenberg D, Fakhry C, et al. The role of positron emission tomography/computed tomography in the management of recurrent papillary thyroid carcinoma. Laryngoscope 2005;115(2):237–43.
138. Helal BO, Merlet P, Toubert ME, et al. Clinical impact of ^{18}F-FDG PET in thyroid carcinoma patients with elevated thyroglobulin levels and negative ^{131}I scanning results after therapy. J Nucl Med 2001;42(10):1464–9.
139. Chin BB, Patel P, Cohade C, et al. Recombinant human thyrotropin stimulation of fluoro-D-glucose positron emission tomography uptake in well-differentiated thyroid carcinoma. J Clin Endocrinol Metab 2004;89(1):91–5.
140. Leboulleux S, Schroeder PR, Busaidy NL, et al. Assessment of the incremental value of recombinant thyrotropin stimulation before 2-[^{18}F]-Fluoro-2-deoxy-D-glucose positron emission tomography/computed tomography imaging to localize residual differentiated thyroid cancer. J Clin Endocrinol Metab 2009; 94(4):1310–6.
141. Soon PS, Magarey CJ, Campbell P, et al. Serum intact parathyroid hormone as a predictor of hypocalcaemia after total thyroidectomy. ANZ J Surg 2005;75(11): 977–80.
142. Kronenberg H, Williams RH. Williams textbook of endocrinology. 11th edition. Philadelphia: Saunders/Elsevier; 2008.
143. Winer KK, Yanovski JA, Cutler GB Jr. Synthetic human parathyroid hormone 1-34 vs calcitriol and calcium in the treatment of hypoparathyroidism. JAMA 1996;276(8):631–6.
144. Winer KK, Yanovski JA, Sarani B, et al. A randomized, cross-over trial of once-daily versus twice-daily parathyroid hormone 1–34 in treatment of hypoparathyroidism. J Clin Endocrinol Metab 1998;83(10):3480–6.
145. Winer KK, Sinaii N, Peterson D, et al. Effects of once versus twice-daily parathyroid hormone 1-34 therapy in children with hypoparathyroidism. J Clin Endocrinol Metab 2008;93(9):3389–95.

Reoperation for Recurrent/Persistent Well-Differentiated Thyroid Cancer

Sara I. Pai, MD, PhD[a,b], Ralph P. Tufano, MD[a,*]

KEYWORDS

- Recurrent/persistent papillary thyroid cancer
- Well-differentiated thyroid cancer
- Reoperative surgery • Algorithm

The incidence of thyroid cancer in the United States has been increasing over the past several decades. Some attribute this increase to improved detection rates of small papillary cancers with the widespread use of high-resolution ultrasonography in combination with fine-needle aspiration (FNA) biopsy of subcentimeter thyroid nodules.[1,2] Most well-differentiated thyroid cancers (WDTC) have a favorable prognosis with excellent long-term overall survival. The American Thyroid Association has generated guidelines that help to clarify posttreatment surveillance strategies for patients diagnosed with WDTC.[3] Similar to the observed trend of increased detection rates of smaller papillary cancers, sensitive assays including ultrasonography and monitoring of serum thyroglobulin levels have ushered in a new era in which clinicians are diagnosing small volume recurrent/persistent disease in lymph nodes of the neck. The effect of nodal recurrence/persistence on prognosis and survival is unclear, especially when it is in the form of small volume disease. Nonetheless, identification of recurrent/persistent disease requires critical thinking as to what, if any, intervention should be performed to control the disease while minimizing morbidity. This presentation discusses the preoperative and technical considerations in reoperative surgery for recurrent/persistent WDTC within the central and/or lateral necks.

PREOPERATIVE EVALUATION

When evaluating a patient in the reoperative setting for recurrent/persistent WDTC, a thorough preoperative evaluation is warranted to minimize the increased operative

[a] Department of Otolaryngology-Head and Neck Surgery, Johns Hopkins Medical Institutions, 601 North Caroline Street, JHOC 6th floor, Baltimore, MA 21287, USA
[b] Department of Oncology, Johns Hopkins University School of Medicine, The Sidney Kimmel Comprehensive Cancer Center at Johns Hopkins, Bunting-Blaustein Cancer Research Building II, 1550 Orleans Street, Room 5M03, Baltimore, MD 21231, USA
* Corresponding author.
E-mail address: rtufano@jhmi.edu

Otolaryngol Clin N Am 43 (2010) 353–363
doi:10.1016/j.otc.2010.02.004
0030-6665/10/$ – see front matter © 2010 Elsevier Inc. All rights reserved.

risks and, most importantly, the need for further revision surgeries. A detailed history and physical examination should be performed. It is imperative to review the previous operative reports to determine the extent of surgery performed at the initial operation. The pathology report and/or slides can provide further information regarding the extent of disease, status of the surgical margins, and integrity of the parathyroid glands. In addition, as part of the history and physical examination, it is important to ascertain if there were any associated complications with the previous surgeries. A detailed cranial nerve assessment should be performed including an analysis of vocal fold function before any reoperative surgery in the central neck.[4,5] Laboratory testing should include a serum calcium level and, if low or the patient is requiring calcium supplementation, obtaining an intact parathyroid hormone (PTH) level should be considered.

The cornerstone of postoperative surveillance for these patients is high-resolution ultrasonography of the thyroid bed and lateral neck.[3] Ultrasound can help localize an area suspicious for recurrent/persistent disease and image-guided FNA biopsy can be used to confirm the presence of malignancy. It is important to have a clear understanding of where the disease is located as it relates to vital structures in the neck.[6] The American Head and Neck Society has defined the compartments of the neck and this designation should be used by all practitioners so that disease localization can be clearly communicated (**Fig. 1**).[7] In the setting of recurrent disease in a previously operated lateral neck, a computed tomography (CT) scan of the neck with intravenous contrast can often be useful in delineating compartments that were not addressed at the time of the initial lateral neck dissection. The presence of fatty tissue harboring lymph nodes can easily be visualized in axial cuts of the CT scan; whereas a lack of a plane between the great vessels and the sternocleidomastoid muscle can suggest previous dissection in that area (**Fig. 2**). However, before obtaining a CT scan, discussions with the endocrinologist are encouraged to ensure that this study would not delay postsurgical adjuvant radioactive iodine (RAI) treatment. An alternative study that can be used to delineate areas of previous dissection in the lateral neck but would not interfere with RAI therapy is a magnetic resonance imaging (MRI) scan with gadolinium. However, the costs associated with an MRI scan need to be considered in the context of whether the patient is a candidate for further RAI treatment.

PATTERNS OF RECURRENCE IN THE NECK

Metastasis to the cervical lymph nodes is common in the tumor progression of papillary thyroid cancer (PTC) and is reported to occur in 20% to 50% of patients.[3] Micrometastases occur at an even higher rate with a study reporting involvement in up to 90% of pathologically examined nodes.[8] These high rates of nodal metastases may contribute to the observed persistence and recurrence rates of PTC.[9] It has been reported that 5% to 20% of patients treated with total thyroidectomy develop palpable local recurrence within 10 years.[10–12] Such recurrences have been reported to localize to the cervical lymph nodes in 60% to 75% of cases with the central compartment of the neck being the most frequently involved site.[13] Cervical lymph node involvement has been associated with an increase in overall mortality in select patient populations.[12,14] High-risk patient groups include patients older than 50 years of age with lymph node metastases greater than 3 cm in size.[15,16] Patients with large nodal metastases have been shown to have increased incidence of local recurrence in the neck with involvement of the surrounding soft tissues of the neck including the carotid artery.[16] At the time of primary surgery for WDTC, prophylactic node dissection is controversial; however, clinically positive lymph nodes should be systematically cleared to minimize the recurrence rates and need for reoperation.[17–19] Reports in

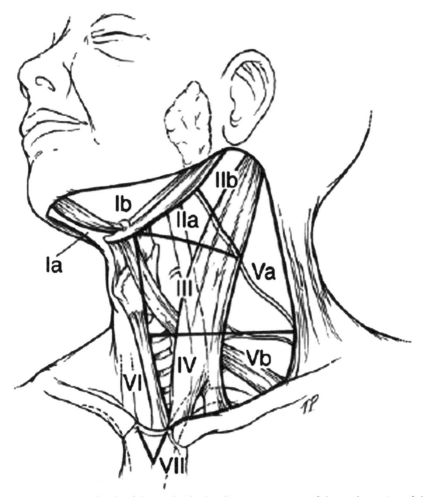

Fig. 1. Compartment levels of the neck. The level Ia compartment of the neck consists of the submental triangle bound by the anterior belly of the digastric muscle and the mylohyoid muscle. Level Ib is the submandibular triangle and is defined by the anterior and posterior bellies of the digastric muscle and body of the mandible. Level II is bound by the lateral border of the sternohyoid muscle, posterior belly of digastric muscle, posterior border of the sternocleidomastoid muscle, skull base, and the level of the carotid bifurcation. Level IIa is anterior to XI and level IIb is posterior to XI. Level III is bound by the lateral border of the sternohyoid muscle, posterior border of the sternoclediomastoid muscle, carotid bifurcation, and omohyoid muscle. Level IV is bound by the lateral border of the sterno-hyoid muscle, posterior border of the sternocleidomastoid muscle, omohyoid muscle, and clavicle. Level V is bound by the posterior border of the sternocleidomastoid muscle, anterior border of the trapezius muscle, and clavicle. Level Va is defined by the lymphatic structures that follow the spinal accessory nerve. Level Vb is defined by the lymphatic structures that lie along the transverse cervical artery. (*From* Pai SI, Tufano RT. Central compartment neck dissection for thyroid cancer: technical considerations. ORL J Otorhinolaryngol Relat Spec 2008;70:292–97; with permission.)

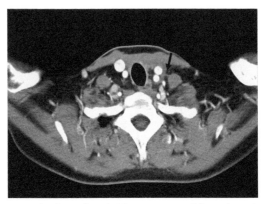

Fig. 2. CT scan of reoperative lateral neck. The presence of fatty tissue harboring lymph nodes can easily be visualized in axial cuts of the CT scan on the right side; whereas, a lack of a plane between the great vessels and the sternocleidomastoid muscle can suggest previous dissection in that area as shown on the left side. Other indications of prior dissection include the presence of soft tissue density surrounding the carotid sheath and presence of fat stranding as depicted by the black arrow.

the literature suggest that comprehensive compartmental resection of the central or lateral neck in the setting of clinically positive lymph nodes can result in better survival and lower recurrence rates.[20]

For recurrent/persistent WDTC cancer, an important element to achieving a successful surgical outcome is to have a systematic approach to the neck, both in surgical technique and extent of lymph node dissection within a defined compartment of the neck. Several studies have shown that for locally recurrent PTC a systematic neck dissection is recommended over simple local resection of recurrent tumors.[21,22] Patients were reported to have a better prognosis after reoperation than those who underwent dissection of local lymph nodes or berry picking. In addition, several studies have demonstrated that patients who develop recurrent tumors within previously dissected areas have a worse outcome than those patients who develop recurrence outside the initial areas of dissection.[22,23]

Although the pattern of cervical lymph node metastases at the time of the initial diagnosis of PTC has been described,[24–26] little is known about the pattern of cervical nodal recurrence in the lateral neck and, subsequently, the extent of surgical intervention required.

Lee and colleagues[27] reported that in the lateral neck, recurrences most frequently occurred in level IV (73.4%), followed by level III (13.3%), and level II (13.3%) and 80% of cases were found ipsilateral to the primary tumor.

Roh and colleagues[28] evaluated the pattern of cervical nodal recurrence by performing a systematic nodal dissection of the ipsilateral central compartment as well as the lateral neck in 22 patients with recurrent/persistent PTC in the lateral neck. They reported that recurrences were common after incomplete resection of the thyroid gland with local recurrence in the remnant thyroid tissue and/or bed in patients who previously underwent partial resection of the gland. Pathologic examination of the removed lymph nodes demonstrated a high incidence (86%) of involved central nodes in patients with lateral nodal neck recurrence. Within the central compartment, the pretracheal and ipsilateral paratracheal sites were commonly involved, whereas, within the lateral compartment, the ipsilateral jugular nodes (levels II, III, and IV) were commonly involved. In contrast, the posterior triangle (level V) and contralateral lateral neck were rarely involved, and skip lesions involving the lateral but not the central lymph nodes were also rare. Because this pattern of nodal recurrence is similar to the pattern of lymph node metastases reported for incidental PTCs, it has been suggested that the lesions may have been present at the time of the initial presentation rather than presenting through altered lymphatic drainage established after the initial surgery to remove the thyroid gland.

Farrag and colleagues[29] evaluated 53 patients with PTC who had undergone therapeutic lateral neck dissection, and 43 of these patients had recurrent/persistent disease. They found that levels IIA, III, and IV were most commonly involved with recurrent/persistent disease. Level IIB was found to harbor disease in less than 10% of patients; however, if level IIA contained metastatic lymph nodes, 100% of patients also harbored disease in level IIB. Therefore, they recommended elective dissection of level IIB only when level IIA is involved based on FNA confirmation or gross involvement intraoperatively. Level VB lymph nodes along the course of the transverse cervical vessels or adjacent to the clavicle were involved in 16 of 40 neck dissection specimens whereas level VA was involved in 0% of specimens. Based on these findings, routine dissection of level VA was not warranted; however, dissection of Level VB should be strongly considered.

Therefore, we can conclude that a reoperative lateral neck dissection should attempt to clear levels II, III, IV, and VB if this was not addressed at a previous surgery. Resection of the recurrent nodal mass alone may be sufficient in those levels of the neck that have undergone previous extensive resection. It is our contention that this formal compartmental approach to clinically positive lymph nodes in the primary or reoperative setting will help to reduce the need for further surgeries.

REOPERATIVE CENTRAL COMPARTMENT DISSECTION

Reoperative surgery of the central compartment places the parathyroid glands and recurrent laryngeal nerves at increased risk for injury compared with primary surgery. Alvarado and colleagues[30] performed a retrospective study and compared 170 patients who had undergone a central lymph node dissection (CLND) as part of their primary surgery with 23 patients who underwent a CLND as a secondary procedure. In this study, the investigators did not find any additional morbidity when the CLND was performed as a secondary procedure; however, other studies have reported an increased morbidity rate associated with reoperative surgery. Furthermore, the overall complication rate, including hypocalcemia and vocal cord paralysis, in patients undergoing bilateral central neck dissections (58%) was found to be significantly higher than those who underwent unilateral central compartment dissection (10%, $P = .031$).[28]

Technical surgical considerations for reoperative central compartment dissection include horizontal transection of the sternothyroid and, if necessary, the sternohyoid muscles. This allows for maximum visualization of the operative field. After the horizontal transection of the strap muscles, the muscle can be separated first medially from the trachea and the dissection carried laterally and superiorly or laterally and inferiorly over the fibrofatty tissue within the central compartment. When separating the superior and inferior limbs of the strap muscles from the paratracheal lymph nodes, the surgeon must be sure that all fibroadipose tissue that may lie immediately posterior to the strap muscle is included as part of the central compartment because metastatic lymph nodes can be adherent to the strap muscles and inadvertently left behind. The surgery can then proceed in a systematic approach to the central compartment.[31] Because the right recurrent laryngeal nerve (RLN) loops around the subclavian artery and ascends away from the tracheoesophageal groove, the right paratracheal lymph nodes can be divided into an anterior and posterior compartment that is separated by the nerve (**Fig. 3**). Recurrent/persistent disease is often localized to the posterior compartment on the right side. Therefore, it is important when performing a reoperation for recurrent/persistent disease in the right central compartment that the right RLN is mobilized and the posterior lymph node compartment removed as part of the dissection. Because the left RLN travels along the tracheoesophageal groove and the esophagus is present immediately posterior to the RLN, dissection of the lymph nodes along the prevertebral fascia and anterior to the left RLN is usually sufficient for the left side (**Fig. 4**).

HYPOPARATHYROIDISM

When performing a reoperation in the central compartment, the parathyroid glands are at increased risk for devascularization or inadvertent removal because of its residence in scar tissue and fibrosis within the thyroid bed. The incidence of temporary hypoparathyroidism following reoperative thyroid surgery ranges between 0.3% and 15%.[32–34] The incidence of permanent hypoparathyroidism following reoperative thyroid surgery ranges between 0% and 3.5%.[33,35] During reoperative surgeries,

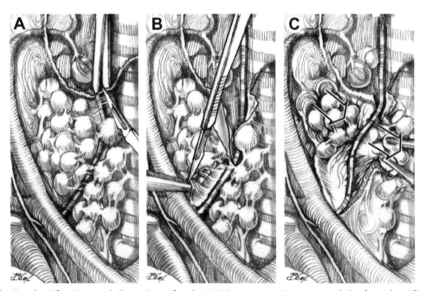

Fig. 3. Identification and dissection of right RLN in reoperative surgery. (*A*) After identification of the RLN low in the neck, typically inferior to the second tracheal ring, the operating surgeon can dissect carefully along the RLN inferiorly to the level of the clavicle with a Crile to allow for atraumatic mobilization from the surrounding lymph node bearing tissue. (*B*) To remove the anterior and posterior lymph node compartments, the right RLN needs to be transposed, which can be achieved without direct retraction of the nerve or without using a nerve hook. (*C*) The posterior compartment lymph nodes can then be mobilized anteriorly and transposed under the nerve. The anterior and posterior lymph node compartments can then be mobilized off the prevertebral fascia and esophagus, and the dissection carried inferiorly to the level of the innominate artery to incorporate the superior mediastinal lymph nodes as part of the central compartment dissection. (*From* Pai SI, Tufano RT. Central compartment lymph node dissection. Oper Tech Otolaryngol Head Neck Surg 2009;20(1):39–43; with permission.)

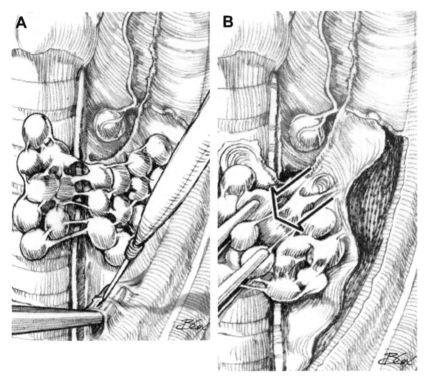

Fig. 4. Dissection of the left RLN in reoperative surgery. (*A*) After identification of the left RLN, the lateral aspect of the paratracheal lymph nodes can be dissected away from the carotid sheath and the dissection extended inferiorly to the innominate artery or brachioce-phalic vein. (*B*) Because the left RLN travels along the tracheoesophageal groove approximating the trachea and esophagus, there is a lack of lymph nodes deep to the left RLN and mobilization of the lymph nodes anterior and posterior to the left RLN without transposition of the nerve itself is usually sufficient for the left side. (*Courtesy of* Pai SI, Tufano RT. Central compartment lymph node dissection. Oper Tech Otolaryngol Head Neck Surg 2009;20(1):39–43; with permission.)

preservation of the inferior thyroid artery is recommended to prevent devascularization of the parathyroid glands. Furthermore, the authors recommend that the superior aspect of the central lymph node packet be defined by the inferior thyroid artery because metastatic lymph nodes are rarely found cephalad to the artery and this approach minimizes risk of injury to the superior parathyroid glands. If recurrent/persistent lymph nodes are present above the inferior thyroid artery, high-resolution ultrasonography is particularly helpful in the reoperative scenario in localizing the metastatic lymph node in the absence of a thyroid shadow. Fibrosis and multiple positive lymph nodes in the reoperative central compartment specimen can make identification and confirmation of parathyroid tissue difficult in situ. Therefore, after dissection of the central compartment packet, the specimen should be carefully examined for the presence of parathyroid tissue. If identified, a biopsy of the gland should be performed for histologic confirmation by frozen-section histopathologic analysis before reimplantation into muscle. Reimplantation of the parathyroid glands of questionable viability into the sternocleidomastoid muscle at the time of the revision surgery also diminishes the risk of long-term permanent hypoparathyroidism. In patients with extensive extracapsular lymph node spread and multiple involved lymph nodes, reimplantation must be performed with caution such that the surgeon does not inadvertently reimplant tumor with parathyroid tissue.

RECURRENT LARYNGEAL NERVE INJURY

The RLN is vulnerable to increased risk of injury in reoperative surgeries for thyroid cancer due to the displacement of the nerve from its normal position secondary to scar tissue as well as increased manipulation when performing a central compartment dissection. The incidence of permanent RLN injury in primary thyroid surgeries has been reported to range between 0 to 5.6%.[36–38] This risk increases to 1 to 12% in reoperative cases.[39–41] Routine early identification of the RLN with subsequent visualization of the nerve during dissection in the central compartment has been found to considerably reduce the risk of injury and, therefore, is regarded as the gold standard of care in thyroid surgery.[42–44] Recent studies have demonstrated that intraoperative nerve monitoring can assist in the identification of the RLN, particularly in the reoperative setting.[44,45] However, the visual identification of the nerve remains the basis for protecting the integrity of the nerve and the nerve monitoring system serves only as an adjunct in its identification. Avoidance of nerve injury can be achieved by early identification during the surgery, dissection with the nerve in view, and the careful use of electro-cautery away from the nerve. Several strategies may be employed to identify the RLN. The RLN can be identified low in the neck typically distant from previous areas of dissection. On the right this usually can be accomplished at the level of the common carotid artery, innominate artery, and subclavian artery junction where the RLN courses deep to this intersection to enter the central neck. The left RLN will course in a more ventral position compared with the right and can be found inferiorly in the tracheoesophageal groove inferior to the second tracheal ring. Other potential approaches include a lateral approach which allows identification of the nerve in a previously undissected area.[39,46] This method may be especially helpful when there have been multiple central neck reoperations.

SUMMARY

At the time of the initial thyroid surgery, a primary goal is to remove the thyroid gland and associated cervical metastatic disease when present. Therefore, any patient with a FNA-confirmed WDTC should undergo an ultrasound of the neck to evaluate for any suspicious lymph nodes that may need to be addressed at the time of the initial surgery.[3] If nodal disease is present within the neck, a formal compartmental therapeutic nodal dissection should be performed. Removal of the primary thyroid cancer and involved regional lymph nodes in this way will likely lessen the need for reoperation. Currently, up to 20% of patients require reoperative surgery for recurrent/persistent disease. When performing a reoperation for WDTC, the algorithm that the authors have elucidated should be used to minimize any associated increased surgical risks and need for further revision surgery.

REFERENCES

1. Davies L, Welch HG. Increasing incidence of thyroid cancer in the United States, 1973–2002. JAMA 2006;295:2164.
2. Surveillance, Epidemiology, and End Results (SEER) Program. April 2006. SEER State Database: Incidence–SEER 9 Regs Public-Use, Nov 2005 Sub (1973–2003), National Cancer Institute, DCCPS, Surveillance Research Program,

Cancer Statistics Branch, released. Available at: http://www.seer.cancer.gov. Accessed November 20, 2009.

3. Cooper DS, Doherty GM, Haugen BR, et al. Revised American Thyroid Association management guidelines for patients with thyroid nodules and differentiated thyroid cancer. Thyroid 2009;19(1):1167–214.

4. Farrag TY, Samlan RA, Lin FR, et al. The utility of evaluating true vocal fold motion before thyroid surgery. Laryngoscope 2006;116(20):235–8.

5. Randolph GW, Kamani D. The importance of pre-operative laryngoscopy in patients undergoing thyroidectomy: voice, vocal cord function, and the preoperative detection of invasive thyroid malignancy. Surgery 2006;139(3):357–62.

6. Farrag TY, Agrawal N, Sheth S, et al. Algorithm for safe and effective reoperative thyroid bed surgery for recurrent/persistent papillary thyroid carcinoma. Head Neck 2007;29(12):1069–74.

7. Robbins KT, Shaha AR, Medina JE, et al. Committee for neck dissection classification, American Head and Neck Society. Consensus statement on the classification and terminology of neck dissection. Arch Otolaryngol Head Neck Surg 2008; 134(5):536–8.

8. Arturi F, Russo D, Giuffrida D, et al. Early diagnosis by genetic analysis of differentiated thyroid cancer metastases in small lymph nodes. J Clin Endocrinol Metab 1997;82:1638–41.

9. Machens A, Hinze R, Thomusch O, et al. Pattern of nodal metastasis for primary and reoperative thyroid cancer. World J Surg 2002;26:22–8.

10. Coburn M, Teates D, Wanebo JH. Recurrent thyroid cancer. Role of surgery versus radioactive iodine (I131). Ann Surg 1994;219:587–93.

11. Schlumberger MJ. Diagnostic follow-up of well-differentiated thyroid carcinoma: historical perspective and current status. J Endocrinol Invest 1999;22:3–7.

12. Grant CS, Hay ID, Gough IR, et al. Local recurrence in papillary thyroid carcinoma: is extent of surgical resection important? Surgery 1988;104: 954–62.

13. Mazzaferri EL, Jhiang SM. Long-term impact of initial surgical and medical therapy on papillary and follicular thyroid cancer. Am J Med 1994;97:418–28.

14. Lundgren CI, Hall P, Dickman PW, et al. Clinically significant prognostic factors for differentiated thyroid carcinoma: a population-based, nested case-control study. Cancer 2006;106:524–31.

15. Lin JD, Liou MJ, Chao TC, et al. Prognostic variables of papillary and follicular thyroid carcinoma patients with lymph node metastases and without distant metastases. Endocr Relat Cancer 1999;6:109–15.

16. Sugitani I, Kasai N, Fujimoto Y, et al. A novel classification system for patients with PTC: addition of the new variables of large (3 cm or greater) nodal metastases and reclassification during the follow-up period. Surgery 2004;135: 139–48.

17. Kouvaraki MA, Lee JE, Shapiro SE, et al. Preventable reoperations for persistent and recurrent papillary thyroid carcinoma. Surgery 2004;136:1183–91.

18. Simon D, Goretzki PE, Witte J, et al. Incidence of regional recurrence guiding radicality in differentiated thyroid carcinoma. World J Surg 1996;20:860–6.

19. Carty SE, Cooper DS, Doherty GM, et al. Consensus statement on the terminology and classification of central neck dissection for thyroid cancer. The American Thyroid Association Surgery Working Group with Participation from the American Association of Endocrine Surgeons, American Academy of Otolaryngology-Head and Neck Surgery and American Head and Neck Society. Thyroid 2009;19(11):1153–8.

20. Scheumann GF, Gimm O, Wegener G, et al. Prognostic significance and surgical management of locoregional lymph node metastases in papillary thyroid cancer. World J Surg 1994;18:559–68.
21. Uchino S, Noguchi S, Yamashita H, et al. Modified radical neck dissection for differentiated thyroid cancer: operative technique. World J Surg 2004;28: 1199–203.
22. Uruno T, Miyauchi A, Shimizu K, et al. Prognosis after reoperation for local recurrence of papillary thyroid carcinoma. Surg Today 2004;34:891–5.
23. Kohara N, Furui J, Tomioka T, et al. Surgical treatment of recurrent thyroid carcinoma after primary resection. Nippon Geka Gakkai Zasshi 1993;94:847–52.
24. Sivanandan R, Soo KC. Pattern of cervical lymph node metastases from papillary carcinoma of the thyroid. Br J Surg 2001;88:1241–4.
25. Kupferman ME, Patterson M, Mandel SJ, et al. Patterns of lateral neck metastasis in papillary thyroid carcinoma. Arch Otolaryngol Head Neck Surg 2004;130:857–60.
26. Caron NR, Tan YY, Ogilvie JB, et al. Selective modified radical neck dissection for papillary thyroid cancer–is level I, II and V dissection always necessary? World J Surg 2006;30:833–40.
27. Lee YH, Lee NJ, Kim JH, et al. US diagnosis of cervical recurrence in patients operated on thyroid cancer: sonographic features and clinical significance. Auris Nasus Larynx 2007;34:213–9.
28. Roh JL, Park JY, Rha KS, et al. Is central neck dissection necessary for the treatment of lateral cervical nodal recurrence of papillary thyroid carcinoma? Head Neck 2007;29:901–6.
29. Farrag T, Lin F, Brownlee N, et al. Is routine dissection of level IIB and VA necessary in patients with papillary thyroid cancer undergoing lateral neck dissection for FNA-confirmed metastases in other levels. World J Surg 2009;33:1680–3.
30. Alvardo R, Sywak MS, Delbridge L, et al. Central lymph node dissection as a secondary procedure for papillary thyroid cancer: is there added morbidity? Surgery 2009;145:514–8.
31. Pai SI, Tufano RP. Central compartment neck dissection for thyroid cancer: technical considerations. ORL J Otorhinolaryngol Relat Spec 2008;70(5):292–7.
32. Shaha AR, Jaffe BM. Parathyroid preservation during thyroid surgery. Am J Otol 1998;109:568–74.
33. Wingert DJ, Friesen SR, Illiopoulos JI, et al. Post-thyroidectomy hypocalcemia: incidence and risk factors. Am J Surg 1986;152:606–10.
34. Levin KE, Clark AH, Duh QY, et al. Reoperative thyroid surgery. Surgery 1992; 111:604–7.
35. Chao TC, Jeng LB, Lin JD, et al. Reoperative thyroid surgery. World J Surg 1997; 21:644–7.
36. Moley JF, Lairmore TC, Doherty GM, et al. Preservation of the recurrent laryngeal nerves in thyroid and parathyroid reoperations. Surgery 1999;125:673–9.
37. Kasemsuwan L, Nubthuenetr S. Recurrent laryngeal nerve paralysis: a complication of thyroidectomy. J Otolaryngol 1997;26:365–7.
38. Wagner HE, Seiler C. Recurrent laryngeal nerve palsy after thyroid gland surgery. Br J Surg 1994;81:226–8.
39. Tisell L, Hansson G, Jansson S, et al. Reoperation in the treatment of asymptomatic metastasizing medullary thyroid carcinoma. Surgery 1986;99:60–6.
40. Goretzki P, Simon D, Frilling A, et al. Surgical reintervention for differentiated thyroid cancer. Br J Surg 1993;80:1009–12.
41. Patou CA, Norton JA, Brennan MF. Hypocalcemia following thyroid surgery: incidence and prediction of outcome. World J Surg 1998;22:718–24.

42. Dralle H, Sekulla C, Haerting J, et al. Risk factors of paralysis and functional outcome after recurrent laryngeal nerve monitoring in thyroid surgery. Surgery 2004;136:1310–22.
43. Randolph GW. Surgical anatomy of the recurrent laryngeal nerve. In: Randolph GW, editor. Surgery of the thyroid and parathyroid glands. Philadelphia: WB Saunders; 2003. p. 300–42.
44. Snyder SK, Hendricks JC. Intraoperative neurophysiology testing of the recurrent laryngeal nerve: plaudits and pitfalls. Surgery 2005;138:1183–92.
45. Dralle H, Sekulla C, Lorenz K, et al. Intraoperative monitoring of the recurrent laryngeal nerve in thyroid surgery. World J Surg 2008;32:1358–66.
46. Moley JF, Wells SA, Dilley WG, et al. Reoperation for recurrent or persistent medullary thyroid cancer. Surgery 1993;114:1090–5.

The Surgical Management of Medullary Thyroid Cancer

Alan P.B. Dackiw, MD, PhD

KEYWORDS

- Medullary thyroid cancer • Treatment guidelines
- Evidence-based treatment • Surgical techniques
- DNA testing • Prognosis • Thyroidectomy

Medullary thyroid cancer (MTC), accounts for approximately 5% to 10% of all thyroid cancers and arises from the parafollicular thyroid C cells, neuroendocrine cells that produce calcitonin, and carcinoembryonic antigen. MTC may occur either as a sporadic event (75%) or secondary to a germline mutation of the RET proto-oncogene (25%) with an autosomal dominant pattern of inheritance and almost complete penetrance. Critical to treatment of this disease is complete surgical resection because MTC cells do not take up iodine and thus iodine-131 therapy is ineffective.[1] Total thyroidectomy is the recommended treatment in all patients with MTC. Because lymph node metastases frequently occur in the central compartment of the neck, central neck dissection, defined as removal of all fibrofatty and lymphatic tissue from the hyoid bone to the innominate vessels, between the internal jugular veins is indicated.

Over the last decade, significant advances in the understanding of the biology and clinical outcomes of MTC have been made, culminating most recently in the publication of treatment guidelines by the American Thyroid Association.[2] The MTC expert panel followed an evidence-based approach because the lack of randomized clinical trial data for MTC limits the ability to form strong consensus recommendations on key issues.

Recommendation levels followed by this esteemed panel include;

"A" STRONGLY RECOMMENDS

The recommendation is based on good evidence that the service or intervention can improve important health outcomes. Evidence includes consistent results from well-designed, well-conducted studies in representative populations that directly assess effects on health outcomes.

Division of Endocrine and Oncologic Surgery, Department of Surgery, Section of Endocrine Surgery, Johns Hopkins Hospital, Johns Hopkins University School of Medicine, 600 North Street, Blalock 606, Baltimore, MD 21287, USA
E-mail address: adackiw1@jhmi.edu

Otolaryngol Clin N Am 43 (2010) 365–374
doi:10.1016/j.otc.2010.01.006
0030-6665/10/$ – see front matter © 2010 Published by Elsevier Inc.

oto.theclinics.com

"B" RECOMMENDS

The recommendation is based on fair evidence that the service or intervention can improve important health outcomes. The evidence is sufficient to determine effects on health outcomes, but the strength of the evidence is limited by the number, quality, consistency of the individual studies, generalizability to routine practice, or indirect nature of the evidence on health outcomes.

"C" RECOMMENDS

The recommendation is based on expert opinion alone.

Among the most important, recommendations 61 to 64 address the extent of surgery in typical cases of MTC.

RECOMMENDATION 61

Patients with known or highly suspected MTC with no evidence of advanced local invasion by the primary tumor, no evidence cervical lymph node metastases on physical examination and cervical ultrasound, and no evidence of distant metastases should undergo total thyroidectomy and prophylactic central compartment (level VI) neck dissection (Grade B recommendation).

Prophylactic lateral neck dissection was omitted (Recommendation 61, Grade B). In discussion, the panel recognized a minority view that considers prophylactic ipsilateral modified neck dissection as a possible option. The data supporting this treatment recommendation are discussed later in further detail. Results of preoperative neck ultrasound and biopsy strongly influence the extent of surgery.

RECOMMENDATION 62

Patients who have MTC with suspected limited local metastatic disease to regional lymph nodes in the central compartment (with a normal ultrasound examination of the lateral neck compartments) in the setting of no distant (extracervical) metastases or limited distant metastases should typically undergo a total thyroidectomy and level VI compartmental dissection. A minority of the Task Force favored prophylactic lateral neck dissection when lymph node metastases were present in the adjacent paratracheal central compartment (Grade B recommendation).

Hence, the finding of positive central and negative lateral nodes typically would be treated with total thyroidectomy and level VI dissection only (Recommendation 62, Grade B).

There is some controversy as to the recommended extent of lymph node dissection in patients presenting with a palpable nodule diagnosed on fine needle aspiration (FNA) cytology to be MTC. In a recent report, more than 80% of patients referred with persistent or recurrent MTC were judged to have had an inadequate initial operation.[3] More than 50% of patients have persistently elevated calcitonin levels after initial surgery for MTC.[4,5] As noted earlier, standard surgical treatment for patients diagnosed with MTC is total thyroidectomy and central compartment lymph node dissection. Controversy exists as to the requirement for a unilateral lateral neck lymph node dissection or bilateral lateral neck lymph node dissection.

In general, for patients with familial or sporadic MTC with clinical evidence of regional metastatic disease, compartment-oriented neck dissection in a systematic fashion is advocated.[6] In patients with familial MTC and an elevated basal calcitonin level or a thyroid nodule palpable on physical examination or visualized on ultrasonography, total thyroidectomy with central compartment lymphadenectomy and bilateral

lateral neck dissection may be performed. In patients with presumed sporadic MTC, and importantly when the primary mass is large (> 2 cm) or when paratracheal nodes are involved, an ipsilateral lateral neck dissection on the side of the lesion may also be indicated. In patients with palpable cervical lymphadenopathy a bilateral lateral neck dissection may also be performed. This approach maximizes local regional tumor control while minimizing the need for reoperation.[7] With improvement in preoperative imaging, specifically high sensitivity ultrasound, operation in the contralateral lateral neck may be performed when cytologically proven disease by FNA is documented.

Moley recently analyzed the distribution of nodal metastases in patients where MTC presented as a palpable thyroid mass. These data indicate a significant incidence of disease in the contralateral lateral neck when patients presented with palpable MTC. In patients with unilateral palpable primary tumors, there was a 47% incidence of positive *contralateral* nodes in Levels II, III, and IV.[8] These authors recommend a bilateral modified neck dissection in patients with palpable MTC. If this can indeed be performed safely, bilateral neck dissection would seem to maximize local tumor control even further. This dissection is controversial as noted earlier in the ATA recommendations.

RECOMMENDATION 63

Patients who have MTC with suspected limited local metastatic disease to regional lymph nodes in the central and lateral neck compartments (with ultrasound-visible lymph node metastases in the lateral neck compartments) in the setting of no distant metastases or limited distant metastases should typically undergo a total thyroidectomy, central (level VI), and lateral neck (levels IIA, III, IV, V) dissection (Grade B recommendation).

Thus, the presence of abnormal central and lateral nodes typically would lead to total thyroidectomy with central compartment dissection, and lateral neck dissection involving levels IIa, III, IV, and V.

RECOMMENDATION 64

In the presence of distant metastatic disease, less aggressive neck surgery may be appropriate to preserve speech, swallowing, and parathyroid function while maintaining locoregional disease control to prevent central neck morbidity (Grade C recommendation).

Thus, less aggressive neck surgery may be appropriate in the setting of extensive metastatic disease (Recommendation 64, Grade C).

TECHNICAL DETAILS OF CENTRAL AND MODIFIED NECK DISSECTION

The extent of central neck dissection includes all thyroid tissue and all nodal tissue from the hyoid bone superiorly to the innominate vessels inferiorly.[7] Central nodal tissue on the anterior surface of the trachea is resected and the superior surface of the innominate vein behind the sternal notch is exposed. Fibrofatty tissue between the carotid sheaths and trachea is removed including the paratracheal nodes along the recurrent laryngeal nerves. This dissection is continued inferiorly on the right to the point at which the junction of the innominate artery and carotid is exposed and to a comparable level on the left behind the head of the clavicle. This systematic compartment oriented lymphadenectomy approach to the surgical management of medullary thyroid cancer has been shown to improve local-regional control and suggested to improve survival (**Fig. 1**).[8,9]

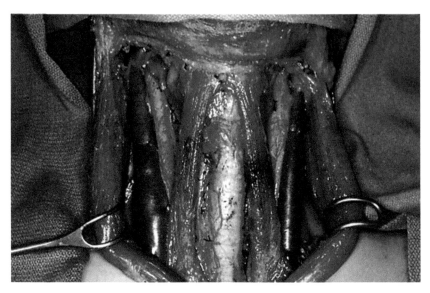

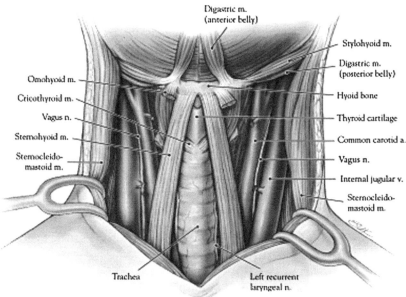

Fig. 1. Intraoperative and schematic sketch following total thyroidectomy, central compartment lymph node dissection, and modified lateral neck dissection in a patient with MEN 2A. (*Adapted from* Fleming JB, Lee JE, Bouvet M, et al. Surgical strategy for the treatment of medullary thyroid carcinoma. Ann Surg 1999;230(5):697–707; with permission.)

A lateral neck lymph node dissection involves removal of lymph nodes anterior and posterolateral to the jugular vein. Defined limits are the posterior belly of the digastric muscle superiorly, the spinal accessory nerve posterolaterally, and the thoracic inlet and clavicle inferiorly. The sternocleidomastoid muscle, jugular vein, carotid artery, and vagus nerve are preserved (see **Fig. 1**). If the jugular vein or sternocleidomastoid muscle are involved with tumor, these are resected as a part of the specimen. If a bilateral dissection is indicated and the jugular vein has been resected on one side, this is best done as a two-stage procedure. If flow in the jugular vein is interrupted on the contralateral side, severe facial edema will result.

There is also some controversy as to how the parathyroid glands should be managed in these patients. Total parathyroidectomy with parathyroid autotransplantation[8] and parathyroid preservation procedures[10–12] have both been advocated. A strong argument can be made in this disease that it may not be possible to perform an adequate nodal clearance unless at least the inferior parathyroid glands are removed. The parathyroid glands may also be devascularized during the course of the central lymph node dissection. Thus, Moley and colleagues advocate total parathyroidectomy with autotransplantation as a part of total thyroidectomy and central nodal clearance in MTC.[3,8–10] Alternatively, an attempt may be made to preserve in situ the superior parathyroid glands (usually located just superior and posterior to the junction of the recurrent laryngeal nerve and inferior thyroid artery).[7] As suggested earlier, the inferior parathyroids are usually inseparable from the central compartment lymph nodes and the thymic horn that extends from the lower pole of the thyroid gland. Thus, the inferior parathyroids should be identified when possible, confirmed histologically to avoid autografting a lymph node metastasis, and then autografted into either the sternocleidomastoid muscle in the neck (and marked with a clip to facilitate identification if hyperparathyroidism was to develop) or into the non-dominant forearm.

There are, of course, other management issues of importance to consider in the overall surgical management of patients with MTC including

1. Work-up preoperatively for pheochromocytoma
2. The surgical management of coexisting endocrinopathies in patients with multiple endocrine neoplasia (MEN) IIA AND MEN IIB
3. The timing and extent of surgery in patients carrying the RET proto-oncogene mutation.

PREOPERATIVE PHEOCHROMOCYTOMA WORK-UP

All patients with a diagnosis of MTC should be investigated for the possibility of a concurrent pheochromocytoma, which may occur in patients with MEN 2A and MEN 2B. A history of hypertension should be sought, associated with the triad of symptoms consisting of headache, palpitations, and diaphoresis. Other symptoms may include anxiety and tremor. Some patients may report panic attacks, and may have been previously diagnosed with an anxiety disorder.

The diagnosis of pheochromocytoma in patients with a history suggestive of this disorder is then based on biochemical tests and the demonstration of elevated catecholamines or catecholamine breakdown products. The diagnostic standard in these patients is a 24-hour collection of urine for determination of catecholamines, vanillylmandelic acid, and metanephrine levels. Plasma catecholamine and metanephrine levels may also be used. Abdominal imaging with three-dimensional CT, and in some circumstances metaiodobenzylguanidine, identifies the anatomic location of the pheochromocytoma.

SURGICAL MANAGEMENT OF COEXISTING ENDOCRINOPATHIES IN PATIENTS WITH MULTIPLE ENDOCRINE NEOPLASIA IIA AND MULTIPLE ENDOCRINE NEOPLASIA IIB

All patients with MTC should have a detailed history taken to determine a family history of any thyroid, parathyroid, or adrenal disorders. As noted earlier, in patients with hereditary MTC there is essentially complete penetrance of MTC; all patients who inherit the mutant allele will develop MTC. Other endocrinopathies in the MEN 2 syndromes demonstrate incomplete penetrance patterns. Specifically, in MEN 2A, approximately 40% of patients inheriting the mutant allele will develop pheochromocytomas and 30% of patients will have hyperparathyroidism.[13] In MEN 2B, approximately 50% of patients will develop pheochromocytomas, and complete penetrance of neural gangliomas (lips, tongue, digestive tract) is observed. Hyperparathyroidism does not occur in MEN 2B. These patients also have a distinct clinical phenotype with a marfanoid habitus, skeletal abnormalities, and the potential for development of megacolon.

All patients with a preoperative diagnosis of MTC should be screened for pheochromocytoma with a 24-hour urine collection for metanephrine, vanillylmandelic acid, and free catecholamines. Hyperparathyroidism is assessed by the measurement of serum calcium levels and intact parathyroid hormone levels. Blood should also be drawn for RET oncogene analysis.

The parathyroid lesion in MEN 2A, like that in MEN 1, is a generalized but asymmetric hyperplasia that often may not result in hypercalcemia. For MEN 2A patients with hypercalcemia, either subtotal parathyroidectomy or total parathyroidectomy with thymectomy and parathyroid autotransplantation may be performed.

Patients from MEN 2 families should undergo yearly screening for pheochromocytoma beginning at 5 to 10 years of age.[14] In contrast to the aggressive behavior of MTC, if not treated early, pheochromocytoma in MEN 2 is rarely malignant. The adrenal glands in patients with MEN 2 should ideally be removed when a pheochromocytoma develops, before the onset of symptoms of excess catecholamines.[9] Evidence suggests that *unilateral* adrenalectomy be performed as the initial procedure in patients who have MEN 2 with a unilateral adrenal abnormality on CT scan. Approximately one third of patients who undergo a unilateral adrenalectomy will ultimately require a subsequent operation for a contralateral tumor. However, this may not occur for many years and patients are not left Addisonian and steroid dependent in the interim. In patients that requires bilateral adrenalectomy, cortical sparing techniques may prevent the need for exogenous steroid replacement.[15]

TIMING AND EXTENT OF SURGERY IN PATIENTS CARRYING THE RET PROTO-ONCOGENE MUTATION

The recent American Thyroid Association treatment guidelines also address this critical issue and reaffirm the importance of germline DNA testing for RET mutations in all patients with MTC whether or not they have a positive family history This is a Grade "A" recommendation and based on the classic "Brandi paper" as reported as a part of the Gubbio International Consensus.[16] This paper is highly recommended reading for clinicians involved in the care of patients with MTC. The Gubbio International Consensus clarified the genotype: phenotype correlations observed in patients with specific RET oncogene mutations and recommended appropriate timing for thyroidectomy in these patients and their families (**Fig. 2**).

Gubbio International Consensus

Level 3 (Highest Risk)
1. Children with MEN 2B and RET codon 883, 918, 922 mutations
2. Total thyroidectomy in first 6 months of life with central compartment nodal dissection.

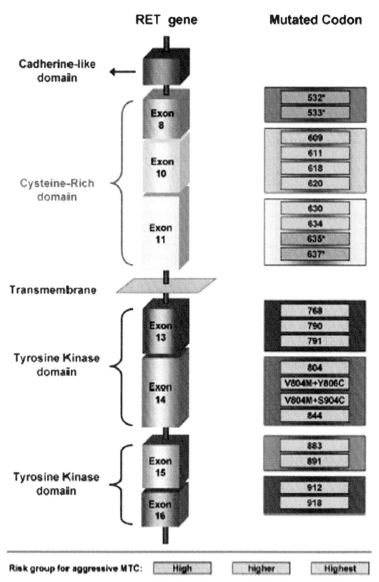

Fig. 2. The RET proto-oncogene and genotype-phenotype correlation in MTC. (*From* Kouvaraki MA, Shapiro SE, Perrier ND, et al. RET proto-oncogene: a review and update of genotype-phenotype correlations in hereditary medullary thyroid cancer and associated endocrine tumours. Thyroid 2005;15:531–44; with permission.)

Level 2 (Higher Risk)
  1. Children with RET codon 611, 618, 620, 634 mutations
  2. Total thyroidectomy before 5 years of age
  3. Central compartment nodal dissection (no consensus).
Level 1 (High Risk)
  1. Children with RET codon 609,768,790,791,804,891 mutations

2. Total thyroidectomy recommended
3. No consensus at what age.

PROGNOSTIC FACTORS

Stage of disease at diagnosis most accurately predicts length of patients' survival. Long-term survival (>10 years) is common (60% to 90%) in patients without metastatic disease or unresectable local-regional disease. Patients with metastatic disease, however, have 5-year survival rates of approximately 50%.[17-20] Thus, prognosis for patients with medullary thyroid cancer falls between those patients with well-differentiated thyroid tumors and anaplastic thyroid cancer. Adverse prognostic factors also include patient age greater than 50 years and MEN 2B. Seventy percent of patients with MEN 2B have metastasis at the time of diagnosis and less than 5% survive 5 years.

The degree of primary tumor invasiveness has also been determined to be an important prognostic variable.[21,22] In these series, primary tumor invasiveness was the only parameter that correlated with a failure to reduce postoperative calcitonin levels to the normal range in patients who were reoperated for recurrent or persistent MTC.

INDICATIONS FOR REOPERATIVE SURGERY

Following primary surgical treatment for MTC, up to 50% of patients have persistently elevated serum calcitonin levels. Initial evaluation of these patients should follow two important principles:

1. Determine the extent and adequacy of the primary surgery that has been performed.
2. Consider and systematically evaluate sites of potential disease recurrence: cervical and mediastinal lymph nodes, thyroid bed, liver, lung and bone.

Reoperative lymphadenectomy should be performed as a part of a standardized diagnostic and treatment algorithm.[7] In a recent series Fleming and colleagues[23] reported the MD Anderson Cancer Center results and surgical strategy for medullary thyroid cancer. In this series, 40 subjects underwent surgery for MTC and were divided into three groups based on whether they had undergone previous thyroidectomy and on the results of standardized staging studies. Group 1 subjects had not had previous surgery and consisted of 11 individuals. Group 2 subjects (13) had undergone thyroidectomy before referral and had elevated calcitonin levels but no radiologic evidence of loco-regional or distant metastatic disease. Finally, group 3 consisted of 16 subjects who underwent thyroidectomy before referral but now had an elevated calcitonin with radiologic evidence of local-regional recurrence. Twenty-nine percent of subjects in groups 1 and 2 achieved normal calcitonin levels postoperatively, whereas only 6% of subjects (one subject) in group 3 achieved normal calcitonin levels with a much higher incidence of postoperative hypoparathyroidism. The authors thus advocate that compartment oriented lymphadenectomy be performed early in the course of MTC.

EXTENT OF REOPERATIVE SURGERY

In patients who have evidence of elevated serum calcitonin levels after previous thyroidectomy, meticulously performed reoperative surgery may result in biochemical cure in 20% to 30% of patients and may improve survival. After the adequacy of the initial surgery is assessed, the subsequent operation is planned. Compartmental cervical nodal dissection is now indicated if it had not been performed previously and is guided by neck and mediastinal imaging. The central compartment of the neck including the thyroid bed is re-explored with a unilateral or bilateral lateral neck dissection. Mediastinal lymphadenectomy is generally performed only when imaging studies suggest recurrent tumor in the Level VII nodes.

The goal of lymphadenectomy for asymptomatic calcitonin elevations is the removal of microscopic metastatic nodal disease to prevent dissemination.[7] However, a number of case series have shown that only a minority of patients actually achieve a biochemical cure following reoperative regional lymphadenectomy.[9,11,12,21,22]

In a recent series from Moley and colleagues,[22] an improved ability to normalize postoperative serum calcitonin levels was found compared with an earlier series.[21] Calcitonin levels were normalized in 17 out of 45 subjects at reoperative surgery. The authors note that improved subject selection was an important factor in these improved results including the use of staging laparoscopy.

ROLE OF DIAGNOSTIC LAPAROSCOPY

Laparoscopy has been advocated for the diagnosis of subclinical hepatic metastases before reoperative surgery. Because of the hypervascular nature of MTC hepatic metastases, these tumors are poorly visualized on CT, and are generally not seen on MRI until they approach 1 cm in size. Tung and colleagues[24] reported that in a series of 44 subjects, metastatic MTC lesions were detected in 10 of these subjects and 9 of these 10 subjects had negative preoperative CT or MRI. These lesions may have a miliary appearance with multiple, small, white raised lesion on the liver surface (1–5 mm in diameter) or a small subcapsular lesion may be detected appearing as a small mass on the surface of the liver. Unfortunately, laparoscopy will detect only these surface metastases; laparoscopic hepatic sonography may be useful in detection of hepatic parenchymal lesions.

In summary, significant advances in the understanding of the biology and clinical outcomes of MTC have been made over the last decade, resulting most recently in the publication of treatment guidelines by the American Thyroid Association.[2] This scholarly work is strongly recommended to the reader to gain further understanding and in-depth insight in the management of patients with medullary thyroid cancer.

REFERENCES

1. Saad MF, Guido JJ, Samaan NA. Radioactive iodine in the treatment of medullary carcinoma of the thyroid. J Clin Endocrinol Metab 1983;57(1):124–8.
2. Kloos RT, Eng C, Evans DB, et al. Medullary thyroid cancer: management guidelines of the American Thyroid Association. Thyroid 2009;19:565–612.
3. Chi DD, Moley JF. Medullary thyroid carcinoma: genetic advances, treatment recommendations, and the approach to the patient with persistent hypercalcitoninemia. Surg Oncol Clin N Am 1998;7(4):681–706.
4. Block MA, Jackson CE, Tashjian AH. Management of occult medullary thyroid carcinoma: evidenced only by serum calcitonin level elevations after apparently adequate neck operations. Arch Surg 1978;113(4):368–72.
5. Block MA, Jackson CE, Greenawald KA, et al. Clinical characteristics distinguishing hereditary from sporadic medullary thyroid carcinoma. Treatment implications. Arch Surg 1980;115(2):142–8.
6. Tisell LE, Hansson G, Jansson S, et al. Reoperation in the treatment of asymptomatic metastasizing medullary thyroid carcinoma. Surgery 1986;99(1):60–6.
7. Evans DB, Fleming JB, Lee JE, et al. The surgical treatment of medullary thyroid carcinoma. Semin Surg Oncol 1999;16(1):50–63.

8. Moley JF, DeBenedetti MK. Patterns of nodal metastases in palpable medullary thyroid carcinoma: recommendations for extent of node dissection. Ann Surg 1999;229(6):880–7 [discussion: 887–8].

9. Dralle H, Damm I, Scheumann GF, et al. Compartment-oriented microdissection of regional lymph nodes in medullary thyroid carcinoma. Surg Today 1994;24(2): 112–21.

10. Kebebew E, Kikuchi S, Duh QY, et al. Long-term results of reoperation and localizing studies in patients with persistent or recurrent medullary thyroid cancer. Arch Surg 2000;135(8):895–901.

11. Gimm O, Dralle H. Reoperation in metastasizing medullary thyroid carcinoma: is a tumor stage-oriented approach justified? Surgery 1997;122(6):1124–30 [discussion: 1130–1].

12. Gimm O, Ukkat J, Dralle H. Determinative factors of biochemical cure after primary and reoperative surgery for sporadic medullary thyroid carcinoma. World J Surg 1998;22(6):562–7 [discussion: 567–8].

13. Howe JR, Norton JA, Wells SA. Prevalence of pheochromocytoma and hyperparathyroidism in multiple endocrine neoplasia type 2A: results of long-term follow-up. Surgery 1993;114(6):1070–7.

14. Gagel RF, Tashjian AH, Cummings T, et al. The clinical outcome of prospective screening for multiple endocrine neoplasia type 2a. An 18-year experience. N Engl J Med 1988;318(8):478–84.

15. Lee JE, Curley SA, Gagel RF, et al. Cortical-sparing adrenalectomy for patients with bilateral pheochromocytoma. Surgery 1996;120(6):1064–70 [discussion: 1070–1].

16. Brandi ML, Gagel RF, Angeli A, et al. Guidelines for diagnosis and therapy of MEN type 1 and type 2. J Clin Endocrinol Metab 2001;86:5658–71.

17. Kallinowski F, Buhr HJ, Meybier H, et al. Medullary carcinoma of the thyroid–therapeutic strategy derived from fifteen years of experience. Surgery 1993;114(3): 491–6.

18. Dottorini ME, Assi A, Sironi M, et al. Multivariate analysis of patients with medullary thyroid carcinoma. Prognostic significance and impact on treatment of clinical and pathologic variables. Cancer 1996;77(8):1556–65.

19. Fuchshuber PR, Loree TR, Hicks WL, et al. Medullary carcinoma of the thyroid: prognostic factors and treatment recommendations. Ann Surg Oncol 1998;5(1): 81–6.

20. Schroder S, Bocker W, Baisch H, et al. Prognostic factors in medullary thyroid carcinomas. Survival in relation to age, sex, stage, histology, immunocytochemistry, and DNA content. Cancer 1988;61(4):806–16.

21. Moley JF, Wells SA, Dilley WG, et al. Reoperation for recurrent or persistent medullary thyroid cancer. Surgery 1993;114(6):1090–5 [discussion: 1095–6].

22. Moley JF, Dilley WG, DeBenedetti MK. Improved results of cervical reoperation for medullary thyroid carcinoma. Ann Surg 1997;225(6):734–40 [discussion: 740–3].

23. Fleming JB, Lee JE, Bouvet M, et al. Surgical strategy for the treatment of medullary thyroid carcinoma. Ann Surg 1999;230(5):697–707.

24. Tung WS, Vesely TM, Moley JF. Laparoscopic detection of hepatic metastases in patients with residual or recurrent medullary thyroid cancer. Surgery 1995;118(6): 1024–9 [discussion: 1029–30].

Minimally Invasive Thyroid and Parathyroid Surgery: Where Are We Now and Where Are We Going?

Melanie W. Seybt, MD, David J. Terris, MD*

KEYWORDS

• Thyroid surgery • Parathyroid surgery
• Minimally invasive • Robotic

ORIGINS OF MINIMALLY INVASIVE AND ENDOSCOPIC THYROID AND PARATHYROID SURGERY

Minimally invasive endocrine neck surgery has evolved considerably over the past decade, after a somewhat humble origin. Michel Gagner performed the first endoscopic parathyroidectomy in 1996 at the Cleveland Clinic.[1] Surgery lasted more than 5 hours and the patient developed massive subcutaneous emphysema. Concerns were subsequently raised regarding sustained intravascular absorption and subcutaneous emphysema from long duration of exposure to CO_2 insufflation.[2] In 1998, Miccoli and his team in Pisa pioneered an endoscopic technique that used a 15- to 20-mm central neck incision and only 3 to 4 minutes of CO_2 insufflation to create an operative pocket.[3] Once the working space was created, visualization was maintained using external retractors. The procedure continued to develop and eventually involved no use of CO_2 insufflation. The operative pocket was created by minimal dissection through the anterior neck incision and visualization of the operative field was obtained using a 5-mm 30-degree high-resolution endoscope. Randomized controlled studies comparing endoscopic parathyroidectomy with conventional bilateral neck exploration confirmed decreased operative times, improved cosmesis, and reduced postoperative pain in the endoscopic group with 100% cure rates in both groups.[4]

MCG Thyroid Center, Department of Otolaryngology, Medical College of Georgia, 1120 Fifteenth Street, BP-4109, Augusta, GA 30912-4060, USA
* Corresponding author.
E-mail address: dterris@mcg.edu

Endoscopic and minimally invasive thyroid surgery evolved from these original investigations in parathyroid surgery. Paolo Miccoli in Pisa[5] and Rocco Bellantone in Rome[6] essentially simultaneously developed similar minimally invasive video-assisted approaches to performing thyroid surgery. The fundamentals developed by these surgeons have carried forth through this decade, and consist of a small single central incision, use of advanced energy devices to maintain hemostasis in a small space, and endoscopic guidance primarily for the management of the vasculature of the thyroid gland and the identification and preservation of the recurrent laryngeal nerves and parathyroid glands. These procedures are accomplished without the need for drainage, and are routinely performed on an outpatient basis in the United States.[7]

EVOLUTION OF MINIMALLY INVASIVE AND ENDOSCOPIC THYROID AND PARATHYROID SURGERY

The most widely practiced variation of minimally invasive thyroid surgery is the Miccoli technique, likely because of the relative ease of performance, combined with substantial advantages to the patient. Several investigators across Europe,[8] in parts of Asia,[9] and now in the United States[10,11] have demonstrated that this technique can be readily performed by high-volume thyroid surgeons. As a further endorsement of this technique, several publications have appeared that clarify the oncologic safety of the procedure,[12] demonstrate the profound cosmetic[13] and even functional superiority relative to conventional surgery,[14] and confirm the compatibility with other technologies such as nerve monitoring or the use of ultrasonic energy (**Fig. 1**).[15]

Miccoli accomplished a compelling prospective randomized trial comparing minimally invasive video-assisted thyroidectomy with conventional thyroidectomy for the management of thyroid cancer,[12] which served to alleviate concerns regarding the thoroughness of resection in thyroid malignancy. Postoperative measures of serum thyroglobulin level and radioactive iodine uptake confirmed that the endoscopic technique yielded a thorough thyroid removal compared with conventional thyroidectomy. In addition, prospective trials were conducted by the Miccoli[13] and Bellantone[14] groups in which the cosmetic and functional advantages of the endoscopic technique were validated. In a comparison between minimally invasive video-assisted thyroidectomy and conventional surgery, patients described greater satisfaction with their scar outcome and reduced pain with the minimally invasive technique.[13] After describing

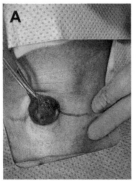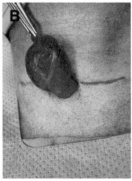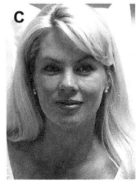

Fig. 1. The combination of advanced energy devices and high-resolution technology have prompted the possibility of using very small incisions to safely deliver diseased thyroid glands (*A, B*). The cosmetic outcomes are superior (*C*) and valued by the population of patients who often develop thyroid problems (young women).

a large North American multi-institutional application of this technique,[11] Terris and colleagues[15] subsequently highlighted the complementary application of endoscopic surgery and laryngeal nerve monitoring, which helps to compensate for the inherently reduced surgical aperture associated with minimally invasive surgery. A low rate of even transient nerve dysfunction was achieved. The magnified visualization of the recurrent laryngeal nerves likely contributes to the excellent functional outcomes.

The emergence of robust nuclear imaging (^{99m}Tc-sestamibi) and high-resolution ultrasonography have facilitated a focused approach in parathyroidectomy. Possibly the most important adjunct in the evolution of minimally invasive parathyroidectomy was the advent of a highly sensitive, rapid, parathyroid hormone assay. In 1988, Nussbaum reported the first successful use of intraoperative parathyroid hormone (IOPTH) in 12 patients undergoing parathyroidectomy.[16] This assay has become widely available since its introduction and allows a focused surgery to be performed, with confidence that all hyperfunctioning parathyroid tissue has been removed before exiting the operating room.[17] Although no universal algorithm has been uniformly endorsed for optimal timing of IOPTH acquisition, the generally accepted criteria is at least 50% reduction in the 10-minute postexcision level compared with the baseline level.[18–21] We advocate obtaining 5-, 10-, and 15-minute postexcision levels with preincision level as baseline, supported by our finding that a 5-minute postexcision level may facilitate earlier termination of focused parathyroidectomy in more than 60% of cases.[22] Traditionally, endoscopic and minimally invasive parathyroidectomy techniques have been used predominantly in the case of a single adenoma (**Fig. 2**). However, as experience with the techniques increases, the indications will likely broaden. For example, recent reports suggest endoscopic bilateral neck exploration is feasible with patients with hyperparathyroidism.[23]

THE FUTURE OF MINIMALLY INVASIVE THYROID AND PARATHYROID SURGERY

With improvements in technology, there seems to be little doubt that endoscopic surgery will continue to evolve. There are 3 likely directions of this evolution: expanded indications for the minimally invasive video-assisted thyroidectomy and parathyroidectomy, the further development of remote access surgery via several different routes, and the application of robotics to further assist the surgeon in accomplishing these

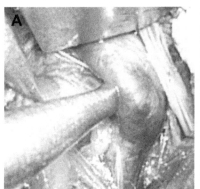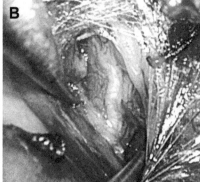

Fig. 2. Identification of adenomatous parathyroid glands (*A*) is facilitated by endoscopic guidance. Visualization of other critical structures in the central compartment is also enhanced, for example the recurrent laryngeal nerves (*B*).

techniques (see the article by F. Christopher Holsinger elsewhere in this issue for further exploration of this topic).

There are already early reports of the expansion of indications for endoscopic surgery. Miccoli and colleagues[23,24] have described the use of this procedure for carriers of the ret proto-oncogene and for bilateral neck exploration. Bellantone and colleagues[25] have published on endoscopic lymph node dissection in the central compartment and in the lateral compartment.[26] In the United States, Lai and colleagues[27] have described at least a small number of cases in which thyroid nodules greater than 3 cm are removed through a minimal access approach. As instrumentation improves, and as retrieval of the gland is facilitated, ever larger glands and lesions may be removed through ever smaller incisions.

There have been numerous reports of remote access thyroidectomy using surgical ports placed in several locations including the anterior chest wall,[28] subclavicular region,[29] or axillary region.[30] The axillary region has proved to be one of the most feasible approaches, although it requires patience and a particularly sophisticated skill set.

To facilitate ease of remote access thyroid surgery and avoid the need for insufflation, the application of robotics in thyroid surgery has emerged. Originally released for human application nearly a decade ago, it is only in the last 2 years that the daVinci surgical robotic system has been used for endocrine applications. An initial report by Wright and Lobe[31] reflected the feasibility of combining an axillary approach with robotic technology to facilitate removal of the thyroid gland. Although this was accomplished in a small number of patients, the Chang group[32] in Korea has been able to apply this approach in a large series of patients, and recently reported on more than 100 robotic thyroidectomies. The Asian culture is such that avoidance of a cervical neck scar may justify the expense of technological investment combined with a lengthy procedure to approach the thyroid compartment remotely. As a result, this technique may not find as much applicability in other parts of the world. Nevertheless, we have pursued cautious implementation of this technique in our practice in Augusta (**Fig. 3**). We offer this approach to patients with anticipated benign pathology in whom a lobectomy only

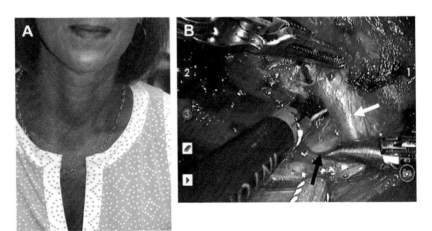

Fig. 3. The robotic approach to the thyroid compartment has as the most appealing feature the complete elimination of a neck scar (A) by virtue of the remote access used (axillary). In addition, the technology affords a true three-dimensional view of the field (B), tremor filtration, and wristed instrumentation. The black arrow indicates the recurrent laryngeal nerve, passing just deep to the inferior thyroid artery (*white arrow*).

has been recommended, and we have combined it with laryngeal nerve monitoring to add a measure of safety. The early results have been satisfactory.

SUMMARY

After nearly a century of performing thyroidectomy essentially the way it was described by Theodore Kocher in the nineteenth century, the technique has quickly evolved. Parathyroidectomy has advanced as biochemical assays and physiologic imaging have become available. Minimally invasive and endoscopic thyroidectomy and parathyroidectomy can now be performed in many patients who benefit from the reduced dissection and smaller incisions associated with these approaches. Although many of the cosmetic, quality of life, and functional improvements have been proved, a better understanding of the procedure and the appropriate indications for its application will continue to develop even as the technique itself evolves, and as new approaches emerge.

REFERENCES

1. Gagner M. Endoscopic subtotal parathyroidectomy in patients with primary hyperparathyroidism. Br J Surg 1996;83(6):875.
2. Gottlieb A, Sprung J, Zheng XM, et al. Massive subcutaneous emphysema and severe hypercarbia in a patient during endoscopic transcervical parathyroidectomy using carbon dioxide insufflation. Anesth Analg 1997;84:1154–6.
3. Miccoli P, Bendinelli C, Conte M, et al. Endoscopic parathyroidectomy by a gasless approach. J Laparoendosc Adv Surg Tech A 1998;8(4):189–94.
4. Miccoli P, Bendinelli C, Berti P, et al. Video-assisted versus conventional parathyroidectomy in primary hyperparathyroidism: a prospective randomized study. Surgery 1999;126(6):1117–21.
5. Miccoli P, Berti P, Conte M, et al. Minimally invasive surgery for thyroid small nodules: preliminary report. J Endocrinol Invest 1999;22:849–51.
6. Bellantone R, Lombardi CP, Raffaelli M, et al. Minimally invasive, totally gasless video-assisted thyroid lobectomy. Am J Surg 1999;177(4):342–3.
7. Terris DJ, Moister B, Seybt MW, et al. Outpatient thyroid surgery is safe and desirable. Otolaryngol Head Neck Surg 2007;136(4):556–9.
8. Miccoli P, Bellantone R, Mourad M, et al. Minimally invasive video-assisted thyroidectomy: multiinstitutional experience. World J Surg 2002;26(8):972–5.
9. Chan CP, Yang LH, Chang HC, et al. An easier technique for minimally invasive video-assisted thyroidectomy. Int Surg 2003;88(2):109–13.
10. Terris DJ, Chin E. Clinical implementation of endoscopic thyroidectomy in selected patients. Laryngoscope 2006;116(10):1745–8.
11. Terris DJ, Angelos P, Steward DL, et al. Minimally invasive video-assisted thyroidectomy: a multi-institutional North American experience. Arch Otolaryngol Head Neck Surg 2008;134(1):81–4.
12. Miccoli P, Elisei R, Materazzi G, et al. Minimally invasive video-assisted thyroidectomy for papillary carcinoma: a prospective study of its completeness. Surgery 2002;132:1070–3.
13. Miccoli P, Berti P, Raffaelli M, et al. Comparison between minimally invasive video-assisted thyroidectomy and conventional thyroidectomy: a prospective randomized study. Surgery 2001;130:1039–43.
14. Lombardi CP, Raffaelli M, D'alatri L, et al. Video-assisted thyroidectomy significantly reduces the risk of early postthyroidectomy voice and swallowing symptoms. World J Surg 2008;32(5):693–700.

15. Terris DJ, Anderson SK, Watts TL, et al. Laryngeal nerve monitoring and minimally invasive thyroid surgery: complementary technologies. Arch Otolaryngol Head Neck Surg 2007;133(12):1254–7.
16. Nussbaum SR, Thompson AR, Hutcheson KA, et al. Intraoperative measurement of parathyroid hormone in the surgical management of hyperparathyroidism. Surgery 1988;104:1121.
17. Barczynski M, Konturek A, Cichon S, et al. Intraoperative parathyroid hormone assay improves outcomes of minimally invasive parathyroidectomy mainly in patients with a presumed solitary parathyroid adenoma and missing concordance of preoperative imaging. Clin Endocrinol 2007;66:878–85.
18. Miura D, Wada N, Arici C, et al. Does intraoperative quick parathyroid hormone assay improve the results of parathyroidectomy? World J Surg 2002;26:926–30.
19. Pelleteri PK. Directed parathyroid exploration: evolution and evaluation of this approach in a single-institution review of 346 patients. Laryngoscope 2003;113: 1857–69.
20. Siperstein A, Berber E, Mackey R, et al. Prospective evaluation of sestamibi scan, ultrasonography, and rapid PTH to predict the success of limited exploration for sporadic primary hyperparathyroidism. Surgery 2004;136:872–80.
21. Irvin GL III, Prudhomme DL, Deriso GT, et al. A new approach to parathyroidectomy. Ann Surg 1994;219:574–9.
22. Seybt MW, Loftus KA, Mulloy AL, et al. Optimal use of intraoperative PTH levels in parathyroidectomy. Laryngoscope 2009;119:1331–3.
23. Miccoli P, Berti P, Materazzi G, et al. Endoscopic bilateral neck exploration versus quick intraoperative parathormone assay (qPTHa) during endoscopic parathyroidectomy: a prospective randomized trial. Surg Endosc 2008;22(2):398–400.
24. Miccoli P, Elisei R, Berti P, et al. Video assisted prophylactic thyroidectomy and central compartment nodes clearance in two RET gene mutation adult carriers. J Endocrinol Invest 2004;27(6):557–61.
25. Bellantone R, Lombardi CP, Raffaelli M, et al. Central neck lymph node removal during minimally invasive video-assisted thyroidectomy for thyroid carcinoma: a feasible and safe procedure. J Laparoendosc Adv Surg Tech A 2002;12(3): 181–5.
26. Lombardi CP, Raffaelli M, Princi P, et al. Minimally invasive video-assisted functional lateral neck dissection for metastatic papillary thyroid carcinoma. Am J Surg 2007;193(1):114–8.
27. Lai SY, Walvekar RR, Ferris RL. Minimally invasive video-assisted thyroidectomy: expanded indications and oncologic completeness. Head Neck 2008;30(11): 1403–7.
28. Cho YU, Park IJ, Choi KH, et al. Gasless endoscopic thyroidectomy via an anterior chest wall approach using a flap-lifting system. Yonsei Med J 2007;48(3): 480–7.
29. Sasaki A, Nakajima J, Ikeda K, et al. Endoscopic thyroidectomy by the breast approach: a single institution's 9-year experience. World J Surg 2008;32(3): 381–5.
30. Ikeda Y, Takami H, Sasaki Y, et al. Clinical benefits in endoscopic thyroidectomy by the axillary approach. J Am Coll Surg 2003;196(2):189–95.
31. Miyano G, Lobe TE, Wright SK. Bilateral transaxillary endoscopic total thyroidectomy. J Pediatr Surg 2008;43(2):299–303.
32. Kang SW, Jeong JJ, Yun JS, et al. Robot-assisted endoscopic surgery for thyroid cancer: experience with the first 100 patients. Surg Endosc 2009 Mar 5 [Epub ahead of print].

Robotic Thyroidectomy: Operative Technique Using a Transaxillary Endoscopic Approach Without CO$_2$ Insufflation

F. Christopher Holsinger, MD[a],*, David J. Terris, MD[b],
Ronald B. Kuppersmith, MD, MBA[c]

KEYWORDS

• Thyroid • Thyroidectomy • Robot • Robotic • Endoscopic

In recent years, several new techniques in thyroid surgery have been developed to improve visualization, reduce risk of complications, and shorten the length of neck incisions.[1–4] In the United States, minimally invasive approaches have been shown to be feasible and safe, and are becoming more widely adopted by surgeons.[5,6]

More recently, there have been several reports from Asia of endoscopic transaxillary approaches to the thyroid.[7–15] Among these is a large series of patients, reported by a group from Seoul, Korea,[16,17] who have undergone transaxillary robotic thyroidectomy incorporating the da Vinci Surgical System (Intuitive Surgical, Sunnyvale, CA, USA). This approach eliminates the need for any cervical incisions, which increases patient satisfaction relative even to the small incisions used in minimally invasive video-assisted techniques.[12] Although patient satisfaction alone may not justify the use of new technology, there may be other issues to consider.

From the surgeon's perspective, the application of the da Vinci Surgical System to thyroid surgery may provide several advantages. The three-dimensional environment

[a] Department of Head and Neck Surgery, The University of Texas MD Anderson Cancer Center, 1400 Hermann Pressler Drive, Unit 1445, Houston, TX 77030, USA
[b] Department of Otolaryngology, Thyroid Center, Medical College of Georgia, 1120 15th Street BP 4109, Augusta, GA 30912, USA
[c] Texas Institute for Thyroid and Parathyroid Surgery, Texas ENT and Allergy, 1730 Birmingham Drive, College Station, TX 77845, USA
* Corresponding author.
E-mail address: holsinger@mdanderson.org

Otolaryngol Clin N Am 43 (2010) 381–388
doi:10.1016/j.otc.2010.01.007
0030-6665/10/$ – see front matter © 2010 Elsevier Inc. All rights reserved.

oto.theclinics.com

created with binocular 30° optics may improve visualization. Wristed instrumentation and 540° rotation increase the surgeon's operative dexterity. With these advantages, robotic assistance may facilitate the endoscopic approach to the thyroid with no increased risk of injury to the parathyroids, and optimize recurrent and superior laryngeal nerve preservation.

Open thyroidectomy is a safe, effective, and time-honored approach. For this reason, many people may be skeptical of the value of using the robot for thyroid surgery. The same skepticism heralded the advent of robotic-assisted prostatectomy when this technique was introduced just 5 years ago. In the United States, 70% to 80% of radical prostatectomies are now performed using the da Vinci Surgical System (Intuitive Surgical, Sunnyvale, CA, USA).

This article introduces the da Vinci Surgical System, describes the technique of robotic thyroidectomy with specific considerations for North American patients, and suggests a training paradigm for surgeons interested in adopting this technique.

DA VINCI SURGICAL SYSTEM

The da Vinci Surgical System, introduced in 1999 by Intuitive Surgical, is a surgical robotic system that has been widely adopted for urologic and gynecologic surgery. The system is composed of 3 components: a surgeon's console, a patient cart, and a video tower.

The surgeon's console allows the surgeon to have a three-dimensional high-definition view of the surgical field using a 0° or 30° stereo endoscope. This setup allows for magnification and enhanced visualization. In addition to controlling the endoscope, the console also allows the surgeon to control up to 3 additional instruments. Most instruments have 7° of freedom, allowing them to be maneuvered into locations that a surgeon normally cannot reach with conventional instruments. In addition, the motions can be scaled and any tremor is filtered out. Perhaps the most important advance is that the surgeon can operate with 2 hands in a large working space. Thus, fundamental and time-honored surgical principles of traction and countertraction, comprehensive exposure, and controlling the wound can be implemented in this robotic-assisted endoscopic approach. One limitation to the system is that the instruments do not provide tactile (haptic) feedback to the surgeon, as the surgeon would normally have when performing endoscopic surgery.

The patient cart is the portion of the system that docks to the patient and has the instruments and stereo endoscope attached to it. This portion is prepared with sterile drapes and typically a technician or nurse will attend to it during surgery.

TECHNIQUE

Like any surgical procedure, a robotic thyroidectomy requires preparation followed by a series of steps for successful completion. The essential steps of the procedure include patient positioning, marking the patient, creation of a surgical working space, docking the robot, performing a lobectomy or total thyroidectomy using the robotic instruments, and closing the wounds.

Room Setup

These cases require a significant amount of equipment to be present in the room, and therefore it is important for the surgeon to determine the best way to organize the room before the procedure. The shape and size of the specific operating room (OR) are aspects that typically cannot be modified and may provide limitations on where equipment can be placed. The positioning of the equipment may also need to be changed depending on whether the surgical incision is being performed on the left side or right side of the patient. Ideally, the operating table will be oriented so that the anesthesia provider is at the head of the table and has access to the patient's airway, head, and neck. The patient cart portion of the robotic surgical system should be covered with sterile drapes and positioned on the contralateral side of the operating table. Initially, it will need to be away from the table, as an assistant will need to stand on the contralateral side to help create the working space and to place the retractor. An assistant or technician will be on the ipsilateral side with the instrument table. The video cart portion of the robotic system or an additional video monitor should be placed so that the assistant on the ipsilateral side can visualize it during the procedure and provide assistance. The surgeon's console portion of the robotic surgical system is typically located in the OR.

Patient Positioning

The patient is positioned in a supine position on a small shoulder roll. The patient's ipsilateral arm is placed in an arm board extended cephalad to expose the axilla. The arm should not be secured in place until after the patient's incision is marked. The patient's contralateral arm is tucked adjacent to the patient's body. It is crucial to place adequate padding around bony prominences on the arm, under the neck, shoulder, and small of the back. Good positioning is essential for exposure in this procedure, so patients with limited range of shoulder or cervical motion require careful positioning and, in severe cases, may not be candidates for this procedure. In addition, morbidly obese patients may pose significant challenges regarding positioning, dissection, and placement of the retractor needed to keep the working space open.

Marking the Patient

A vertical line is marked from the sternal notch to the hyoid in the midline. A 5- to 6-cm line is marked in the axilla at the posterior aspect of the pectoralis muscle (**Fig. 1**). The

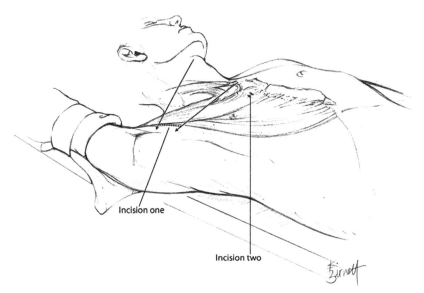

Fig. 1. Skin markings showing the incision within medial axillary fold and location of robotic instrumentation. (*Courtesy of* Marina Medical Instruments, Inc, Sunrise, FL; with permission.)

arm is placed into its natural position to confirm that the incision marked will be hidden in the axilla postoperatively. The arm can then be secured in place. A line is then drawn from the superior aspect of the axillary incision line to the superior aspect of the midline marking, and from the inferior aspect of the axillary incision line to the inferior aspect of the midline marking. These lines define the limits of the dissection.

A small incision on the ipsilateral chest is marked for the placement of the fourth robotic arm. Kang and Chung[16] recommend placement of an 8-mm incision, located 2 cm superior to the right nipple and 6 to 8 cm medial of the right nipple (between the breast and sternum). However, because of differences in body mass index, stature, or breast size in the North American population, the location of this incision may need to be modified to ensure that port placement will allow the instrument to reach the working space.

Placement of the Nerve Monitor

Before preparing the patient, the laryngeal nerve monitor grounding electrode is inserted. The electrode can be placed slightly off the midline to the contralateral side, inserted into the field, and secured with a clear sterile adhesive dressing before starting the procedure.

Creation of the Working Space

An incision is made along the line marked in the axilla and carried down to the level of the pectoralis muscle. Dissection is performed with electrocautery above the pectoralis major muscle to create a space using serially longer retractors to elevate the skin, subcutaneous tissue, and platysma by the contralateral assistant. Lighted breast retractors or a headlight can be used to see within this space. It is helpful to have suction to evacuate the smoke. The skin markings provide a guide to the extent of the subplatysmal dissection. The dissection is continued over the clavicle to identify the space between the clavicular and sternal head of the sternocleidomastoid muscle. This space is opened superiorly, the omohyoid is retracted superficially and posterolaterally or divided, and the sternohyoid and sternothyroid muscles are elevated off the thyroid gland. The modified Chung thyroid retractor with table mount lift (Marina Medical, Sunrise, FL, USA) is placed under the strap muscles and secured to the table mount lift (**Fig. 2**). The lift is used to ensure an adequate working space with ample visualization of the thyroid, and should be at least 4 cm in height at the opening. The anesthesiologist should ensure that the patient has adequate padding around the neck and shoulders after the retractor is secured.

An 8-mm paramedian vertical incision is then made on the chest wall. A tract is created using hemostats and then a blunt-tipped trocar is placed and tunneled into the working space. This trocar will be used to place the third arm of the robot and later the ProGrasp instrument.

Docking the Robot

Once the space has been created and the retractor is in place, the patient cart of the da Vinci Surgical System is moved to a position adjacent to the table and the arms are oriented to insert the instruments. A 30° down stereoscopic endoscope, 8-mm Harmonic curved shears, and a 5-mm Maryland dissector are placed in the ports that enter through the axillary incision. The Harmonic curved shears are placed in the position that would correspond with the surgeon's dominant hand. The angles with which these instruments are placed are essential to prevent conflict within the wound. The camera, which is in the middle, should be low outside the wound and high inside the wound. In this way it is oriented with a view down on the thyroid and

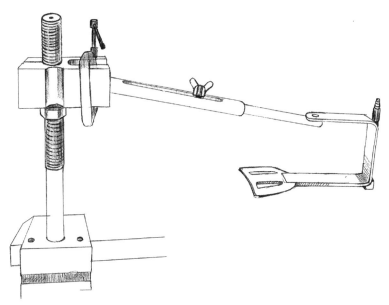

Fig. 2. Chung retractor and table. (*Courtesy of* Marina Medical Instruments, Inc, Sunrise, FL; with permission.)

out of the way of the instruments. The instruments should enter high in the wound and be angled to a low position, so that they are under the camera.

An 8-mm ProGrasp forceps is placed in the port that enters through the chest incision, and is typically used to retract the thyroid and other tissues during the procedure.

Removing the Ipsilateral Thyroid Lobe

The superior pole of the ipsilateral thyroid lobe is retracted with the ProGrasp forceps and the superior thyroid pole is dissected from the cricothyroid muscle and other surrounding tissues. It is then transected with the Harmonic shears. The inferior aspect of the thyroid is also dissected from the trachea using the Harmonic shears. The thyroid is then retracted medially and ventrally, away from the trachea and paratracheal groove, using the ProGrasp forceps. In so doing, the recurrent laryngeal nerve and both parathyroids are identified and preserved. The thyroid lobe is then dissected off the trachea to the midline and divided using the Harmonic shears.

Removing the Contralateral Lobe

Kang and colleagues[17] have demonstrated the technique and advocated for total thyroidectomy via a single transaxillary incision. If a total thyroidectomy is to be performed, the contralateral superior pole is retracted using the ProGrasp forceps and transected using the Harmonic shears. A subcapsular dissection is performed between the deep aspect of the thyroid and the trachea using the Maryland forceps and Harmonic shears. However, exposure of the nerve in the contralateral paratracheal groove is technically more challenging because of limited visualization. Dr Chung (personal communication) recommends that the robotic-assisted endoscopic surgeon demonstrate significant competency with a robotic thyroidectomy before attempting total thyroidectomy via unilateral transaxillary incision.

Closure

After hemostasis is obtained, a closed suction drain is placed, and the incisions are closed by the surgeon's preferred method.

Postoperative Care

Patients are treated postoperatively by the surgeon's usual protocols for managing drains, hypocalcemia, and inpatient observation. Because the working space created is much larger than in conventional thyroid surgery, the risk of postoperative airway compression from a hematoma is low, and therefore it is plausible that these patients could be discharged on the same day.

SUGGESTED TRAINING PARADIGM

For surgeons currently in practice there is no definitive training algorithm for incorporating robot-assisted techniques into their surgical practice. For experienced thyroid surgeons, using the da Vinci Surgical System to perform thyroid surgery represents the application of a new tool to anatomy already well understood to perform an existing surgical procedure. This situation is not dissimilar from the progression from open techniques to the application of the endoscope to sinus surgery. However, many of the surgeons in Asia now embracing robotic-assisted approaches in thyroid surgery have a long experience of nonrobotic totally endoscopic thyroidectomy. A learning curve undoubtedly exists but has yet to be defined.

During mentorship and training for robotic surgery, the surgeon should consult with their local hospital credential committee to understand requirements and to follow recommendations on how to acquire and validate privileges for specific new procedures. Because the da Vinci Surgical System is complex and the surgeon is ultimately responsible for its operation, it is essential that surgeons undergo thorough training before performing this procedure on patients.

In addition to learning how to use the robot and its instruments, it is recommended that surgeons become familiar with the use and tissue effects of the Harmonic shears before using the robot. At present, the Harmonic shears are the primary cutting and coagulation instrument used in the procedure. One blade oscillates at 55,000 Hz and although the other is insulated, which partially protects surrounding soft tissues and neurovascular structures from thermal injury and neuropraxia. However, because the Harmonic oscillation requires a unique mechanical architecture, the 540° wristed instrumentation found in other da Vinci instruments is lacking. This omission creates certain limitations for its use. Alternatives include the Maryland forceps with bipolar cautery.

Critical activities to learning this technique include:

- da Vinci Surgical System Training. All surgeons must undergo online and hands-on robotic training as recommended by Intuitive Surgical. This training will allow surgeons to understand the components, functions, and controls of the robotic surgical system.
- Live case observation. Surgeons should consider observing robotic thyroidectomy in a live setting with an experienced surgeon. This process will be helpful in visualizing the room setup, patient positioning, the surgical approach, OR staff use, and positioning of the robot.
- Video case observation. Obtaining a video of the robotic portion of the procedure to study the steps involved before performing the procedure is helpful. Surgeons should also record their own cases and review the videos after completing the operation to look for opportunities for improvement.

- Cadaver dissection. In the laboratory, surgeons can practice positioning the patient, marking the patient, performing the surgical approach, docking the robot, and removing the thyroid using the robot in a fresh cadaver model. One suggested method would be to perform the transaxillary dissection and approach on one side, then use the robot to perform a thyroid lobectomy. After completing the lobectomy, the robot could be removed from the field; then the contralateral transaxillary dissection and approach can be repeated. After performing the second approach, the robot could be redocked on the ipsilateral side so that a total thyroidectomy can be performed. This method will enhance the surgeon's ability to understand the transaxillary approach as well as the technique for ipsilateral lobectomy and contralateral lobectomy.
- Proctored cases. Surgeons could benefit from, and hospitals may require, having an experienced robotic surgeon proctor cases, particularly if the surgeon does not have live experience using the robot in other settings.

SUMMARY

Based on the experience of the group in Korea, our case observation in Korea, and the performance of this procedure on cadavers and patients, this technique seems to be safe and feasible. However, there are many unanswered questions including the benefits of the application of this technology relative to its costs, and whether the technology will provide additional benefits to patients and surgeons, particularly as new innovations are added to the system.

REFERENCES

1. Gagner M. Endoscopic subtotal parathyroidectomy in patients with primary hyperparathyroidism. Br J Surg 1996;83:875.
2. Huscher C, Chiodini S, Napolitano C, et al. Endoscopic right thyroid lobectomy. Surg Endosc 1997;11:877.
3. Miccoli P, Berti P, Conte M, et al. Minimally invasive video-assisted parathyroidectomy: lesson learned from 137 cases. J Am Coll Surg 2000;191:613–8.
4. Kuppersmith R, Salem A, Holsinger F. Advanced approaches for thyroid surgery. Otolaryngol Head Neck Surg 2009;141:340–2.
5. Hunter JG. Minimally invasive surgery: the next frontier. World J Surg 1999;23: 422–4.
6. Terris DJ. Minimally invasive thyroidectomy: an emerging standard of care. Minerva Chir 2007;62:327–33.
7. Ikeda Y, Takami H, Sasaki Y, et al. Endoscopic neck surgery by the axillary approach. J Am Coll Surg 2000;191:336–40.
8. Kim JS, Kim KH, Ahn CH, et al. A clinical analysis of gasless endoscopic thyroidectomy. Surg Laparosc Endosc Percutan Tech 2001;11:268–72.
9. Ikeda Y, Takami H, Niimi M, et al. Endoscopic thyroidectomy and parathyroidectomy by the axillary approach. A preliminary report. Surg Endosc 2002;16:92–5.
10. Shimizu K, Kitagawa W, Akasu H, et al. Video-assisted endoscopic thyroid and parathyroid surgery using a gasless method of anterior neck skin lifting: a review of 130 cases. Surg Today 2002;32:862–8.
11. Shimizu K, Tanaka S. Asian perspective on endoscopic thyroidectomy – a review of 193 cases. Asian J Surg 2003;26:92–100.
12. Ikeda Y, Takami H, Sasaki Y, et al. Are there significant benefits of minimally invasive endoscopic thyroidectomy? World J Surg 2004;28:1075–8.

13. Lobe TE, Wright SK, Irish MS. Novel uses of surgical robotics in head and neck surgery. J Laparoendosc Adv Surg Tech A 2005;15:647–52.

14. Yoon JH, Park CH, Chung WY. Gasless endoscopic thyroidectomy via an axillary approach: experience of 30 cases. Surg Laparosc Endosc Percutan Tech 2006; 16:226–31.

15. Cho YU, Park IJ, Choi KH, et al. Gasless endoscopic thyroidectomy via an anterior chest wall approach using a flap-lifting system. Yonsei Med J 2007;48:480–7.

16. Kang SW, Jeong JJ, Yun JS, et al. Robot-assisted endoscopic surgery for thyroid cancer: experience with the first 100 patients. Surg Endosc 2009. [Epub ahead of print].

17. Kang SW, Jeong JJ, Yun JS, et al. Gasless endoscopic thyroidectomy using trans-axillary approach; surgical outcome of 581 patients. Endocr J 2009;56: 361–9.

Evaluation of Hypercalcemia in Relation to Hyperparathyroidism

Phillip K. Pellitteri, DO

KEYWORDS

- Hypercalcemia • Primary hyperparathyroidism
- Parathyroid hormone • 1,25-Dihydroxyvitamin D

Hypercalcemia has been reported as occurring in approximately 1% to 4% of the adult population in general, and anywhere from 0.5% to 3% of hospitalized adult populations.[1] Patients with hypercalcemia may present with clinical symptoms that vary across a wide spectrum, depending on the severity of the level of excess serum calcium found. Most commonly, mild hypercalcemia is relatively asymptomatic or minimally symptomatic, but severe hypercalcemia may be accompanied by significant and potentially life-threatening symptoms, especially when the serum calcium exceeds 14 mg/dL.

The definition of hypercalcemia is predominantly dependent on the range of normal serum calcium. Most assays will report this normal range as being 8.5 to 10.5 mg/dL; however, there appears to be significant variation in the normal range reported by different laboratories depending on assay differences to detect serum calcium levels. Serum calcium within the circulation is predominantly bound to proteins (approximately 45%), primarily albumin, and complexes to circulating ions such as bicarbonate, phosphate, citrate, or sulfate (approximately 10%). The remainder of serum calcium as found as the free ionized form (approximately 45%), which is solely responsible for exerting the physiologic effects of calcium in the body. It is the ionized form of serum calcium that represents the major regulator of parathyroid hormone secretion.

The level of serum calcium reflects the balance between calcium influx into and calcium efflux from extracellular fluid. The influx of calcium into the extracellular fluid is principally derived from intestinal absorption, skeletal resorption, and renal reabsorption. The efflux of calcium from the extracellular fluid is determined by intestinal secretion, renal excretion, and skeletal uptake. Hypercalcemia usually results when the rate of calcium influx into the extracellular fluid exceeds the rate of calcium efflux

Section of Head, Neck & Endocrine Surgery, Department of Otolaryngology/Head & Neck Surgery, Geisinger Health System, Temple University School of Medicine, 100 North Academy Avenue, Geisinger Medical Center, Danville, PA 17822-1333, USA
E-mail address: ppellitteri@geisinger.edu

Otolaryngol Clin N Am 43 (2010) 389–397
doi:10.1016/j.otc.2010.02.006
0030-6665/10/$ – see front matter © 2010 Published by Elsevier Inc.

from the extracellular fluid. Under most pathologic conditions hypercalcemia results from increased skeletal resorption or intestinal absorption with normal or decreased renal excretion; however, it may also result from normal calcium influx into the extracellular fluid, with decreased renal excretion or defective skeletal mineralization. Increased skeletal resorption is usually caused by accelerated osteoclast recruitment and activation, most often under the influence of parathyroid hormone (PTH), parathyroid hormone-related protein (PTHrP), or 1,25-dyhdroxyvitamin D.[2] The increased intestinal absorption of calcium is a less frequent cause of hypercalcemia, although this may occur with increased 1,25-dyhoroxyvitamin D production by extrarenal 1α-hydroxylase activity or absorptive hypercalciuria. Under most normal physiologic circumstances associated with increased calcium influx into extracellular fluid, the kidneys normally compensate appropriately by increasing urinary calcium excretion. Serum calcium levels do not typically increase unless the kidneys fail to clear the filtered calcium load.

Other factors indirectly affecting serum calcium levels include increased levels of PTH or PTHrP directly stimulating renal tubular absorption of filtered calcium, thereby decreasing renal calcium excretion to some degree. Nausea and vomiting directly resulting from hypercalcemia may lead to further hemoconcentration. Any condition that results in significant volume depletion may eventually limit renal calcium excretion. Immobilization resulting in prolonged bed rest may directly increase bone resorption caused by decreased gravitational biomechanical effects on the skeleton.

EVALUATION OF HYPERCALCEMIA

Hypercalcemia may result in a wide variety of clinical symptoms. Even in minimally symptomatic patients, subtle neurologic dysfunction is often reported, and may range from subtle cognitive impairment or drowsiness to mild depression. Worsening hypercalcemia may result in frank confusion, delirium, or obtundation. Minimally symptomatic patients may also manifest muscle weakness particularly if the hypercalcemia becomes more severe. Constipation may be commonly reported together with anorexia with severe hypercalcemia, prompting nausea, vomiting, and other gastrointestinal symptoms. The hypercalcemia associated with primary hyperparathyroidism has frequently resulted in the development of pancreatitis and peptic ulcer disease; however, the pathophysiologic mechanism of this association remains uncertain. Frequent urination and thirst are not uncommon with moderate hypercalcemia, and result from the increased renal water clearance necessary to excrete the filtered calcium load. Persistent hypercalcemia may result in the development of renolithiasis or nephrocalcinosis. Cardiac manifestations of hypercalcemia include decreased repolarization time associated with shortened QT interval, bradycardia, first-degree atrioventricular block, and other cardiac dysrhythmias. Chronic hypercalcemia eventually may be associated with osteopenia or osteoporosis and subsequent increased fracture risk. Most patients with hypercalcemia will remain asymptomatic or minimally symptomatic unless the serum calcium increases beyond a threshold of approximately 12 mg/dL or in the event the serum calcium undergoes a rapid increase over a short period of time. All patients essentially will become symptomatic when the serum calcium exceeds 14 mg/dL.

DIFFERENTIAL DIAGNOSIS

The differential diagnosis of hypercalcemia is quite broad. The most common cause of outpatient hypercalcemia remains primary hyperparathyroidism, whereas the most common cause of hypercalcemia in hospitalized patients is malignancy. In most cases, the differential diagnosis of hypercalcemia may be broadly divided into PTH-mediated and non-PTH–mediated hypercalcemia (**Tables 1–3**).

PTH-mediated hypercalcemia is associated most frequently with primary hyperparathyroidism (see **Table 1**). However, it may be caused by physiologic secondary hyperparathyroidism, defined as hyperparathyroidism caused by a recognized physiologic effect without associated renal insufficiency, or pathologic secondary hyperparathyroidism, with associated chronic renal failure. Tertiary hyperparathyroidism may occur in patients with long-standing renal insufficiency or chronic renal failure.

Physiologic secondary hyperparathyroidism can occur in patients with insufficient calcium intake, decreased intestinal calcium absorption, insufficient vitamin D intake or malabsorption, or renal hypercalciuria, and represents the homeostatic attempt to maintain normal serum calcium levels by any physiologic means. It is important to distinguish physiologic secondary hyperparathyroidism from primary hyperparathyroidism before approaching primary hyperparathyroidism surgically. This distinction is discussed later when considering the diagnosis of primary hyperparathyroidism. It is thought that the hyperparathyroidism associated with both pathologic secondary hyperparathyroidism and tertiary hyperparathyroidism results from subtle ionized hypocalcemia persisting over months to years, resulting in chronic stimulation of the parathyroid glands. Eventually, after long-standing renal insufficiency or failure, parathyroid glands may become autonomous and no longer respond to regulation by serum ionized calcium, and develop tertiary hyperparathyroidism.

Familial hypocalciuric hypercalcemia (FHH) may mimic the serum biochemical appearance of primary hyperparathyroidism and should not be confused with that entity, as this may result in unnecessary parathyroid surgery. FHH represents an autosomal dominant disorder, linked to chromosomes 3q, 13 p, and 19q, and is largely caused by inactivating mutations in the parathyroid cell calcium sensing receptor (CaSR) linked to chromosome 3q.[3] This entity results in mild hypercalcemia associated with high normal or mildly increased intact PTH levels. Patients with FHH have a low 24-hour urinary calcium excretion relative to their hypercalcemia. The best physiologic study to distinguish FHH from primary hyperparathyroidism is the 24-hour urinary calcium to creatinine clearance ratio.[4] The calculation of this ratio requires knowledge of the 24-hour urinary calcium and creatinine, with simultaneously measured serum calcium and creatinine levels. Patients with FHH typically have ratios of less than 0.01, whereas patients with primary hyperparathyroidism have ratios that exceed 0.01.

The second most frequent cause of hypercalcemia is that of malignancy (see **Table 2**). Malignancy-associated hypercalcemia is most commonly caused by

Table 1
Causes of PTH-mediated hypercalcemia
Primary hyperparathyroidism
Parathyroid adenoma
Parathyroid lipoadenoma
Parathyroid hyperplasia
Parathyroid carcinoma
Neck or mediastinal parathyroid cyst
Secondary hyperparathyroidism
Tertiary hyperparathyroidism

Table 2 Causes of hypercalcemia of malignancy	
PTHrP secretion by:	Cancers: Lung, Esophagus, Head and Neck, Renal cell, Ovary, Bladder, Pancreatic, Thymic carcinoma, Islet cell carcinoma, Carcinoid, Sclerosing hepatic carcinoma
Ectopic PTH secretion by:	Cancers: Small cell lung, Small cell ovarian, Squamous cell lung, Ovarian adenocarcinoma, Thymoma, Papillary thyroid carcinoma, Hepatocellular carcinoma, Undifferentiated neuroendocrine tumor
Ectopic 1,25-dihydroxyvitamin D production by:	B-cell lymphoma, Hodgkin disease, Lymphomatoid granulomatosis
Lytic bone metastases caused by:	Multiple myeloma, Lymphomas, Breast cancer, Invasive sarcoma
Tumor production of other cytokines by:	T-cell lymphomas/leukemias, non-Hodgkin lymphoma, Other hematologic malignancies

humoral hypercalcemia of malignancy (HHM), which occurs as a result of excessive PTHrP secretion by tumors of various types.[5] A wide range of solid tumors have been reported to secrete excessive PTHrP including those of the lung, esophagus, head and neck, kidney, ovary, bladder, breast, and pancreas. Further, thymic carcinoma, islet cell carcinomas, malignant carcinoid tumors, and sclerosing hepatic carcinomas have been reported to also secrete this hormone. PTHrP production in excess has further been associated with adult T-cell leukemia or lymphoma, or B-cell lymphoma.[6,7]

Ectopic PTH secretion has been documented in single cases of small cell lung cancer, small cell ovarian carcinoma, squamous cell lung carcinoma, ovarian adeno-carcinoma, thymoma, papillary thyroid carcinoma, hepatocellular carcinoma, and undifferentiated neuroendocrine tumor.[8] In addition, ectopic 1,25-dihdroxyvitamin D may be produced in excess by B-cell lymphomas, Hodgkin disease, or lymphomatoid granulomatosis.[9–11]

The hypercalcemia caused by malignancy may occur as a result of extensive lytic bone metastases due to multiple myeloma, lymphomas, breast cancer, or invasive sarcomas.[12] In these cases, where extensive bone destruction is the mechanism, patients are usually late in the course of their malignancy and the underlying diagnosis is generally not in doubt.

Many nonmalignant causes of non-PTH–mediated hypercalcemia are known (see **Table 3**). Certain benign tumors, including those of ovarian dermoid cysts or uterine fibroids, may occasionally secrete PTHrP or other bone resorbing cytokines.[13] Non-PTH–mediated hypercalcemia may be caused by a variety of endocrine disorders including thyrotoxicosis (resulting from increased bone resorption), pheochromocy-toma, adrenal insufficiency or crisis, and VIPomas.[14–16]

Granulomatous diseases will often cause hypercalcemia when malignancy or endo-crine disorders are not present, especially when occurring in younger and middle-aged adults, and may occasionally present with hypercalcemia as the presenting finding. Case reports of hypercalcemia caused by overproduction of 1,25-dihydroxy-vitamin D have come from patients with sarcoidosis, Wegener granulomatosis,

Table 3
Causes of non-PTH–mediated, nonmalignant hypercalcemia

Benign tumors: PTHrP-secreting ovarian dermoid cyst or uterine fibroid

Endocrine disease
  Thyrotoxicosis
  Pheochromocytoma
  Addison's disease
  Islet cell pancreatic tumors
  VIPoma

Granulomatous disorders
  Sarcoidosis
  Wegener granulomatosis
  Berylliosis
  Silicone- and paraffin-induced granulomatosis
  Eosinophilic granuloma
  Tuberculosis (focal, disseminated, MAC in AIDS)
  Histoplasmosis
  Coccidioidomycosis
  Candidiasis
  Leprosy
  Cat-scratch disease

Drugs
  Vitamin D excess (oral or topical)
  Vitamin A excess
  Thiazide diuretics
  Lithium
  Estrogens and antiestrogens
  Androgens
  Aminophylline, theophylline
  Gancyclovir
  Recombinant growth hormone treatment of AIDS patients
  Foscarnet
  8–Chlorocyclic AMP

Miscellaneous
  Familial hypocalciuric hypercalcemia
  Immobilization with or without Paget disease of bone
  End-stage liver failure
  Total parenteral nutrition
  Milk-alkali syndrome
  Hypophosphatasia
  Systemic lupus erythematosus
  Juvenile rheumatoid arthritis
  Recent hepatitis B vaccination
  Gaucher disease with acute pneumonia
  Aluminum intoxication (chronic hemodialysis)
  Manganese intoxication
  Primary oxalosis

Abbreviations: AMP, adenosine monophosphate; MAC, *Mycobacterium avium* complex.

berylliosis, silicone- or paraffin-induced granulomatosis, eosinophilic granuloma, focal or disseminated tuberculosis, and histoplasmosis, as well as coccidiomycosis and cat-scratch disease.[17–20]

Medications are a well-known cause of hypercalcemia occurring as a consequence of a variety of physiologic mechanisms. Excess vitamin D intake may stimulate intestinal calcium absorption, and thiazide diuretics may directly inhibit renal calcium excretion. Lithium therapy may interfere with the ability of calcium to interact with parathyroid and renal CaSRs, thereby increasing PTH secretion by the parathyroid glands. Vitamin A excess may stimulate bone resorption by as yet undetermined mechanisms, and a variety of other agents, including estrogens, antiestrogens or androgens, aminophylline or theophylline, ganciclovir, recombinant growth hormone in AIDS patients, as well as others may affect other physiologic mechanisms, resulting in hypercalcemia.

DIAGNOSIS OF PRIMARY HYPERPARATHYROIDISM

The incidence of primary hyperparathyroidism is estimated to be 1 in 1000 in men and 2 to 3 in 1000 in women. Primary hyperparathyroidism may occur at all ages, but is most commonly noted in postmenopausal women in the sixth decade of life. Primary hyperparathyroidism is caused by the inappropriate secretion or oversecretion of PTH relative to the serum calcium level. Solitary parathyroid adenomas are responsible for primary hyperparathyroidism in 80% to 85% if the cases, whereas 4-gland hyperplasia is responsible in 15% to 20% of cases, and parathyroid cancer in less than 0.5% of cases. The majority of single adenomas represent sporadic disease, whereas 4-gland hyperplasia may imply a familial disorder, most commonly multiple endocrine neoplasia types 1 or 2A. Parathyroid adenomas are thought to secrete excess PTH because of loss of feedback control of PTH secretion by extracellular calcium at the cellular level, caused by an increased set point for suppression of PTH secretion. Hyperplastic parathyroid glands are thought to secrete excess PTH because of the increased number of parathyroid cells, with each parathyroid cell maintaining a normal calcium set point for suppression of PTH secretion.

The etiology of sporadic primary hyperparathyroidism is not well understood. Parathyroid adenomas represent clonal expansion of a single or several abnormal cells, caused by a genetic abnormality leading to either stimulation of cell proliferation or loss of inhibition of cell proliferation.[21] A small number of adenomas have been found with a PRAD1 (cyclin D1) proto-oncogene rearrangement, in which the PRAD1 gene was inserted adjacent to PTH gene enhancer elements, resulting in stimulation of parathyroid cell division whenever PTH secretion was stimulated by hypocalcemia. PRAD1 protein expression has been reported to be increased in about 20% of parathyroid adenomas. Up to 17% of parathyroid adenomas have been found to have mutations in the MEN-1 (menin) gene. The MEN-1 gene normally functions as a tumor suppressor gene, and it is thought that mutations in this gene result in the loss of control of parathyroid cell division.

Most patients currently diagnosed with primary hyperparathyroidism present with either asymptomatic or minimally symptomatic mild hypercalcemia, typically with serum calcium levels in the 10.0 to 11.0 mg/dL range. Many patients have a diagnosis of osteopenia, which may be caused predominantly by age or menopausal status. More severely affected patients may have classic bone features, including osteitis fibrosis cystica, with distal phalangeal subperiosteal bone resorption, distal clavicular resorption, "salt and pepper" skull, bone cysts, and long bone brown tumors, or osteoporosis, predominantly at cortical sites such as the mid or distal one-third radius.

Classic osteitis fibrosis cystica, once a common abnormality in hyperparathyroidism, is currently recognized in fewer than 5% of patients. Kidney disease, including renal insufficiency caused by a chronic or relatively acute hypercalcuria, nephrocalcinosis, or calcium-containing nephrolithiasis, may be seen in up to 20% of patients. Neuropsychiatric dysfunction is a commonly reported symptom, typically manifesting as mild fatigue or weakness with subtle cognitive impairment. Previously reported associations with peptic ulcer disease or pancreatitis are probably not causally related to hypercalcemia, unless they are associated with the MEN syndromes. More symptomatic patients may manifest cardiovascular symptoms including mild hypertension, coronary artery or cardiovalvular calcifications, or septal and left ventricular hypertrophy.

The diagnosis of primary hyperparathyroidism is usually straightforward, based on minimal criteria involving the serum total calcium and intact PTH levels. The classically diagnosed patient presents with increased serum total calcium with increased or inappropriately high normal PTH levels. Some patients with surgically proven primary hyperparathyroidism present with high normal serum total calcium, with inappropriately high normal or increased PTH levels. It is important to recognize that patients with primary hyperparathyroidism will almost uniformly have documented increased serum total or ionized calcium levels at some time during their course, even with some variation in the overall serum calcium levels over time.

The possibility of physiologic secondary hyperparathyroidism may represent an obstacle in diagnosing certain patients with documentation of serum calcium levels over time to be mostly in the mid to lower normal range, even if they are found to have increased intact PTH levels. Patients with mid to lower normal serum calcium levels associated with increased intact PTH levels should be further evaluated to ensure that they do not have low calcium or vitamin D intake, calcium or vitamin D malabsorption, inability to convert 25-hydroxyvitamin D to biologically active 1,24-dihydroxyvitamin D, or significant hypercalcuria. Each of these situations, either independently or in combination, could explain the findings of a mid to low normal serum calcium and increased intact PTH levels. Patients with low calcium intake of less than 600 mg/d or intestinal calcium malabsorption will usually maintain serum total calcium in the normal range at the expense of skeletal calcium, and have normal serum 25-hydroxyvitamin D levels, but have 24-hour urinary calcium levels of less than 100 mg/d, often less than 50 mg/d. Patients with low vitamin D intake or intestinal vitamin D malabsorption will usually have serum 25-hydroxyvitamin D levels of less than 20 ng/mL (normal range 14–80 ng/mL) and often have low 24-hour urinary calcium values. Patients who are unable to convert serum 25-hydroxyvitamin D to biologically active 1,25-dihydroxyvitamin D because of renal insufficiency or specific inhibitors of renal 1α-hydroxylase activity typically have normal serum 25-hydroxyvitamin D but low or undetectable serum 1,25-dihydroxyvitamin D levels (normal range to 15–60 pg/mL). Patients with idiopathic hypercalcuria typically have 24-hour urinary calcium values in excess of 400 mg/d. Thus it may be difficult to distinguish patients with true primary hyperparathyroidism from those with idiopathic hypercalcuria and high normal serum total calcium levels, as patients with primary hyperparathyroidism are expected to have at least relative hypercalciuria.

Patients with primary hyperparathyroidism usually have serum phosphate in the low normal to mildly decreased range. Patients with simultaneously high normal or increased serum calcium and high normal or increased serum phosphate should be investigated further for intestinal hyperabsorptive states or vitamin D excess.

There is no cross-reactivity between PTH and PTHrP in current assays, making the distinction between primary hyperparathyroidism and PTHrP-mediated hypercalcemia of malignancy certain. Patients with primary hyperparathyroidism almost always have suppressed PTHrP levels when checked, and patients with PTHrP-mediated hypercalcemia of malignancy almost always have suppressed intact PTH levels. Patients who have been treated with thiazide diuretics or lithium may have mild hypercalcemia and increased intact PTH levels without coexisting primary hyperparathyroidism, so it is essential to discontinue these medications for at least 1 month before reassessing the levels of serum total calcium and intact PTH to make the correct diagnosis. Hypercalcemic patients treated with thiazides or lithium who have coexisting primary hyperparathyroidism will have persistent hypercalcemia and increased intact PTH after discontinuing these medications.

Once the diagnosis of primary hyperparathyroidism is secured, surgical intervention is usually necessary in patients with symptomatic primary hyperparathyroidism and in many patients who are asymptomatic but at risk for developing problems later in life. This topic is discussed elsewhere in this issue.

Patients with symptomatic hypercalcemia unable to tolerate surgery have limited options for medical treatment. These patients usually do best by maintaining adequate hydration and remaining physically active. Thiazide diuretics and lithium should generally be avoided. Dietary calcium intake of 800 to 1000 mg/d is usually advised to minimize bone loss and to avoid aggravation of the persistent hypercalcemia or hypercalciuria. Oral bisphosphonates, such as alendronate or risedronate, or intravenous pamidronate, may potentially be beneficial in women not able to take postmenopausal estrogen, or in men unable to undergo surgery. Calcium-sensing receptor agonists (calcimimetics) have been used for some patients with excessive hypercalcemia, in those patients with renal failure induced secondary hyperparathyroidism, and in those with parathyroid carcinoma. It is uncertain as to whether these medications represent a long-term effective modality for medical treatment of primary hyperparathyroidism.

REFERENCES

1. Frolich A. Prevalence of hypercalcemia in normal and hospitalized populations. Dan Med Bull 1998;45:436–9.
2. Mundy FR, Guise TA. Hormonal control of calcium homeostasis. Clin Chem 1999; 45:1347–52.
3. Brown EM, Pollak M, Seidman CE, et al. Calcium-ion-sensing cell-surface receptors. N Engl J Med 1995;333:234–40.
4. Marx SJ, Attie MF, Levine MA, et al. The hypercalciuric or benign variant of familial hypercalcemia: clinical and biochemical features of in fifteen kindreds. Medicine 1981;60:397–412.
5. Grill V, Ho P, Body JJ, et al. Parathyroid hormone-related protein: elevated levels in both humoral hypercalcemia of malignancy and hypercalcemia complicating metastatic breast cancer. J Clin Endocrinol Metab 1991;73:1309–15.
6. Ikeda K, Ohno H, Hane M, et al. Development of a sensitive two-site immunoradiometric assay for parathyroid hormone-related peptide: evidence for elevated levels in plasma from patients with adult T-cell leukemia/lymphoma and B-cell lymphoma. J Clin Endocrinol Metab 1994;79:1322–7.
7. Nagai Y, Yamato H, Akogi K, et al. Role of interleukin 6 in uncoupling of bone in vivo in a human squamous carcinoma co-producing PTHrp and interleukin 6. J Bone Miner Res 1998;13:664–72.

8. Breslau NA, McGuire JL, Zerwekh JE, et al. Hypercalcemia associated with increased serum calcitriol levels in three patients with lymphoma. Ann Intern Med 1984;100:1–7.

9. Rosenthal NR, Insogna KL, Godsall JW, et al. Elevations in circulating 1,25(OH)2D in three patients with lymphoma-associated hypercalcemia. J Clin Endocrinol Metab 1985;60:29–33.

10. Adams JS, Fernandez M, Gacad MA, et al. Vitamin D metabolite mediated hypercalcemia and hypercalciuria in patients with AIDS and non-AIDS-associated lymphoma. Blood 1989;73:235–9.

11. Seymour JF, Gagel RF. Calcitriol: the major humoral mediator of hypercalcemia in Hodgkin's disease and non-Hodgkin's lymphomas. Blood 1993;82:1383–94.

12. Mundy GR, Yoneda T, Guise TA. Hypercalcemia in hematologic malignancies and in solid tumors associated with extensive localized bone destruction. In: Favus MJ, editor. Primer on metabolic bone diseases and disorders of mineral metabolism. 4th edition. Philadelphia: Lippencott Williams and Wilkins; 1999. p. 183–7.

13. Knecht TP, Behling CA, Burton DW, et al. The humoral hypercalcemia of benignancy. A newly appreciated syndrome. Am J Clin Pathol 1996;105:487–92.

14. Burman KD, Monchick JM, Earll JM, et al. Ionized and total serum calcium and parathyroid hormone in hyperparathyroidism. Ann Intern Med 1976;84:668–71.

15. Stewart AF, Hoecker J, Segre GV, et al. Hypercalcemia in pheochromocytoma: evidence for a novel mechanism. Ann Intern Med 1985;102:776–9.

16. Mune T, Katakami H, Kato Y, et al. Production and secretion of parathyroid hormone-related protein in pheochromocytoma: participation of an α-adrenergic mechanism. J Clin Endocrinol Metab 1993;76:757–62.

17. Adams JS, Singer FR, Gacad MA, et al. Isolation and structural identification of 1,25-dihyroxyvitamin D3 produced by cultured alveolar macrophages in sarcoidosis. J Clin Endocrinol Metab 1985;60:960–6.

18. Edelson GW, Talpos GB, Bone HG III. Hypercalcemia associated with Wegener's granulomatosis and hyperparathyroidism: etiology and management. Am J Nephrol 1993;13:275–7.

19. Stoeckle JD, Hardy HL, Weber AL. Chronic beryllium disease: long-term follow-up of sixty cases and selective review of the literature. Am J Med 1969;46:545–61.

20. Parker MS, Dokoh S, Woolfenden JM, et al. Hypercalcemia in coccidioidomycosis. Am J Med 1983;74:721–4.

21. Tominaga Y, Takagi H. Molecular genetics of hyperparathyroidism disease. Curr Opin Nephrol Hypertens 1996;5:336–41.

Imaging of Parathyroid Glands

David Chien, MD, Heather Jacene, MD*

KEYWORDS

• Parathyroid • Sestamibi • Scintigraphy
• Nuclear medicine • PET • Imaging

Parathyroidectomy is the treatment of choice for patients with primary hyperparathyroidism and may be indicated in patients with secondary or tertiary hyperparathyroidism if they do not respond to medical therapy.[1] Preoperative imaging studies have an important role in facilitating successful localization of adenomas for surgeons. Their use has increased and parallels the recent growth of minimally invasive parathyroidectomy.

A variety of anatomic and functional imaging techniques can be used to localize parathyroid adenomas, including ultrasound, MRI, CT, and scintigraphy (nuclear medicine). Surgeons may rely on one or a combination of modalities for planning an operation. In many studies, scintigraphy is reported to have the highest accuracy for localization of adenomas when compared with anatomic imaging techniques.[2–5] This article discusses the current role and limitations of imaging, with a focus on scintigraphy, in the evaluation of patients before surgery for hyperparathyroidism.

SCINTIGRAPHY WITH SINGLE-PHOTON EMITTERS

Parathyroid scintigraphy can be accomplished with several different radiopharmaceuticals and techniques. Selenium-75–methionine, an amino acid analog of methionine, and thallium-201/technetium-99m (^{99m}Tc)–pertechnetate subtraction imaging are of historical interest and were abandoned because of poor image quality and technical limitations that led to suboptimal accuracy. ^{99m}Tc-sestamibi is the current radiotracer of choice for parathyroid scintigraphy.

^{99m}Tc-sestamibi is a lipophilic cation that is ultimately sequestered in mitochondria because of transmembrane electrical gradients in the cell and mitochondria. Accumulation of ^{99m}Tc-sestamibi is probably related to increased vascularity and a higher number of mitochondria-rich oxyphil cells in adenomas.[6] Slower release of the tracer

---

Division of Nuclear Medicine, The Russell H. Morgan Department of Radiology and Radiological Science, Johns Hopkins University School of Medicine, 601 North Caroline Street, JHOC 3235, Baltimore, MD 21287, USA
* Corresponding author.
E-mail address: hjacene1@jhmi.edu

Otolaryngol Clin N Am 43 (2010) 399–415
doi:10.1016/j.otc.2010.01.008
0030-6665/10/$ – see front matter © 2010 Elsevier Inc. All rights reserved.

from adenomas compared with normal surrounding tissues (parathyroid and thyroid) allows for distinction between the two by imaging (**Fig. 1**).[7]

The sensitivity of ^{99m}Tc-sestamibi parathyroid scintigraphy for detecting and localizing a single adenoma in patients with primary hyperparathyroidism ranges from 54% to 96%.[4,8–16] Few of the studies reported specificity with ranges from 83% to 99%.[4,12,15] A meta-analysis, including 20,225 patients with primary hyperparathyroidism, reported an overall 88% sensitivity for detecting a solitary adenoma.[17] Sensitivities were lower for detecting double adenomas (30%) or parathyroid hyperplasia (45%).[17] In patients with tertiary hyperparathyroidism, ^{99m}Tc-sestamibi parathyroid scintigraphy performs well with a sensitivity of approximately 76%.[18]

Various imaging techniques can be used for ^{99m}Tc-sestamibi parathyroid scintigraphy and this is the likely reason for its wide range of diagnostic performance in the literature. Imaging can be performed at 1 or 2 time points after radiotracer injection (single- vs dual-phase imaging) and using 2-D planar versus 3-D single-photon emission computed tomography (SPECT) imaging techniques. Specific protocols are determined in part by the nuclear medicine cameras available at an imaging center.

A few studies have directly compared planar with SPECT imaging for detection of parathyroid adenomas. These studies have demonstrated a higher sensitivity of SPECT for detecting and localizing parathyroid adenomas compared with planar imaging.[8,19–23] The false-negative rate is reported to be lower for SPECT,[22,23] and SPECT detects small parathyroid adenomas immediately posterior to the thyroid gland better than planar imaging.[8]

Hybrid SPECT/CT imaging has been a recent focus and studies have demonstrated an advantage of this technique over conventional ones for localization of adenomas,[12,24–26] especially in patients with ectopic glands.[26] SPECT/CT allows visualization of corresponding anatomy for differentiation of thyroidal from nonthyroidal tissue and the relationship of the adenoma to adjacent structures (**Fig. 2**). Mediastinal and intrathyroidal adenomas can be precisely localized, all aiding in the surgical approach (**Fig. 3**). The precise localization is important because ectopic adenomas can be located in the paraesophageal region (28%), mediastinum (26%), intrathymic

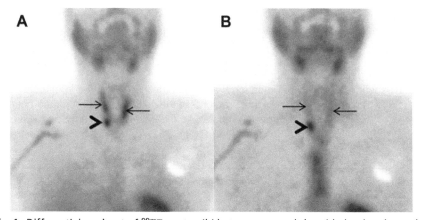

Fig. 1. Differential washout of ^{99m}Tc-sestamibi between normal thyroid gland and parathyroid adenoma. Early images (*A*) demonstrate physiologic uptake of ^{99m}Tc-sestamibi throughout the thyroid gland (*arrows*), which washes out on subsequent delayed images (*B*). There is a persistent focus of uptake inferior to the right lower pole of the thyroid gland on early and delayed images (*arrowheads*), which represents a parathyroid adenoma.

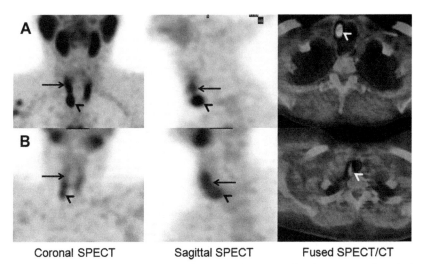

Coronal SPECT   Sagittal SPECT   Fused SPECT/CT

Fig. 2. This figure demonstrates the use of SPECT and SPECT/CT for determining the relationship of parathyroid adenomas to adjacent structures and differentiating ectopic superior from true inferior adenomas. In the case in the top row (A), a focus of uptake (*arrowhead*) is seen inferior to the lower pole of the right thyroid gland (*arrow*). Early SPECT/CT images localize this focus to the anterior paratracheal region. At surgery, this was determined to be a true right inferior parathyroid adenoma. In the case in the bottom row (B), a focus of uptake (*arrowhead*) is seen inferior and posterior to the lower pole of the right thyroid gland (*arrow*). Early SPECT/CT images localize this focus to the right tracheoesophageal groove. At surgery, this was determined to be an ectopic right superior parathyroid adenoma.

region (24%), intrathyroidal region (11%), carotid sheath region (9%), and high cervical positions (2%).[27] The accuracy of adenoma localization may continue to improve as CT components with higher resolution are incorporated into SPECT/CT cameras.

Another consideration in protocol design is single-phase versus dual-phase imaging. Higher sensitivities are reported for dual-phase imaging protocols. The advantage of the dual-phase technique is 2-fold: (1) distinction between abnormal parathyroid tissue and normal parathyroid or thyroid tissue by differential washout between early and late images and (2) localization of a focus of uptake in relation to thyroid tissue on early images. Dual-phase images may also help identify adenomas with very fast washout rates that might be missed on delayed imaging alone.

Lavely and colleagues[12] performed a comprehensive study of ^{99m}Tc-sestamibi parathyroid scintigraphy in 110 patients with primary hyperparathyroidism and no prior neck surgery. Patients underwent planar and SPECT/CT imaging at 15 minutes and 2 hours after injection of ^{99m}Tc-sestamibi. Early and delayed planar, SPECT, and SPECT/CT images were evaluated individually for each patient. Paired image sets (eg, early and delayed planar and early planar and delayed SPECT) were also evaluated. A total of 19 different combinations of imaging technique was evaluated for each patient. Early SPECT/CT with any delayed imaging emerged as the best methodology for preoperative parathyroid adenoma localization (sensitivity approximately 73%, specificity approximately 99%, accuracy approximately 86%, positive predictive value 86%–91%, and negative predictive value approximately 98%). In the absence of SPECT/CT, dual-phase studies with planar or SPECT imaging was the second best technique (sensitivity approximately 58%–66%, specificity approximately 98%,

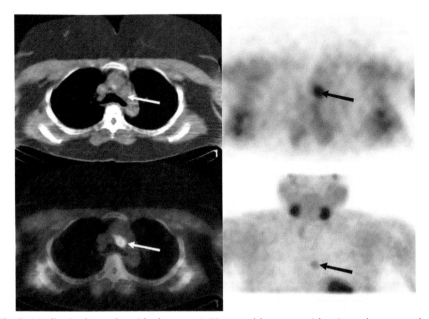

Fig. 3. Mediastinal parathyroid adenoma. A 52-year-old woman with primary hyperparathyroidism (calcium level 12.2 mg/dL, parathyroid hormone level 145 pg/mL). Delayed SPECT/CT images demonstrate no abnormal foci of ^{99m}Tc-sestamibi uptake in the neck, but there is focal uptake fusing to the left tracheobronchial region (*arrows*). Frozen histopathologic analysis during surgery demonstrated parathyroid tissue within the focus and intraoperative parathyroid hormone level decreased from 117 pg/mL at baseline to 30 pg/mL after excision confirming removal of a hyperfunctioning parathyroid gland.

accuracy approximately 78%–82%, positive predictive value approximately 80%–83%, and negative predictive value approximately 97%).

More recent studies have also confirmed the benefit of hybrid SPECT/CT imaging. Neumann and colleagues[25] compared dual isotope iodine-123 (^{123}I)/^{99m}Tc-sestamibi SPECT with SPECT/CT. In the patients with primary hyperparathyroidism, the sensitivity (approximately 70%) for localizing an adenoma was not improved with SPECT/CT; however, anatomic localization significantly improved specificity (96% for SPECT/CT vs 48% for SPECT alone, $P<.006$). In a study of 23 patients,[24] hybrid SPECT/CT accurately localized an adenoma within 19 mm of its intraoperative location in 95% of cases. In addition, the median time from skin incision to adenoma localization was 14 minutes for single adenomas.[24]

Other techniques to optimize preoperative localization of parathyroid adenomas continue to be investigated in the absence of SPECT/CT. Pinhole imaging, which provides a magnified image, has better diagnostic performance versus parallel-hole collimator imaging and SPECT.[28–30] Pinhole SPECT is also being investigated and early results are encouraging.[20]

Parathyroid scintigraphy with ^{99m}Tc-tetrofosmin, a tracer similar to ^{99m}Tc-sestamibi, has been investigated. Comparisons of the diagnostic accuracy of the two ^{99m}Tc-labeled agents have yielded mixed results. Several studies have shown that ^{99m}Tc-tetrofosmin performs at least as well as ^{99m}Tc-sestamibi,[4,31–34] but others have found discordant results with ^{99m}Tc-sestamibi performing better.[35–38] Nearly all studies have shown that the differential washout of ^{99m}Tc-tetrofosmin from the thyroid gland is slower than that of ^{99m}Tc-sestamibi, resulting in lower adenoma to thyroid/background ratios. For this reason, ^{99m}Tc-sestamibi has remained the radio-pharmaceutical of choice in most nuclear medicine imaging centers.

Limitations of Scintigraphy

The most common cause for a false-positive ^{99m}Tc-sestamibi study is accumulation of the tracer in thyroid adenomas (**Fig. 4**).[11,14,16] Other causes of false-positive results are thyroid carcinoma, inflammatory thyroid disease (such as chronic lymphocytic thyroiditis [**Fig. 5**]), and inflammatory or malignant cervical lymphadenopathy. Subtraction imaging with a thyroid imaging agent in combination with ^{99m}Tc-sestamibi or hybrid SPECT/CT can reduce false-positive results.[11,39,40] In the subtraction technique, images with agents that concentrate solely in the thyroid gland (for example, ^{99m}Tc-pertechnetate and ^{123}I) are subtracted from those obtained with ^{99m}Tc-sestamibi (which accumulates in thyroid tissue and parathyroid adenomas). The resulting

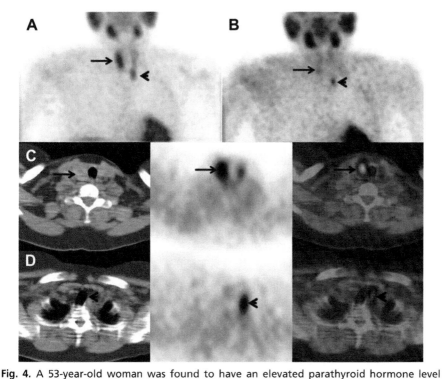

Fig. 4. A 53-year-old woman was found to have an elevated parathyroid hormone level after presenting with an elevated calcium level on routine laboratory work-up. (*A*) Early SPECT/CT images demonstrate asymmetrically increased uptake of ^{99m}Tc-sestamibi in the right thyroid gland versus the left (*arrow*) and a focus of uptake inferior to the left inferior thyroid gland (*arrowhead*). (*B*) The delayed images showed persistent uptake in both locations, although much less on the right (*arrow*) than the left (*arrowhead*). (*C*) The early SPECT/CT images show that the uptake on the right fuses to the thyroid gland. At the time of surgery, a right lower-pole thyroid nodule was found. (*D*) The early SPECT/CT images show that the focal uptake on the left fuses in the anterior left paratracheal region inferior to the left thyroid gland. At the time of surgery, a 1.7-g left inferior parathyroid adenoma was excised.

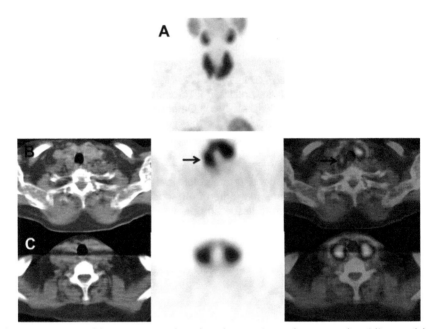

Fig. 5. A 74-year-old woman was found to have primary hyperparathyroidism and her history also included Hashimoto thyroiditis for which she was taking levothyroxine. Early (not shown) and delayed ^{99m}Tc-sestamibi parathyroid scintigraphy (A) showed diffuse uptake of the tracer throughout the thyroid gland. Transaxial slices through the inferior poles of the thyroid gland (B) demonstrated more focal uptake fusing to lower-pole hypodense nodule in the right inferior lower pole (arrow). The rest of the uptake (C) corresponded to an enlarged thyroid gland and no additional imaging findings were consistent with a parathyroid adenoma. The patient underwent a 4-gland parathyroid exploration. At surgery, there was thyroiditis and the thyroid gland had multiple nodules, including a right exophytic lower-pole thyroid nodule. After further exploration, a 467-mg left superior parathyroid adenoma was resected. This case demonstrates false-positive results from a thyroid adenoma as well as some of the challenges in image interpretation in the setting of background thyroid disease.

subtraction image can then localize the parathyroid adenoma. A major limitation of the subtraction technique is potential artifact generated on the digitally subtracted images due to patient motion during image acquisition.[40]

Some investigators have tried to identify factors that may affect the sensitivity of scintigraphy for detecting a parathyroid adenoma. Scintigraphy has a better sensitivity for detecting large-sized adenomas and single-gland disease.[41–43] Higher preoperative parathyroid hormone and calcium levels and decreased vitamin D levels are associated with improved sensitivity in some studies.[42,44,45] In addition, thyroid suppression has been associated with increased sensitivity for detecting adenomas,[46] whereas decreased sensitivity has been reported with the use of calcium channel blockers, high P-glycoprotein levels, and multidrug resistance proteins.[47–50] The cohorts investigated in the various studies, however, were fairly specific and the results cannot be generalized to all patients undergoing ^{99m}Tc-sestamibi scintigraphy.

Given the various techniques available for performing parathyroid scintigraphy, it is important for referring physicians to be aware of the imaging technique used for their individual patients as it may have impact on the diagnostic performance of the test.

Collaboration between surgeons and nuclear medicine physicians/radiologists may also help to improve the accuracy of gland localization.[51]

Recurrent Primary Hyperparathyroidism

A persistently elevated parathyroid hormone level after curative therapy may be due to progression of underlying disease after response to bone mineralization or initial surgery failure. Failure to recognize and adequately resect multigland disease at initial surgery is one of the most common causes for failed initial surgery.[27,52,53] This remains a challenge because detection of multigland disease is a limitation of ^{99m}Tc-sestamibi parathyroid scintigraphy.[43]

Another significant cause of failed initial surgery is lack of detection of an ectopically located gland (**Fig. 6**).[27] The frequency of multiple or ectopic glands, often coexisting, as the cause for recurrence ranges from 44% to 70%.[52,54] In one study, ^{99m}Tc-sestamibi parathyroid imaging was reported to have a sensitivity of 65% for localizing these recurrences.[54] Jaskowiak and colleagues[55] reported that the most common site of a missed ectopic adenoma is the tracheoesophageal grove (**Fig. 7**). Lavely and colleagues[12] reported that the advantage of combined SPECT/CT seems to be its ability to differentiate ectopic superior glands in the tracheoesophageal groove (located inferior and posterior to the thyroid gland) from true inferior glands (see **Fig. 2**). Wider use of this technique in the future may prove to decrease recurrence rates due to failed initial surgeries.

Patients with a prior history of thyroid or parathyroid surgery were included in several studies evaluating parathyroid scintigraphy and the technique seems equally sensitive for localizing and detecting parathyroid adenomas regardless of the surgical status of the neck. Civelek and colleagues[10] reported sensitivities of 87% versus 92% for delayed ^{99m}Tc-sestamibi SPECT imaging in those with (N = 51) versus without (N = 287) a prior history of neck surgery. Similarly, Billotey and colleagues[8] reported 91% overall sensitivity for adenoma detection in all patients and 87% sensitivity for 39 patients undergoing reoperation. In the reoperative setting, ^{99m}Tc-sestamibi parathyroid imaging was superior to anatomic imaging modalities.[5,8,9,54–57]

In 3% of cases, persistent or recurrent hyperparathyroidism may be due to regrowth of previously resected tumor or remnant tissue.[27] Additionally, when surgery for secondary or tertiary hyperparathyroidism is performed, one-half of a gland is often reimplanted into a graft site and recurrence can occur due to hyperfunctional activity within the reimplanted parathyroid tissue. In these cases, it is imperative for an imaging physician to know the location of the reimplanted tissue so directed imaging can be performed. When patients with secondary hyperparathyroidism recur, ^{99m}Tc-sestamibi imaging is useful to determine if the failure is due to a hyperfunctioning graft or an ectopic fifth gland, necessitating a change in management.[56] Itoh and Ishizuka[58] confirmed the high sensitivity (100% in this study) of ^{99m}Tc-sestamibi for the preoperative localization of hyperfunctioning parathyroid glands in patients with persistent or recurrent hyperparathyroidism after 4-gland parathyroidectomy with autoimplantation of parathyroid tissue.

RADIOGUIDED PARATHYROIDECTOMY

Radioguided parathyroidectomy is a technique that involves the injection of ^{99m}Tc-sestamibi before surgery and intraoperative use of a gamma probe that can help localize the parathyroid adenoma for the surgeon. Several approaches to radioguided parathyroidectomy are reported.[59–63] Some groups administer the radiotracer, obtain imaging studies, and then perform surgery within a 2- to 3-hour time frame on the

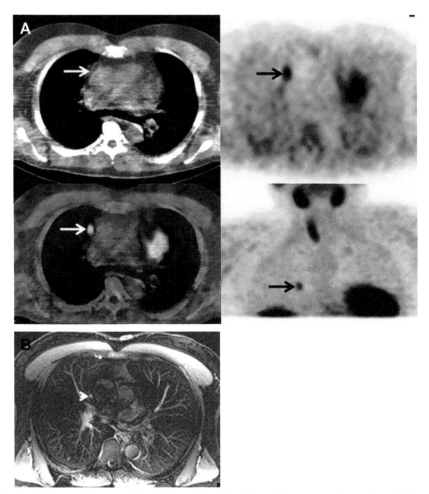

Fig. 6. A 54-year-old man with a history of left hemithyroidectomy and parathyroidectomy for a suspicious thyroid nodule and hypercalcemia presented with persistent hypercalcemia. At the initial surgery, bilateral normal superior parathyroid glands were found, a small right inferior adenoma was removed, but the left inferior parathyroid gland was not identified. The patient presented with persistent hypercalcemia and was referred for parathyroid scintigraphy. Early SPECT/CT images (A) demonstrated ^{99m}Tc-sestamibi uptake in the remaining right thyroid gland and focal uptake in the right prevascular region (*arrows*). MRI (B) of the thorax subsequently confirmed a corresponding nodule lateral to the ascending aorta (*arrowhead*) and the patient underwent a median sternotomy and resection of a 1153-mg parathyroid gland from this location.

same day whereas others omit the imaging on the day of surgery and inject the tracer before the start of the operation and only use the gamma probe intraoperatively. For both approaches, localization of the adenoma is performed by scintigraphy or other imaging modalities before surgery. A small amount of radioactivity is required when using the gamma probe as compared with imaging studies; therefore, an advantage of not obtaining images on the day of surgery is that the surgical team is exposed to less radiation. Another advantage is that the shorter time interval between tracer

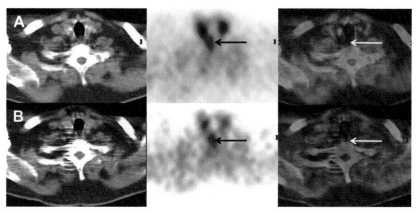

Fig. 7. A 65-year-old man presented with persistent hyperparathyroidism after a left para-thyroidectomy. Prior parathyroid scan (uncertain technique) reportedly demonstrated an adenoma on the left and a MRI concurred with this finding. At surgery, a 1.8-g left parathy-roid gland was resected. No intraoperative parathyroid hormone level measurements were obtained. Postoperatively, the patient continued to have elevated calcium and parathyroid hormone levels. Early (A) and delayed (B) ^{99m}Tc-sestamibi SPECT/CT images demonstrate a persistent focus of uptake in the right tracheoesophageal groove (arrows) consistent with a parathyroid adenoma. At surgery, a 330-mg ectopic right superior parathyroid adenoma was resected. His intraoperative parathyroid hormone level declined from 106 pg/mL at baseline to 22 pg/mL at 20 minutes after resection consistent with biochemical resolution of his hyperparathyroidism.

injection and surgery may enhance a surgeon's ability to detect those adenomas that have rapid washout of radiotracer.

The operative technique for using the gamma probe is reviewed by Mariani and colleagues.[64] In general, a parathyroid-to-thyroid count ratio of greater than 1.5 is suggestive of a parathyroid adenoma. Once removed, an ex vivo count rate of at least 20% greater than thyroid background (counted in vivo) confirms the resection of an adenoma. The reported accuracy for distinguishing adenoma from multigland hyper-plasia was 100% in the initial studies describing the "greater than 20% rule."[65]

Subsequent studies have shown ex vivo count rates of greater than 20% in thyroid nodules and hyperplasia limiting the application of the initial observation.[62,66–68] Rubello and colleagues[62] suggested that an explanation for this might be that the timing between the ^{99m}Tc-sestamibi injection and surgery was longer (2–3 hours) in the initial studies, which allowed for additional washout from nonadenomas. The optimal timing to surgery may vary from patient to patient and a patient-specific, optimal time-to-surgery protocol has been described.[59] Surgery is performed based on the timing of peak adenoma-to-background ratio as determined by dynamic imaging.[59]

The usefulness of radioguided parathyroidectomy in patients with negative preop-erative ^{99m}Tc-sestamibi imaging studies is unclear. In 2005, Rubello and colleagues[62] reported that from a surgeon's perspective, use of the gamma probe was not helpful in 20 patients with negative scans. Forty percent (8/20) of these patients demonstrated multigland disease. More recently, however, Chen and colleagues[69] found equivalent cure rates and major complication rates using radioguided parathyroidectomy in patients with negative (n = 134) versus positive (n = 635) preoperative ^{99m}Tc-sesta-mibi scans. In the scan-negative group, there was a higher rate of multigland disease and the parathyroid gland weight was lower. Both of these are known to cause false-negative results on scintigraphy. The in vivo and ex vivo count rates were also lower in the scan-negative versus scan-positive patients but significantly greater than background counts in both instances.[69]

Proposed guidelines for radioguided minimally invasive parathyroidectomy include its use for patients with a high probability of a solitary adenoma and a normal thyroid gland.[64] Other considerations are optimizing the preoperative scintigraphy protocols based on all available information, minimizing radiation exposure to the surgical team, and determining the completeness of surgical resection based on in vivo and ex vivo gamma counting data as well as a documented decline in intraoperative parathyroid hormone levels.[64]

ANATOMIC IMAGING
Ultrasound

Ultrasound offers detailed anatomic imaging of the neck and does not expose patients to radiation. Parathyroid adenomas typically appear as hypoechoic homogenous well-demarcated masses, which contrast with adjacent hyperechoic thyroid glands. Ultrasound can provide excellent images of enlarged inferior and superior parathyroid glands located adjacent to the inferior poles of the thyroid, in the thyrothymic ligament or upper cervical portion of the thymus, and just posterior to the thyroid gland (**Fig. 8**). Certain locations of the parathyroid adenoma limit ultrasound localization, however, such as lesions within the thyroid that may be confused with a thyroid adenoma and those in the tracheoesophageal groove, retroesophageal region, mediastinum, or other ectopic locations.[70,71] Ultrasound only demonstrates enlargement of parathyroid glands but does not provide functional information. In these scenarios, scintigraphic imaging of the parathyroid adenoma may be beneficial.

A range of sensitivities (51% to 78%) and specificities (67% to 96%) is reported for the ability of ultrasound to detect and localize parathyroid adenomas.[4,20,31,72] Comparisons between ultrasound and scintigraphy also vary in the literature and are highly dependent on the skill of the ultrasonographer and the scintigraphic method used. Studies comparing scintigraphy with ultrasound have generally reported a higher accuracy with scintigraphy. There is a general consensus that the combination of ultrasonography and scintigraphy, however, offers significant superiority in sensitivity and accuracy in the detection and localization of functional parathyroid adenomas.[31,72–76] Some clinical practices use the combination of ultrasonography and scintigraphy to maximize the likelihood of success of minimally invasive surgeries and video-assisted parathyroidectomy.[77,78] One recent study of 144 patients suggested that scintigraphy may be reserved for those patients with a negative ultrasound performed by a radiologist.[72]

MRI

Normal parathyroid glands are not usually visualized on MRI. Parathyroid adenomas are identified as soft tissue masses that have indeterminate signal intensity on T1-weighted images and high signal intensity on T2-weighted images, and this may depend on histologic composition.[79,80] When gadolinium is administered, the signal intensity of parathyroid adenomas significantly increases compared with the adjacent thyroid gland and skeletal muscle on T1-weighted images.[81]

The sensitivity of planar ^{99m}Tc-sestamibi/^{123}I thyroid subtraction parathyroid imaging is higher than MRI and ultrasound in detecting abnormal parathyroid glands, including single adenomas, multiple adenomas, and 4-gland hyperplasia.[82] Studies

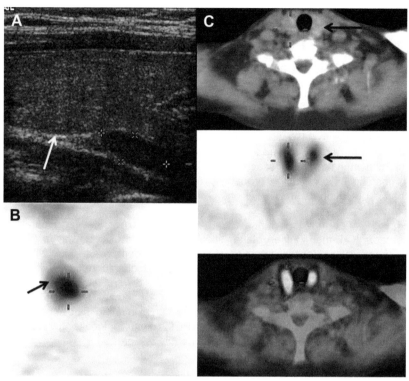

Fig. 8. A 58-year-old woman presented with primary hyperparathyroidism. Ultrasound (*A*) showed a hypoechoic nodule (*crosshairs*) posterior to the right lobe of the thyroid gland (*arrow*). Sagittal SPECT images (*B*) demonstrated a focus of ^{99m}Tc-sestamibi uptake (*crosshairs*) posterior to the thyroid gland (*arrow*). Transaxial SPECT/CT images (*C*) demonstrated that the focus of uptake fused just posterior (*crosshairs*) to the right midpole of the thyroid gland (*arrows*). At surgery, a 760-mg ectopic right superior parathyroid adenoma was resected. Her intraoperative parathyroid hormone level declined from 103 pg/mL at baseline to 30 pg/mL at 10 minutes after resection consistent with biochemical resolution of her hyperparathyroidism.

comparing MRI with ^{99m}Tc-sestamibi SPECT parathyroid imaging demonstrate an 86% sensitivity rate in localizing adenomas with SPECT scintigraphy as compared with 71% sensitivity obtained with MRI.[83] Ruf and colleagues[83] reported added value of software fusing ^{99m}Tc-sestamibi SPECT and MRI in 7 of 17 patients with primary hyperparathyroidism. The MRI provided anatomic localization in 5 patients and scintigraphy improved inconclusive MRI findings in 2 patients. Again, no direct comparisons of MRI with hybrid SPECT/CT have yet been performed.

CT

CT alone is not commonly used for preoperative localization of parathyroid adenomas. The sensitivity of CT for detecting parathyroid adenomas ranges between 40% and 70% in the unoperated neck and is lower (25%–55%) in the postoperative neck.[3,84–86] In combination with SPECT, however, CT is helpful for precise localization of suspected adenomas.[12]

CT characterization depends on density measurements of the parathyroid adenoma to differentiate it from lymph nodes and normal thyroid tissue and is dependent on the timing after the injection of contrast material. Typically, the parathyroid adenomas enhance faster and to a greater extent and have faster washout rates compared with lymph nodes.[87]

SCINTIGRAPHY WITH POSITRON EMITTERS (POSITRON EMISSION TOMOGRAPHY)

The role of 2-[^{18}F]-fluoro-2-deoxy-D-glucose (FDG), a glucose analog, and positron emission tomography (PET) for the detection of parathyroid adenomas or hyperplasia remains uncertain. A few studies over the past 2 decades have yielded sensitivities ranging from 13% to 94%.[88,89] Early studies showed promising results, particularly in patients with primary hyperparathyroidism with no prior history of neck surgery. One study demonstrated higher sensitivity of FDG-PET versus dual-phase ^{99m}Tc-sestamibi imaging (86% vs 43%)[89] probably due to a higher resolution of the PET images and better detection of smaller lesions. These early results have not been reliably reproduced.

PET with ^{11}C-L-methionine has also been evaluated for localizing parathyroid adenomas. ^{11}C-L-methionine uptake reflects amino acid use. Similar to FDG, the range of sensitivities for the detection of parathyroid adenomas is wide with ^{11}C-L-methionine (54%–95%).[90–92] The detection rates seem higher for patients with primary hyperparathyroidism and elevated calcium levels.[92] Several studies have shown a benefit of using ^{11}C-L-methionine in patients with nonprimary hyperparathyroidism and hypercalcemia when conventional ^{99m}Tc-sestamibi imaging is nonlocalizing.[93,94] There may be a subgroup of patients in whom PET is useful for localizing a parathyroid adenoma, but further studies are needed to identify this group.

REFERENCES

1. Marx SJ. Hyperparathyroid and hypoparathyroid disorders. N Engl J Med 2000; 343(25):1863–75.
2. Geatti O, Shapiro B, Orsolon PG, et al. Localization of parathyroid enlargement: experience with technetium-99m methoxyisobutylisonitrile and thallium-201 scintigraphy, ultrasonography and computed tomography. Eur J Nucl Med 1994; 21(1):17–22.
3. Ishibashi M, Nishida H, Hiromatsu Y, et al. Localization of ectopic parathyroid glands using technetium-99m sestamibi imaging: comparison with magnetic resonance and computed tomographic imaging. Eur J Nucl Med 1997;24(2): 197–201.
4. Ishibashi M, Nishida H, Hiromatsu Y, et al. Comparison of technetium-99m-MIBI, technetium-99m-tetrofosmin, ultrasound and MRI for localization of abnormal parathyroid glands. J Nucl Med 1998;39(2):320–4.
5. Peeler BB, Martin WH, Sandler MP, et al. Sestamibi parathyroid scanning and preoperative localization studies for patients with recurrent/persistent hyperparathyroidism or significant comorbid conditions: development of an optimal localization strategy. Am Surg 1997;63(1):37–46.
6. Melloul M, Paz A, Koren R, et al. 99mTc-MIBI scintigraphy of parathyroid adenomas and its relation to tumour size and oxyphil cell abundance. Eur J Nucl Med 2001;28(2):209–13.
7. Falke THM, Sandler MP, Schipper J. Parathyroid glands. In: Sandler MP, Coleman RE, editors. Diagnostic nuclear medicine. 3rd edition. Baltimore (MD): Williams & Wilkins; 1994. p. 991–1012.
8. Billotey C, Sarfati E, Aurengo A, et al. Advantages of SPECT in technetium-99m-sestamibi parathyroid scintigraphy. J Nucl Med 1996;37(11):1773–8.

9. Blanco I, Carril JM, Banzo I, et al. Double-phase Tc-99m sestamibi scintigraphy in the preoperative location of lesions causing hyperparathyroidism. Clin Nucl Med 1998;23(5):291–7.

10. Civelek AC, Ozalp E, Donovan P, et al. Prospective evaluation of delayed technetium-99m sestamibi SPECT scintigraphy for preoperative localization of primary hyperparathyroidism. Surgery 2002;131(2):149–57.

11. Hindie E, Melliere D, Jeanguillaume C, et al. Parathyroid imaging using simultaneous double-window recording of technetium-99m-sestamibi and iodine-123. J Nucl Med 1998;39(6):1100–5.

12. Lavely WC, Goetze S, Friedman KP, et al. Comparison of SPECT/CT, SPECT, and planar imaging with single- and dual-phase (99m)Tc-sestamibi parathyroid scintigraphy. J Nucl Med 2007;48(7):1084–9.

13. Moka D, Voth E, Dietlein M, et al. Technetium 99m-MIBI-SPECT: a highly sensitive diagnostic tool for localization of parathyroid adenomas. Surgery 2000;128(1):29–35.

14. Perez-Monte JE, Brown ML, Shah AN, et al. Parathyroid adenomas: accurate detection and localization with Tc-99m sestamibi SPECT. Radiology 1996;201(1):85–91.

15. Sfakianakis GN, Irvin GL III, Foss J, et al. Efficient parathyroidectomy guided by SPECT-MIBI and hormonal measurements. J Nucl Med 1996;37(5):798–804.

16. Taillefer R, Boucher Y, Potvin C, et al. Detection and localization of parathyroid adenomas in patients with hyperparathyroidism using a single radionuclide imaging procedure with technetium-99m-sestamibi (double-phase study). J Nucl Med 1992;33(10):1801–7.

17. Ruda JM, Hollenbeak CS, Stack BC Jr. A systematic review of the diagnosis and treatment of primary hyperparathyroidism from 1995 to 2003. Otolaryngol Head Neck Surg 2005;132(3):359–72.

18. Loftus KA, Anderson S, Mulloy AL, et al. Value of sestamibi scans in tertiary hyperparathyroidism. Laryngoscope 2007;117(12):2135–8.

19. Ansquer C, Mirallie E, Carlier T, et al. Preoperative localization of parathyroid lesions. Value of 99mTc-MIBI tomography and factors influencing detection. Nuklearmedizin 2008;47(4):158–62.

20. Carlier T, Oudoux A, Mirallie E, et al. 99mTc-MIBI pinhole SPECT in primary hyperparathyroidism: comparison with conventional SPECT, planar scintigraphy and ultrasonography. Eur J Nucl Med Mol Imaging 2008;35(3):637–43.

21. Jorna FH, Jager PL, Que TH, et al. Value of 123I-subtraction and single-photon emission computed tomography in addition to planar 99mTc-MIBI scintigraphy before parathyroid surgery. Surg Today 2007;37(12):1033–41.

22. Lorberboym M, Minski I, Macadziob S, et al. Incremental diagnostic value of preoperative 99mTc-MIBI SPECT in patients with a parathyroid adenoma. J Nucl Med 2003;44(6):904–8.

23. Sharma J, Mazzaglia P, Milas M, et al. Radionuclide imaging for hyperparathyroidism (HPT): which is the best technetium-99m sestamibi modality? Surgery 2006;140(6):856–63.

24. Harris L, Yoo J, Driedger A, et al. Accuracy of technetium-99m SPECT-CT hybrid images in predicting the precise intraoperative anatomical location of parathyroid adenomas. Head Neck 2008;30(4):509–17.

25. Neumann DR, Obuchowski NA, Difilippo FP. Preoperative 123I/99mTc-sestamibi subtraction SPECT and SPECT/CT in primary hyperparathyroidism. J Nucl Med 2008;49(12):2012–7.

26. Serra A, Bolasco P, Satta L, et al. Role of SPECT/CT in the preoperative assessment of hyperparathyroid patients. Radiol Med 2006;111(7):999–1008.

27. Shen W, Duren M, Morita E, et al. Reoperation for persistent or recurrent primary hyperparathyroidism. Arch Surg 1996;131(8):861–7.
28. Ho Shon IA, Yan W, Roach PJ, et al. Comparison of pinhole and SPECT 99mTc-MIBI imaging in primary hyperparathyroidism. Nucl Med Commun 2008;29(11): 949–55.
29. Nichols KJ, Tomas MB, Tronco GG, et al. Preoperative parathyroid scintigraphic lesion localization: accuracy of various types of readings. Radiology 2008;248(1): 221–32.
30. Tomas MB, Pugliese PV, Tronco GG, et al. Pinhole versus parallel-hole collimators for parathyroid imaging: an intraindividual comparison. J Nucl Med Technol 2008; 36(4):189–94.
31. Alexandrides TK, Kouloubi K, Vagenakis AG, et al. The value of scintigraphy and ultrasonography in the preoperative localization of parathyroid glands in patients with primary hyperparathyroidism and concomitant thyroid disease. Hormones (Athens) 2006;5(1):42–51.
32. Apostolopoulos DJ, Houstoulaki E, Giannakenas C, et al. Technetium-99m-tetrofosmin for parathyroid scintigraphy: comparison to thallium-technetium scanning. J Nucl Med 1998;39(8):1433–41.
33. Fjeld JG, Erichsen K, Pfeffer PF, et al. Technetium-99m-tetrofosmin for parathyroid scintigraphy: a comparison with sestamibi. J Nucl Med 1997;38(6):831–4.
34. Wakamatsu H, Noguchi S, Yamashita H, et al. Technetium-99m tetrofosmin for parathyroid scintigraphy: a direct comparison with (99m)Tc-MIBI, (201)Tl, MRI and US. Eur J Nucl Med 2001;28(12):1817–27.
35. Duarte PS, Domingues FC, Costa MS, et al. Discordant results in Tc-99m tetrofosmin and Tc-99m sestamibi parathyroid scintigraphies. Arq Bras Endocrinol Metabol 2007;51(7):1166–8.
36. Froberg AC, Valkema R, Bonjer HJ, et al. 99mTc-tetrofosmin or 99mTc-sestamibi for double-phase parathyroid scintigraphy? Eur J Nucl Med Mol Imaging 2003; 30(2):193–6.
37. Giordano A, Meduri G, Marozzi P, et al. Differences between 99mTc-sestamibi and 99mTc-tetrofosmin uptake in thyroid and salivary glands: comparison with 99mTc-pertechnetate in 86 subjects. Nucl Med Commun 2003;24(3): 321–6.
38. Harrell RM, Mackman DM, Bimston DN. Nonequivalent results of tetrofosmin and sestamibi imaging of parathyroid tumors. Endocr Pract 2006;12(2):179–82.
39. Lorberboym M, Ezri T, Schachter PP. Preoperative technetium Tc 99m sestamibi SPECT imaging in the management of primary hyperparathyroidism in patients with concomitant multinodular goiter. Arch Surg 2005;140(7):656–60.
40. Palestro CJ, Tomas MB, Tronco GG. Radionuclide imaging of the parathyroid glands. Semin Nucl Med 2005;35(4):266–76.
41. Bergson EJ, Sznyter LA, Dubner S, et al. Sestamibi scans and intraoperative parathyroid hormone measurement in the treatment of primary hyperparathyroidism. Arch Otolaryngol Head Neck Surg 2004;130(1):87–91.
42. Bhatnagar A, Vezza PR, Bryan JA, et al. Technetium-99m-sestamibi parathyroid scintigraphy: effect of P-glycoprotein, histology and tumor size on detectability. J Nucl Med 1998;39(9):1617–20.
43. Katz SC, Wang GJ, Kramer EL, et al. Limitations of technetium 99m sestamibi scintigraphic localization for primary hyperparathyroidism associated with multiglandular disease. Am Surg 2003;69(2):170–5.
44. Kandil E, Tufaro AP, Carson KA, et al. Correlation of plasma 25-hydroxyvitamin D levels with severity of primary hyperparathyroidism and likelihood of parathyroid

adenoma localization on sestamibi scan. Arch Otolaryngol Head Neck Surg 2008;134(10):1071–5.

45. Parikshak M, Castillo ED, Conrad MF, et al. Impact of hypercalcemia and parathyroid hormone level on the sensitivity of preoperative sestamibi scanning for primary hyperparathyroidism. Am Surg 2003;69(5):393–8.

46. Royal RE, Delpassand ES, Shapiro SE, et al. Improving the yield of preoperative parathyroid localization: technetium Tc 99m-sestamibi imaging after thyroid suppression. Surgery 2002;132(6):968–74.

47. Friedman K, Somervell H, Patel P, et al. Effect of calcium channel blockers on the sensitivity of preoperative 99mTc-MIBI SPECT for hyperparathyroidism. Surgery 2004;136(6):1199–204.

48. Gupta Y, Ahmed R, Happerfield L, et al. P-glycoprotein expression is associated with sestamibi washout in primary hyperparathyroidism. Br J Surg 2007;94(12): 1491–5.

49. Pons F, Torregrosa JV, Fuster D. Biological factors influencing parathyroid localization. Nucl Med Commun 2003;24(2):121–4.

50. Yamaguchi S, Yachiku S, Hashimoto H, et al. Relation between technetium 99m-methoxyisobutylisonitrile accumulation and multidrug resistance protein in the parathyroid glands. World J Surg 2002;26(1):29–34.

51. Melton GB, Somervell H, Friedman KP, et al. Interpretation of 99mTc sestamibi parathyroid SPECT scan is improved when read by the surgeon and nuclear medicine physician together. Nucl Med Commun 2005;26(7):633–8.

52. Gough I. Reoperative parathyroid surgery: the importance of ectopic location and multigland disease. ANZ J Surg 2006;76(12):1048–50.

53. Liew V, Gough IR, Nolan G, et al. Re-operation for hyperparathyroidism. ANZ J Surg 2004;74(9):732–40.

54. Rodriquez JM, Tezelman S, Siperstein AE, et al. Localization procedures in patients with persistent or recurrent hyperparathyroidism. Arch Surg 1994; 129(8):870–5.

55. Jaskowiak NT, Sugg SL, Helke J, et al. Pitfalls of intraoperative quick parathyroid hormone monitoring and gamma probe localization in surgery for primary hyperparathyroidism. Arch Surg 2002;137(6):659–68.

56. Chou FF, Lee CH, Chen HY, et al. Persistent and recurrent hyperparathyroidism after total parathyroidectomy with autotransplantation. Ann Surg 2002;235(1): 99–104.

57. Weber CJ, Sewell CW, McGarity WC. Persistent and recurrent sporadic primary hyperparathyroidism: histopathology, complications, and results of reoperation. Surgery 1994;116(6):991–8.

58. Itoh K, Ishizuka R. Tc-99m-MIBI scintigraphy for recurrent hyperparathyroidism after total parathyroidectomy with autograft. Ann Nucl Med 2003;17(4):315–20.

59. Bozkurt MF, Ugur O, Hamaloglu E, et al. Optimization of the gamma probe-guided parathyroidectomy. Am Surg 2003;69(8):720–5.

60. Casara D, Rubello D, Piotto A, et al. 99mTc-MIBI radio-guided minimally invasive parathyroid surgery planned on the basis of a preoperative combined 99mTc-pertechnetate/99mTc-MIBI and ultrasound imaging protocol. Eur J Nucl Med 2000;27(9):1300–4.

61. Casara D, Rubello D, Cauzzo C, et al. 99mTc-MIBI radio-guided minimally invasive parathyroidectomy: experience with patients with normal thyroids and nodular goiters. Thyroid 2002;12(1):53–61.

62. Rubello D, Pelizzo MR, Boni G, et al. Radioguided surgery of primary hyperparathyroidism using the low-dose 99mTc-sestamibi protocol: multiinstitutional

experience from the Italian Study Group on Radioguided Surgery and Immuno-scintigraphy (GISCRIS). J Nucl Med 2005;46(2):220–6.

63. Rubello D, Giannini S, Martini C, et al. Minimally invasive radio-guided parathy-roidectomy. Biomed Pharmacother 2006;60(3):134–8.

64. Mariani G, Gulec SA, Rubello D, et al. Preoperative localization and radioguided parathyroid surgery. J Nucl Med 2003;44(9):1443–58.

65. Murphy C, Norman J. The 20% rule: a simple, instantaneous radioactivity measurement defines cure and allows elimination of frozen sections and hormone assays during parathyroidectomy. Surgery 1999;126(6):1023–8.

66. Chen H, Mack E, Starling JR. Radioguided parathyroidectomy is equally effective for both adenomatous and hyperplastic glands. Ann Surg 2003;238(3):332–7.

67. McGreal G, Winter DC, Sookhai S, et al. Minimally invasive, radioguided surgery for primary hyperparathyroidism. Ann Surg Oncol 2001;8(10):856–60.

68. Perrier ND, Ituarte PH, Morita E, et al. Parathyroid surgery: separating promise from reality. J Clin Endocrinol Metab 2002;87(3):1024–9.

69. Chen H, Sippel RS, Schaefer S. The effectiveness of radioguided parathyroidec-tomy in patients with negative technetium tc 99m-sestamibi scans. Arch Surg 2009;144(7):643–8.

70. Ahuja AT, Wong KT, Ching AS, et al. Imaging for primary hyperparathyroidism—what beginners should know. Clin Radiol 2004;59(11):967–76.

71. Hindie E, Ugur O, Fuster D, et al. 2009 EANM parathyroid guidelines. Eur J Nucl Med Mol Imaging 2009;36(7):1201–16.

72. Tublin ME, Pryma DA, Yim JH, et al. Localization of parathyroid adenomas by sonography and technetium tc 99m sestamibi single-photon emission computed tomography before minimally invasive parathyroidectomy: are both studies really needed? J Ultrasound Med 2009;28(2):183–90.

73. De Feo ML, Colagrande S, Biagini C, et al. Parathyroid glands: combination of (99m)Tc MIBI scintigraphy and US for demonstration of parathyroid glands and nodules. Radiology 2000;214(2):393–402.

74. Loney EL, Dick EA, Francis IS, et al. Localization of parathyroid nodules. Radi-ology 2001;218(3):916–7.

75. Shah S, Win Z, Al-Nahhas A. Multimodality imaging of the parathyroid glands in primary hyperparathyroidism. Minerva Endocrinol 2008;33(3):193–202.

76. Sukan A, Reyhan M, Aydin M, et al. Preoperative evaluation of hyperparathy-roidism: the role of dual-phase parathyroid scintigraphy and ultrasound imaging. Ann Nucl Med 2008;22(2):123–31.

77. Dobrinja C, Trevisan G, Liguori G. Minimally invasive video-assisted parathyroid-ectomy. Initial experience in a general surgery department. J Endocrinol Invest 2009;32(2):130–3.

78. Richard B. [Primary hyperparathyroidism: ultrasonography and scintigraphy]. J Radiol 2009;90(3 Pt 2):397–408 [in French].

79. Auffermann W, Guis M, Tavares NJ, et al. MR signal intensity of parathyroid adenomas: correlation with histopathology. AJR Am J Roentgenol 1989;153(4):873–6.

80. Kabala JE. Computed tomography and magnetic resonance imaging in diseases of the thyroid and parathyroid. Eur J Radiol 2008;66(3):480–92.

81. Seelos KC, DeMarco R, Clark OH, et al. Persistent and recurrent hyperparathy-roidism: assessment with gadopentetate dimeglumine-enhanced MR imaging. Radiology 1990;177(2):373–8.

82. Wakamatsu H, Noguchi S, Yamashita H, et al. Parathyroid scintigraphy with 99mTc-MIBI and 123I subtraction: a comparison with magnetic resonance imaging and ultrasonography. Nucl Med Commun 2003;24(7):755–62.

83. Ruf J, Lopez HE, Steinmuller T, et al. Preoperative localization of parathyroid glands. Use of MRI, scintigraphy, and image fusion. Nuklearmedizin 2004; 43(3):85–90.
84. Harari A, Zarnegar R, Lee J, et al. Computed tomography can guide focused exploration in select patients with primary hyperparathyroidism and negative sestamibi scanning. Surgery 2008;144(6):970–6.
85. Randall GJ, Zald PB, Cohen JI, et al. Contrast-enhanced MDCT characteristics of parathyroid adenomas. AJR Am J Roentgenol 2009;193(2):W139–43.
86. Rotstein L, Irish J, Gullane P, et al. Reoperative parathyroidectomy in the era of localization technology. Head Neck 1998;20(6):535–9.
87. Ernst O. [Hyperparathyroidism: CT and MR findings]. J Radiol 2009;90(3 Pt 2): 409–12 [in French].
88. Neumann DR, Esselstyn CB Jr, MacIntyre WJ, et al. Primary hyperparathyroidism: preoperative parathyroid imaging with regional body FDG PET. Radiology 1994; 192(2):509–12.
89. Neumann DR, Esselstyn CB, MacIntyre WJ, et al. Comparison of FDG-PET and sestamibi-SPECT in primary hyperparathyroidism. J Nucl Med 1996;37(11): 1809–15.
90. Beggs AD, Hain SF. Localization of parathyroid adenomas using 11C-methionine positron emission tomography. Nucl Med Commun 2005;26(2):133–6.
91. Cook GJ, Wong JC, Smellie WJ, et al. [11C]Methionine positron emission tomography for patients with persistent or recurrent hyperparathyroidism after surgery. Eur J Endocrinol 1998;139(2):195–7.
92. Sundin A, Johansson C, Hellman P, et al. PET and parathyroid L-[carbon-11]methionine accumulation in hyperparathyroidism. J Nucl Med 1996;37(11): 1766–70.
93. Otto D, Boerner AR, Hofmann M, et al. Pre-operative localisation of hyperfunctional parathyroid tissue with 11C-methionine PET. Eur J Nucl Med Mol Imaging 2004;31(10):1405–12.
94. Rubello D, Fanti S, Nanni C, et al. 11C-methionine PET/CT in 99mTc-sestamibi-negative hyperparathyroidism in patients with renal failure on chronic haemodialysis. Eur J Nucl Med Mol Imaging 2006;33(4):453–9.

Primary Hyperparathyroidism

Erin A. Felger, MD[a],*, Emad Kandil, MD[b]

KEYWORDS

- Hypercalcemia • Hyperparathyroidism
- Asymptomatic hyperparathyroidism • Sestamibi
- Reoperative parathyroid surgery

Primary hyperparathyroidism (PHPT) has been recognized as a disease process since the 1920s when it was discovered in both Europe and the United States.[1] In 1925, the first parathyroid surgery was performed by Felix Mandl in Vienna, Austria, who showed that by removing the affected gland, the patient had resolution of severe symptoms associated with the disease.[2,3] The first successful parathyroid surgery in the United States was performed by Dr Isaac Olch in 1928 at Barnes Hospital in St Louis.[4] Since that time, the recognition, diagnosis, and treatment of PHPT have evolved because of improved laboratory testing, accurate preoperative localization, and less invasive surgical procedures.

The prevalence of PHPT is in the range of 0.1% to 0.4%, and the incidence increases with age reaching a peak between age 50 and 60 years.[1,5–7] After the introduction of automated serum calcium measurements in the 1970s, the prevalence increased significantly and has since leveled out.[1,5] PHPT has a higher frequency in women and in patients who have a history of neck irradiation.[8–10] Over the last few decades, patients are presenting less frequently with overt or classical symptoms of the disease and more often with vague symptoms, which has prompted the National Institutes of Health (NIH) to publish guidelines for the management of asymptomatic PHPT.[5,11] Once a diagnosis is made and the patient is deemed an appropriate surgical candidate, preoperative localization of the involved gland or glands aids in the choice of operation. With the advent of intraoperative PTH (IOPTH) in addition to prelocalization, minimally invasive techniques for parathyroidectomy have become more popular.

PATHOLOGY AND ETIOLOGY

PHPT is the third most common endocrine disorder and the most common cause of hypercalcemia in the outpatient setting.[5,7] It is defined as hypercalcemia secondary to

[a] Department of Surgery, Washington Hospital Center, 110 Irving Street NW, Room G-247D, Washington, DC 20010, USA
[b] Department of Surgery, Tulane Medical Center, 1430 Tulane Avenue, SL22, New Orleans, LA 70112, USA
* Corresponding author.
E-mail address: erin.a.felger@medstar.net

Otolaryngol Clin N Am 43 (2010) 417–432
doi:10.1016/j.otc.2010.01.009
0030-6665/10/$ – see front matter © 2010 Elsevier Inc. All rights reserved.

overproduction of PTH by one or more parathyroid glands. Normally, increased calcium levels suppress the production of PTH because of a negative feedback mechanism.[7,8] Parathyroid glands detect small changes in serum calcium through the calcium sensing receptor, which results in significant changes in PTH secretion. The goal of this pathway is to normalize serum calcium.[1,8,12] In PHPT, however, the feedback mechanism does not work appropriately so that unregulated PTH production results from elevated serum calcium.[12,13] The effects of this altered feedback loop include increased or inappropriate PTH production, increased renal absorption of calcium, increased synthesis of $1,25(OH)_2D_3$, phosphaturia, and increased resorption of bone.[5]

In patients who present with hypercalcemia and elevated PTH, it is essential to exclude other causes of elevated calcium including chronic renal disease, thiazide diuretic use, lithium use, and familial hypocalciuric hypercalcemia (FHH).[7,8] Once these factors have been ruled out, the next step is to determine the etiology of the patient's PHPT. Most cases are sporadic; however, approximately 5% of cases are familial. Patients can present with single or double adenomas, multigland disease (MGD), or rarely parathyroid cancer. Several studies have shown that most patients have a single adenoma (80%–85%). MGD occurs less frequently (10%–15%) and double adenomas are even more rare (4%–5%). Parathyroid cancer is diagnosed in less than 1% of patients with HPT.[8,14]

Familial syndromes with a PHPT component include multiple endocrine neoplasia (MEN) I, MEN IIA, hyperparathyroidism–jaw tumor syndrome, and neonatal severe PHPT. Prevalence of PHPT and its clinical features differ among the various inherited syndromes.[15–17]

MEN I is an autosomal-dominant disorder caused by an inactivating mutation of the menin gene on chromosome 11q13 with a high penetrance for PHPT, which is usually the initial presentation of the disease (**Box 1**).[17] Approximately 90% to 95% of patients with MEN I develop PHPT, which often presents at a younger age in this population and may be the only manifestation of the syndrome.[18] PHPT presents as MGD most of the time, necessitating a subtotal or total parathyroidectomy with autotransplantation.[15,16] Patients can also have pituitary tumors and pancreatic tumors.

MEN IIA is an autosomal-dominant disorder caused by activating mutations involving the RET proto-oncogene.[15,16] Only 20% to 30% of patients with this disorder have PHPT, which tends to be mild in its course. Patients display single gland disease or MGD, which usually does not require an aggressive surgical approach.[16] MEN IIA patients usually present with medullary thyroid cancer and pheochromocytoma, which can be life threatening. It is imperative to rule out a pheochromocytoma before parathyroidectomy or any invasive procedure.[16]

Hyperparathyroidism–jaw tumor syndrome is another autosomal-dominant disorder caused by an inactivating mutation of HRPT2.[16,18] PHPT is the most common feature of the syndrome and these patients have an increased risk of parathyroid cancer. PHPT presents at an early age as single gland or multigland involvement.[15,16] Surgical options for these patients vary. If parathyroid cancer is present an en bloc resection is required. If cancer is not suspected, all four parathyroid glands should be identified to ensure there is no abnormal-appearing parathyroid tissue. These patients also develop fibro-osseus tumors of the mandible or maxilla and they may have renal pathology.[15,18]

Neonatal severe PHPT is caused by homozygous inactivating mutations of the calcium sensing receptor and can be fatal if not treated immediately with a total parathyroidectomy.[15]

Parathyroid cancer is an extremely rare cause of PHPT accounting for less than 1% of all cases. It is difficult to diagnose preoperatively because there are no definitive

---

Box 1
Association of PHPT with MEN syndromes

MEN I

   Hyperparathyroidism

   Pituitary tumor

   Pancreatic gastrinoma

MEN IIA

   Medullary thyroid carcinoma

   Pheochromocytoma

   Hyperparathyroidism

   Lichen planus amyloidosis

   Hirschsprung disease

MEN IIB

   Medullary thyroid carcinoma

   Pheochromocytoma

   Marfanoid body habitus

   Mucosal neuromas

   Ganglioneuromatosis of the gastrointestinal tract

---

cytologic criteria.[7] These patients present with severe symptomatic hypercalcemia and require hospitalization to correct the high levels of serum calcium; they also have markedly elevated intact PTH levels. Rarely, a palpable neck mass may be found on physical examination, but more often the disease is identified intraoperatively.[10,19] Characteristics of a cancerous parathyroid gland include adherence to and invasion into surrounding tissues including the thyroid and involvement of blood vessels and the recurrent laryngeal nerve (RLN).[5,7] The gland is usually white-gray in color and very firm. En bloc resection of the parathyroid, ipsilateral thyroid lobe, and any adherent or suspicious-appearing soft tissue in the central neck including lymph nodes is the best surgical option for these patients.[19] Postoperatively, a metastatic work-up including CT of the chest and abdomen should be completed. The 5-year survival rate for this cancer is 86%.[10,19]

PRESENTATION AND DIAGNOSIS

Over the last 30 years, a shift has occurred in the presentation of PHPT. Historically, patients presented with clinical findings related to long-standing disease, such as nephrolithiasis, brown tumors, osteitis fibrosa cystic, and muscle atrophy.[1] With the advent of routine serum calcium measurements, patients present with hypercalcemia much earlier and subsequently have fewer, if any, overt symptoms. Up to 80% of patients have been described as asymptomatic; however, many studies have shown these patients actually have vague symptoms that are more difficult to qualify.[6] In one study, there was some benefit to doing neuropsychological testing and evaluation of health-related quality of life to determine the need for surgery in patients with biochemically diagnosed PHPT.[20] Some of these nonspecific symptoms include fatigue, weakness, bony pain, depression, memory loss, decreased concentration, and sleep issues.[1,10] Many patients who do not complain of symptoms before surgery report significant improvement postoperatively, implying that these subtle symptoms are meaningful in terms of patient well-being.[6]

Interestingly, nephrolithiasis is the most common clinical manifestation of PHPT, occurring in 20% of patients presenting with the disease.[1] These patients are often followed for years before they are diagnosed with PHPT because hypercalcemia is not considered as a cause of kidney stones.[21] They are often not diagnosed with PHPT until they have another manifestation of the disease.

Subtle changes on bone densitometry are noted in patients with PHPT. Bone integrity is altered by high bone turnover because of increased PTH resulting in osteopenia, osteoporosis, and increases risk of fracture.[1,8,21] Primarily cortical and cancellous bone loss is seen. Postoperatively, bone loss is often stalled or improved with increased bone density over time.[10]

Various cardiovascular conditions are associated with PHPT including hypertension, valvular calcifications, left ventricular hypertrophy, and cardiovascular mortality.[1,22] Surgery does not affect hypertension in these patients so that most remain on their antihypertensive medication postoperatively.[22] The risk of cardiovascular mortality decreases in patients with severe PHPT who have parathyroidectomy. Unfortunately, studies on cardiovascular mortality in patients with mild PHPT are limited and inconclusive.[22]

The diagnosis of PHPT is usually made biochemically with elevated serum calcium and elevated PTH.[7] Some patients present with normocalcemia, which is within the continuum of the disease. Patients can also have PTH values within the reference range, which reflects an inappropriate response to hypercalcemia. Vitamin D levels should be checked initially in all patients with a diagnosis of PHPT because the presence of vitamin D deficiency can affect the interpretation of the PTH assay resulting in elevated PTH levels.[23] Patients who have vitamin D deficiency should be repleted before diagnosing PHPT.

Other laboratory tests that are useful in making the diagnosis include phosphorous, creatinine clearance, and 24-hour urine calcium level.[1,11] Although a 24-hour urine calcium level is no longer required per the NIH Guidelines for all patients, it is important to have when there is a concern for FHH (**Box 2**). Prior family history is very helpful when FHH is suspected.[8] In this case, urine calcium levels less than 100 make the diagnosis and prevent unnecessary surgery.

Bone densitometry is recommended to measure the effect of hypercalcemia on the bones.[1] A bone density T-score of -2.5 or less at any site in perimenopausal and postmenopausal women and men greater than 50 years old or a Z-score of -2.5 or less in premenopausal women and men less than 50 years old are diagnostic for bone loss resulting in osteopenia or in more advanced cases osteoporosis.[22]

Box 2
NIH guidelines (2008) for surgical treatment of asymptomatic PHPT

- Serum Ca >1 mg/dL above upper limit of normal
- Creatinine clearance <30% of age-matched normal subjects
- Diminished bone density (T score <−2.5) or fragility fracture
- Age <50 years
- Difficult periodic follow-up

Indications for surgery include patients with a biochemical diagnosis of PHPT and overt clinical signs or symptoms, such as kidney stones, decreased bone density, prior fracture, or brown tumors.[11] For patients who have a biochemical diagnosis but are asymptomatic, the NIH has developed a set of guidelines, which were modified in 2008 (see **Box 2**). A 24-hour urine calcium level is no longer indicated per the new guidelines.[11] As previously discussed, patients who have vague symptoms and a biochemical diagnosis should also be strongly considered for surgery. Several studies report overall improvement especially in neurocognitive symptoms and better quality of life for these patients after parathyroidectomy.[6,20,24,25]

Imaging

Preoperative localization of abnormal parathyroid glands has become very important in the era of minimally invasive parathyroid (MIP) surgery. The two most common imaging modalities are ultrasonography and ^{99m}Tc-sestamibi scintigraphy. When these two modalities are used together, the accuracy of localizing the suspect gland increases. CT and MRI are less used but are useful in patients with failed parathyroidectomy or persistent HPT to identify ectopic glands (**Table 1**).[26]

High-resolution ultrasound is a useful modality to locate enlarged parathyroid glands in the neck. Normal parathyroids, which average $5 \times 3 \times 1$ mm in size are usually not visualized on ultrasound.[26,27] One of the benefits of cervical ultrasound is the ability to study the thyroid gland concurrently for any abnormalities. Because MIP surgery limits the surgeon's ability to palpate or visualize the thyroid intraoperatively, sonography is an invaluable preoperative tool.[28] Eighteen percent of patients with PHPT have synchronous thyroid disease with an overall malignancy rate of 2%.[29] Ultrasound is also beneficial because it is inexpensive, it does not use ionizing radiation, and it has a sensitivity in the range of 72% to 85%.[26,27] One downside of ultrasonography is the difficulty in finding glands located in the mediastinum, the retroesophageal space, and other ectopic locations. It is also less helpful in patients who have a multinodular goiter or minimally enlarged parathyroid glands.[27]

On ultrasound, a parathyroid adenoma is hypoechoic, homogenous, and solid with a bean-shaped or oval appearance (**Fig. 1**). There is usually a small branch from the inferior thyroid artery, which enters the gland at one of its poles. It is difficult to distinguish both thyroid nodules and cervical lymph nodes from parathyroid glands, which decreases the accuracy of this modality when used without other imaging.[26,27]

^{99m}Tc-sestamibi is taken up by both parathyroid and thyroid tissue making it a logical choice for preoperative localization in patients with HPT. Adenomatous and hyperplastic parathyorids have more avid and more prolonged uptake than the thyroid tissue.[26] After injection of the radiotracer, one set of images is taken within 15 minutes and then a delayed set is taken at 2 hours. Asymmetry of uptake can be noted on early images, but usually, the delayed images are necessary to locate the focus of radiotracer, which characterizes hyperfunctioning parathyroid (**Figs. 2** and **3**).[26]

Single-photon emission CT (SPECT) can help differentiate parathyroid tissue from thyroid tissue increasing the sensitivity of scintigraphy. For solitary adenomas, there is a sensitivity of 87% when using SPECT. Its sensitivity decreases with double

Table 1				
Positive predictive values for various preoperative diagnostic modalities				
% Ultrasound	% Sestamibi	% CT	% MRI	% Positron Emission Tomography
60–92	78–100	36–100	51–100	70–74

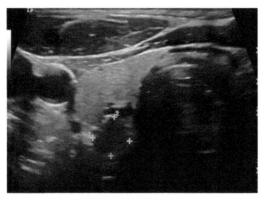

Fig. 1. Ultrasound demonstration of a parathyroid adenoma.

adenomas (30%) and MGD (44%).[26] A hybrid of SPECT and CT used for the early images has also been shown to enhance the accuracy of localization when combined with various delayed imaging methods, particularly dual-phase imaging, which is better than single-phase imaging.[30]

The combination of ultrasound and [99m]TC-sestamibi scintigraphy to localize parathyroid adenomas preoperatively increases the sensitivity to 95% because each modality contributes different data to help determine the gland location.[26] Ultrasonography is more specific for anatomic location of the gland in relation to the thyroid, whereas scintigraphy is better at finding ectopic glands especially in the mediastinum.[26] For double adenomas and MGD, the sensitivity continues to be lower even when these modalities are combined.

For patients with persistent disease, CT with thin cuts from the skull base through the chest can identify contrast-enhanced parathyroid tissue with a sensitivity ranging from 46% to 87%.[26] CT is particularly useful in patients who have altered anatomy or a failed parathyroidectomy (**Fig. 4**). MRIs, which are rarely done, can also identify abnormal parathyroid tissue and are used in patients with recurrent or persistent disease.[26]

IOPTH

PTH is an 84 amino acid peptide hormone produced by the parathyroid glands. PTH first is synthesized as a preproparathyroid hormone with 155 amino acids, and after cleavage of a 25 amino acid sequence and a 6 amino acid sequence, it is converted to intact PTH, an 84 amino acid hormone.[31] Intact PTH has a half-life of less than 5 minutes with most of its metabolism in the liver and the remainder in the kidney. Intact PTH assays detect 1-84 PTH and large c-terminal fragments, which can alter PTH values.[18] Biointact and whole PTH assays use an antibody that is specific for the complete molecule, 1-84 PTH, minimizing the possibility of amino acid fragments from affecting PTH values. These assays are second- and third-generation assays, which have similar sensitivities in diagnosing PHPT.[18,32] Various second- and third-generation assays are available, and they use similar types of analyses with comparable turnaround times between 10 and 15 minutes.[15,31] The QuiCk Intraoperative Bio-Intact PTH Assay By Nichol Institute Diagnostics (now out of business) was first used in 1996, and today there are several commercial IOPTH assays available.[31,33]

IOPTH is used to determine the adequacy of resection of parathyroid tissue to prevent operative failures secondary to missed MGD.[4,34,35] IOPTH levels predict postoperative calcium levels because of the dynamic change in hormone following resection of all

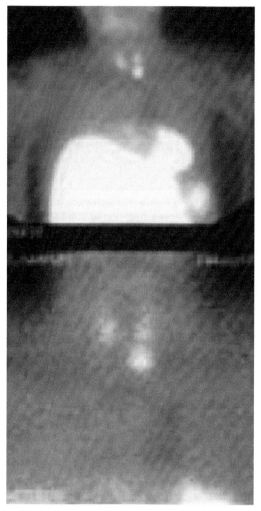

Fig. 2. Sestamibi scan demonstrating radiotracer uptake in the left inferior thyroid bed for a patient with PHPT.

hypersecreting glands. When levels remain elevated after excision of suspected gland, conversion to a bilateral neck exploration (BNE) from a unilateral neck exploration (UNE) may be necessary to locate the remaining hypersecreting tissue.[35]

IOPTH is measured according to a set of criteria first developed in Miami and subsequent modifications of these criteria have been developed by other surgeons.[36] The premise of the Miami criteria is a 50% or greater drop from the highest PTH level drawn to the PTH level measured 10 minutes after gland excision. Specifically, a pre-incision PTH level is drawn and a pre-excision level because of the possibility of gland manipulation with a further increase in PTH from the original baseline value.[34] Because multiple PTH levels are required throughout the procedure, good peripheral access should be obtained preoperatively. Using the Miami criteria, IPOTH has an overall accuracy of 97% even when compared with other IOPTH criteria. Its success is

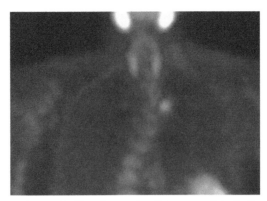

Fig. 3. Sestamibi scan demonstrating aberrant radiotracer uptake in the left superior anterior mediastinum of a persistent primary hyperparathyroid patient. Note the physiologic uptake of radiotracer by normal salivary glands.

caused by fewer false-positive results, which translates to a decrease in operative failures.[36]

Successful parathyroid surgery is determined by both postoperative calcium levels and calcium levels at 6 months that are within normal limits.[34] Using IOPTH in conjunction with preoperative localization facilitates the ability to perform minimally invasive surgery in an ambulatory surgery setting with improved success intraoperatively, decreased costs perioperatively, and increased patient satisfaction postoperatively.[4,31,37]

SURGICAL OPTIONS

Traditionally, parathyroid surgery involved a BNE and identification of all parathyroids before removal of the abnormal gland or glands. With the advent of both improved preoperative localization studies and IOPTH, MIP surgery has emerged as the new standard for most surgeons worldwide.[38] There are several types of MIP surgery based on the size of incision and use of endoscopy. A UNE uses a standard Kocher incision toward the side of the localized gland, and BNE is not done unless the gland cannot be located.[39] UNE has a shorter operative time than BNE with equivalent

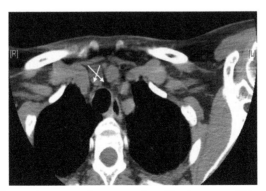

Fig. 4. Contrast CT scan demonstrating a parathyroid adenoma within the thymus, in the anterior mediastinum, of a remedial one-degree HPT patient (*crossed arrows*).

success. Both in UNE and other types of MIP procedures, care must be taken not to rupture the gland on extraction because of the risk of cell spillage and subsequent parathyromatosis.[2]

Another type of MIP surgery involves making a smaller or more focused incision in the central or lateral neck with the premise of doing a directed procedure.[39,40] It has a 97% success rate with minimal morbidity and no procedure-specific complications. Some surgeons believe that the incision for a true MIP procedure cannot exceed 2.5 cm in length.[40] This operation can be performed under general anesthesia, with a cervical block or with local anesthetic and sedation. Preoperative localization is critical in this situation because most of the neck is not explored given the focused nature of the procedure.[39,40] If the gland is not located, the incision should be extended to explore the rest of the neck.

Radioguided surgery using ^{99m}Tc-sestamibi and a gamma probe intraoperatively is advocated by some surgeons.[39,41] A positive sestamibi scan is obtained preoperatively for localization. On the day of surgery the patient receives an injection of ^{99m}Tc-sestamibi approximately 2 hours before surgery. Before making an incision the gamma probe is used to mark the area of uptake potentially by the affected gland.[39,41,42] A small incision is made over this area, and the gland is removed. Background counts are done and a count on the excised gland. With a success rate ranging from 77% to 100% in the literature, this method is not widely used because many surgeons do not find it beneficial.[42]

Endoscopy also plays a role in MIP surgery including a complete endoscopic approach and a video-assisted approach. In a complete endoscopic operation, a minimum of three small port incisions are made and gas insufflation is used to visualize the cervical region, especially the superior pole area.[39,43] In most cases, the dissection is done through a lateral approach and the gland is usually removed through a separate incision.[39,43] Complications specific to this procedure include hypercarbia postoperatively and extensive subcutaneous emphysema, which usually resolves within a few days.[39,43]

In the video-assisted approach, gas insufflation is not necessary because dissection is accomplished using the scope for magnification and instrumentation, such as spatulas that are amenable to small work spaces.[41,44] A 1.5-cm midline incision is made and minimal dissection is performed without elevation of subplatysmal flaps to separate the strap muscles in the midline. After retractors are placed to optimize the small workspace, a 5-mm 30-degree laparoscope is used to visualize the thyroid and other pertinent structures in the neck.[41,45] Once the gland is identified and its arterial supply is ligated, it is removed through the midline incision. Patient selection is an important aspect of this operation just as it also is for the complete endoscopic method. Physical characteristics, such as obesity or an enlarged thyroid gland, are not optimal and having a nonlocalizing study also presents a challenge for this procedure. A video-assisted approach is not recommended for reoperative surgery or for patients with MGD.[41,44,45] Contraindications for videoscopic parathyroidectomy in patients with PHPT include previous cervical surgery, inconclusive preoperative localization, local anesthesia, associated large goiter, and cervical hematoma.

Complications for all of these procedures include persistent hyperparathyroidism, RLN injury, and transient postoperative hypocalcemia.[40,44,46] Adjuncts used to minimize these complications include accurate preoperative localization as previously discussed, intraoperative nerve monitoring, frozen section, and postoperative oral calcium supplementation.[42]

The gold standard for prevention of RLN injury continues to be direct visualization and identification of the nerve.[47] Intraoperative nerve monitoring is used by many surgeons as an additional method for ensuring RLN continuity.[48] Often the nerve is not visualized in MIP surgery because of the location of the parathyroid; one of the benefits of using a scope in these cases is its magnification, which allows easier visualization of the nerve usually with minimal dissection.[41,44] The nerve monitor should be used to document a complete circuit exists after the nerve has been identified; however, there is no evidence to show that it is beneficial in first-time parathyroid surgery where rates of RLN injury are typically less than 1%.[42]

Frozen section in parathyroid surgery is used to differentiate parathyroid tissue from nonparathyroid tissue. Although frozen section is very accurate, it can still be misinterpreted leading to erroneous results and the need for further surgery.[42] IOPTH assay of the tissue aspirate can also be evaluated with reasonable success to determine whether or not the specimen is a parathyroid.[42,49] Both of these methods are helpful when there is a question of a nodule being parathyroid or some other type of tissue. Frozen section should not be used routinely because most parathyroids can be identified by their appearance, consistency, and location in the neck.[42]

Although no protocol exists for calcium supplementation following parathyroid surgery, most surgeons place their patients on some type of oral calcium regimen, which can be weaned over the course of a few weeks.[40,41,44] Placing patients on postoperative oral calcium is especially important when patients are having a MIP procedure and often going home the same day. Approximately 10% of the patients have transient hypocalcemia after removal of a large gland or glands, and it is more challenging to monitor serum calcium levels when they are not hospitalized.[46] If these patients are discharged without a calcium regimen, they often have complaints associated with hypocalcemia, such as perioral and extremity numbness and tingling, which usually stops after oral calcium is begun.

MIP surgery is a feasible, efficacious alternative to the traditional BNE. Although the rates of success are similar between the two approaches, 95% versus 97% respectively, MIP surgery offers a more cosmetic result, less postoperative pain, decreased hospital stays, and lower overall cost compared with BNE.[40,44,45] Operative times for MIP procedures including video-assisted parathyroidectomy are shorter than for BNE.[2,45] Patient satisfaction is also higher after a MIP procedure because of the smaller scar and decreased pain.[40,44]

PERSISTENT AND RECURRENT PHPT

Cure of PHPT is most readily achieved during initial neck exploration. Unfortunately, a subset of patients requires re-exploration for persistent or recurrent disease. Neck re-exploration is technically difficult because of distortion of neck anatomy by fibrosis and frequently obliterated normal tissue planes. Accordingly, reoperative surgery relative to de novo cases carries an increased risk of injury to RLNs and to normal residual parathyroid tissue. Pathologic hyperfunctioning parathyroid tissue is also more frequently ectopic in the reoperative setting and can be difficult to localize. Nonetheless, excision of culprit hyperfunctioning parathyroid tissue continues to be the standard of care for these challenging scenarios.

DIAGNOSTIC APPROACH

Recurrent disease is defined as redevelopment of PHPT more than 6 months after initial curative surgery. Between 1% and 6% of one-degree HPT patients experience persistent disease or develop a recurrence after initial resection.[50] Accordingly, all patients require confirmation of cure following initial exploration.[51]

Initial postoperative serum iPTH levels are commonly elevated in the context of low calcium following curative resection. This is usually a postoperative normal physiologic response caused by relative hypocalcemia and is usually self-limited.[52] In contrast, persistent disease is defined as persistent postoperative elevation of iPTH, in association of rising serum calcium levels. Measurement of a 24-hour urine calcium level can also be helpful, because a value of less than 30 mg is suggestive of FHH, a mild hypercalcemic condition that rarely requires surgical intervention.

INDICATIONS FOR SURGICAL RE-EXPLORATION

Surgical intervention for PHPT in patients with no previous surgical intervention affords a cure rate greater than 95%. There are no data specifically addressing the efficacy of surgical versus nonsurgical interventions for recurrent or persistent asymptomatic disease, however, and it is reasonable to consider similar guidelines when assessing asymptomatic patients with persistent or recurrent disease for surgical referral.

PREOPERATIVE EVALUATION

A careful preoperative assessment is required to optimize outcomes for these challenging patients. A thorough history and physical examination, including laryngoscopic vocal cord evaluation and biochemical verification of PHPT, should be considered in preoperative evaluation. The risk of increased morbidity associated with re-exploration should be discussed with the patient. Asymptomatic patients with persistent or recurrent disease referred for surgical evaluation who have borderline elevation of iPTH and calcium levels may be followed clinically, with operative intervention offered for disease progression. Ectopic parathyroid tissue and supernumerary parathyroid glands are more common and present in as many as 53% of reoperative cases.[53] Preoperative localization imaging assists the surgeon in minimizing the extent and morbidity of re-exploration.

Initial preoperative imaging should be noninvasive and relatively inexpensive, reserving invasive and costly techniques for cases of initial nonlocalizing imaging modalities. The most commonly used studies are ultrasound and sestamibi scans, both of which are inexpensive and readily available. The sensitivity of sestamibi scans can be dramatically enhanced by coimaging with SPECT scanning, which allows three-dimensional localization of parathyroid lesions.[54]

CT scanning and MRI can be also used. They can be useful in localizing ectopic mediastinal lesion that would otherwise be undetectable by ultrasound. Positron emission tomography, which is often combined with CT scanning, is more expensive. In addition, background thyroid signal intensity limits the sensitivity of positron emission tomography for localizing perithyroidal disease. Assessment of PTH levels in parathyroid lesions using fine-needle aspirates under ultrasound guidance can also be used with reported 87% sensitivity and 74% specificity.[55]

Finally, selective arteriography and venous sampling for PTH is an invasive imaging modality that can be used with reported 84% sensitivity and 88% specificity. This technique is expensive, requires considerable technical expertise, and can be associated with groin hematomas and vascular injury. It should be reserved for cases in which other imaging studies fail to localize the culprit for the disease persistence or recurrence.

Recent advances in preoperative localization have led to significant improvements in outcomes after reoperative surgery. It is prudent, however, to reassess the operative indications in patients with persistent negative localization studies to determine if they can be maintained without surgery.

OPERATIVE TECHNIQUES

Hyperfunctioning parathyroid tissue in reoperative PHPT can be usually resected by a cervical incision. Medial approach is the standard approach for exploration, which attempts to use the operative planes explored during the patient's initial surgery. Lateral approach, dissecting the plane between the strap muscles and the sternocleidomastoid muscle, allows avoidance of scarred tissues from previous exploration and allows posterior access to the thyroid bed.[56] Medial approach, however, allows for bilateral cervical exploration.

Most mediastinal disease is accessible by a cervical approach because the culprit is either retroesophageal or intrathymic. Median sternotomy, partial sternal split, or video-assisted thoracic approach, however, may be required.[57]

Intraoperative Adjuncts

Gamma probe detection of radiolabeled sestamibi has been used; however, it has not gained wide acceptance because background signal from normal tissues interferes with directed dissection.[58] A rapid IOPTH assay is reported to be the most useful adjunct in reoperative surgery. The operative definition of a successful resection is at least a 50% fall from the initial baseline and a final value within the normal reference range. Continuous intraoperative electromyographic monitoring of RLN function is recommended to avoid the risk of RLN injury during re-exploration.

Ethanol Ablation

Ultrasound-guided ethanol ablation of culprit parathyroid tissue has been proposed; however, it has a very low cure rate relative to surgical re-exploration. Additionally, RLN injury has been reported. It should be reserved for cases in which surgery cannot be safely performed (Harman, 1998).[59]

POSTOPERATIVE CARE

Cure rates following surgical re-exploration are between 94% and 96% with low complication rates in cases performed by experienced surgeons (Hessman, 2008).[60] These patients require careful postoperative care, however, because they are at risk for RLN injury and postoperative hypocalcemia.

Reoperative surgery for patients with recurrent or persistent PHPT remains a significant challenge. If persistent or recurrent disease is biochemically confirmed, thorough assessment should be carefully performed. Additional new work-up includes a detailed history and physical examination, repeat laryngoscopic evaluation, and preoperative localization studies. Given the increased risk of complications with each repeat cervical exploration, asymptomatic patients having borderline biochemical evidence may be considered for nonoperative management. Nonetheless, surgical re-exploration is required with progressive clinical disease.

SUMMARY

The evolution of PHPT since it was first recognized nearly 100 years ago has been profound because of technologic and biochemical advances that have furthered the knowledge and the ability to effectively treat the disease. Understanding the genetics of the disease also plays a major role in the management of patients with familial syndromes that encompass PHPT. Preoperative localization has revolutionized the surgical decision-making process along with the use of IOPTH assays to determine completeness of resection. Because of these breakthroughs, surgeons have been able to develop new minimally invasive surgical approaches for the treatment of PHPT resulting in low complication rates and high patient satisfaction. Despite the significant challenges associated with reoperative surgery for recurrent and persistent PHPT, excellent outcomes can be reproducibly achieved when proper preoperative, intraoperative, and postoperative management is used.

REFERENCES

1. Ahmad R, Hammond JM. Primary, secondary, and tertiary hyperparathyroidism. Otolaryngol Clin North Am 2004;37:701–13, vii–viii.
2. Reeve TS, Babidge WJ, Parkyn RF, et al. Minimally invasive surgery for primary hyperparathyroidism: systematic review. Arch Surg 2000;135:481–7.
3. Niederle BE, Schmidt G, Organ CH, et al. Albert J and his surgeon: a historical reevaluation of the first parathyroidectomy. J Am Coll Surg 2006;202: 181–90.
4. Irvin GL III. The William H. Harrige memorial lecture: parathormone and the disease. Am J Surg 2007;193:301–4.
5. DeLellis RA, Mazzaglia P, Mangray S. Primary hyperparathyroidism: a current perspective. Arch Pathol Lab Med 2008;132:1251–62.
6. Mack LA, Pasieka JL. Asymptomatic primary hyperparathyroidism: a surgical perspective. Surg Clin North Am 2004;84:803–16.
7. Rodgers SE, Lew JI, Solorzano CC. Primary hyperparathyroidism. Curr Opin Oncol 2008;20:52–8.
8. Fraser WD. Hyperparathyroidism. Lancet 2009;374:145–58.
9. Stephen AE, Chen KT, Milas M, et al. The coming of age of radiation-induced hyperparathyroidism: evolving patterns of thyroid and parathyroid disease after head and neck irradiation. Surgery 2004;136:1143–53.
10. Wheeler MH. Primary hyperparathyroidism: a surgical perspective. Ann R Coll Surg Engl 1998;80:305–12.
11. Bilezikian JP, Khan AA, Potts JT Jr. Guidelines for the management of asymptomatic primary hyperparathyroidism: summary statement from the third international workshop. J Clin Endocrinol Metab 2009;94:335–9.
12. Brown EM. The calcium-sensing receptor: physiology, pathophysiology and CaR-based therapeutics. Subcell Biochem 2007;45:139–67.
13. Brown EM. Clinical lessons from the calcium-sensing receptor. Nat Clin Pract Endocrinol Metab 2007;3:122–33.
14. Ruda JM, Hollenbeak CS, Stack BC Jr. A systematic review of the diagnosis and treatment of primary hyperparathyroidism from 1995 to 2003. Otolaryngol Head Neck Surg 2005;132:359–72.
15. Miedlich S, Krohn K, Paschke R. Update on genetic and clinical aspects of primary hyperparathyroidism. Clin Endocrinol (Oxf) 2003;59:539–54.
16. Carling T, Udelsman R. Parathyroid surgery in familial hyperparathyroid disorders. J Intern Med 2005;257:27–37.
17. Blackburn M, Diamond T. Primary hyperparathyroidism and familial hyperparathyroid syndromes. Aust Fam Physician 2007;36:1029–33.
18. Eastell R, Arnold A, Brandi ML, et al. Diagnosis of asymptomatic primary hyperparathyroidism: proceedings of the third international workshop. J Clin Endocrinol Metab 2009;94:340–50.
19. Okamoto T, Iihara M, Obara T, et al. Parathyroid carcinoma: etiology, diagnosis, and treatment. World J Surg 2009;33(11):2343–54.

20. Coker LH, Rorie K, Cantley L, et al. Primary hyperparathyroidism, cognition, and health-related quality of life. Ann Surg 2005;242:642–50.
21. Mazzaglia PJ, Berber E, Kovach A, et al. The changing presentation of hyperparathyroidism over 3 decades. Arch Surg 2008;143:260–6.
22. Silverberg SJ, Lewiecki EM, Mosekilde L, et al. Presentation of asymptomatic primary hyperparathyroidism: proceedings of the third international workshop. J Clin Endocrinol Metab 2009;94:351–65.
23. Weaver S, Doherty DB, Jimenez C, et al. Peer-reviewed, evidence-based analysis of vitamin D and primary hyperparathyroidism. World J Surg 2009;33:2292–302.
24. Mittendorf EA, Wefel JS, Meyers CA, et al. Improvement of sleep disturbance and neurocognitive function after parathyroidectomy in patients with primary hyperparathyroidism. Endocr Pract 2007;13:338–44.
25. Roman SA, Sosa JA, Mayes L, et al. Parathyroidectomy improves neurocognitive deficits in patients with primary hyperparathyroidism. Surgery 2005;138:1121–8 [discussion: 1128–9].
26. Johnson NA, Tublin ME, Ogilvie JB. Parathyroid imaging: technique and role in the preoperative evaluation of primary hyperparathyroidism. AJR Am J Roentgenol 2007;188:1706–15.
27. Meilstrup JW. Ultrasound examination of the parathyroid glands. Otolaryngol Clin North Am 2004;37:763–78, ix.
28. Monroe DP, Edeiken-Monroe BS, Lee JE, et al. Impact of preoperative thyroid ultrasonography on the surgical management of primary hyperparathyroidism. Br J Surg 2008;95:957–60.
29. Bentrem DJ, Angelos P, Talamonti MS, et al. Is preoperative investigation of the thyroid justified in patients undergoing parathyroidectomy for hyperparathyroidism? Thyroid 2002;12:1109–12.
30. Lavely WC, Goetze S, Friedman KP, et al. Comparison of SPECT/CT, SPECT, and planar imaging with single- and dual-phase (99m)Tc-sestamibi parathyroid scintigraphy. J Nucl Med 2007;48:1084–9.
31. Sokoll LJ. Measurement of parathyroid hormone and application of parathyroid hormone in intraoperative monitoring. Clin Lab Med 2004;24:199–216.
32. Boudou P, Ibrahim F, Cormier C, et al. Third- or second-generation parathyroid hormone assays: a remaining debate in the diagnosis of primary hyperparathyroidism. J Clin Endocrinol Metab 2005;90:6370–2.
33. Sokoll LJ, Donovan PI, Udelsman R. The National Academy of Clinical Biochemistry Laboratory Medicine practice guidelines for intraoperative parathyroid hormone. Point Care 2007;6:253–60.
34. Irvin GL III, Solorzano CC, Carneiro DM. Quick intraoperative parathyroid hormone assay: surgical adjunct to allow limited parathyroidectomy, improve success rate, and predict outcome. World J Surg 2004;28:1287–92.
35. Carneiro-Pla DM, Solorzano CC, Irvin GL III. Consequences of targeted parathyroidectomy guided by localization studies without intraoperative parathyroid hormone monitoring. J Am Coll Surg 2006;202:715–22.
36. Carneiro DM, Solorzano CC, Nader MC, et al. Comparison of intraoperative iPTH assay (QPTH) criteria in guiding parathyroidectomy: which criterion is the most accurate? Surgery 2003;134:973–9 [discussion: 979–81].
37. Shindo M. Intraoperative rapid parathyroid hormone monitoring in parathyroid surgery. Otolaryngol Clin North Am 2004;37:779–87, ix.
38. Sackett WR, Barraclough B, Reeve TS, et al. Worldwide trends in the surgical treatment of primary hyperparathyroidism in the era of minimally invasive parathyroidectomy. Arch Surg 2002;137:1055–9.

39. Lorenz K, Nguyen-Thanh P, Dralle H. Unilateral open and minimally invasive procedures for primary hyperparathyroidism: a review of selective approaches. Langenbecks Arch Surg 2000;385:106–17.
40. Palazzo FF, Delbridge LW. Minimal-access/minimally invasive parathyroidectomy for primary hyperparathyroidism. Surg Clin North Am 2004;84:717–34.
41. Terris DJ, Stack BC Jr, Gourin CG. Contemporary parathyroidectomy: exploiting technology. Am J Otolaryngol 2007;28:408–14.
42. Harrison BJ, Triponez F. Intraoperative adjuncts in surgery for primary hyperparathyroidism. Langenbecks Arch Surg 2009;394:799–809.
43. Naitoh T, Gagner M, Garcia-Ruiz A, et al. Endoscopic endocrine surgery in the neck: an initial report of endoscopic subtotal parathyroidectomy. Surg Endosc 1998;12:202–5 [discussion: 206].
44. Barczynski M, Cichon S, Konturek A, et al. Minimally invasive video-assisted parathyroidectomy versus open minimally invasive parathyroidectomy for a solitary parathyroid adenoma: a prospective, randomized, blinded trial. World J Surg 2006;30:721–31.
45. Miccoli P, Bendinelli C, Berti P, et al. Video-assisted versus conventional parathyroidectomy in primary hyperparathyroidism: a prospective randomized study. Surgery 1999;126:1117–21 [discussion: 1121–2].
46. Shoman N, Melck A, Holmes D, et al. Utility of intraoperative parathyroid hormone measurement in predicting postparathyroidectomy hypocalcemia. J Otolaryngol Head Neck Surg 2008;37:16–22.
47. Jatzko GR, Lisborg PH, Muller MG, et al. Recurrent nerve palsy after thyroid operations: principal nerve identification and a literature review. Surgery 1994;115:139–44.
48. Brennan J, Moore EJ, Shuler KJ. Prospective analysis of the efficacy of continuous intraoperative nerve monitoring during thyroidectomy, parathyroidectomy, and parotidectomy. Otolaryngol Head Neck Surg 2001;124:537–43.
49. Perrier ND, Ituarte P, Kikuchi S, et al. Intraoperative parathyroid aspiration and parathyroid hormone assay as an alternative to frozen section for tissue identification. World J Surg 2000;24:1319–22.
50. Pradeep PV, Mishra A, Agarwal G, et al. Long-term outcome after parathyroidectomy in patients with advanced primary hyperparathyroidism and associated vitamin D deficiency. World J Surg 2008;32:829–35.
51. Heinrich S, Schafer M, Rousson V, et al. Evidence-based treatment of acute pancreatitis: a look at established paradigms. Ann Surg 2006;243:154–68.
52. Mandal AK, Udelsman R. Secondary hyperparathyroidism is an expected consequence of parathyroidectomy for primary hyperparathyroidism: a prospective study. Surgery 1998;124:1021–6 [discussion: 1026–7].
53. Shen W, Duren M, Morita E, et al. Reoperation for persistent or recurrent primary hyperparathyroidism. Arch Surg 1996;131:861–7 [discussion: 867–9].
54. Lorberboym M, Minski I, Macadziob S, et al. Incremental diagnostic value of preoperative 99mTc-MIBI SPECT in patients with a parathyroid adenoma. J Nucl Med 2003;44:904–8.
55. Kiblut NK, Cussac JF, Soudan B, et al. Fine needle aspiration and intraparathyroid intact parathyroid hormone measurement for reoperative parathyroid surgery. World J Surg 2004;28:1143–7.
56. Moley JF, Lairmore TC, Doherty GM, et al. Preservation of the recurrent laryngeal nerves in thyroid and parathyroid reoperations. Surgery 1999;126:673–7 [discussion: 677–9].
57. Chae AW, Perricone A, Brumund KT, et al. Outpatient video-assisted thoracoscopic surgery (VATS) for ectopic mediastinal parathyroid adenoma: a case

report and review of the literature. J Laparoendosc Adv Surg Tech A 2008;18: 383–90.

58. Jaskowiak NT, Sugg SL, Helke J, et al. Pitfalls of intraoperative quick parathyroid hormone monitoring and gamma probe localization in surgery for primary hyperparathyroidism. Arch Surg 2002;137:659–68 [discussion: 668–9].

59. Harman CR, Grant CS, Hay ID, et al. Indications, technique, and efficacy of alcohol injection of enlarged parathyroid glands in patients with primary hyperparathyroidism. Surgery 1998;124:1011–20.

60. Hessman O, Stålberg P, Sundin A, et al. High success rate of parathyroid reoperation may be achieved with improved localization diagnosis. World J Surg 2008;32:774–81.

Parathyroid Surgery in Renal Failure Patients

Vidas Dumasius, MD, Peter Angelos, MD, PhD*

KEYWORDS

- Hyperparathyroidism • Renal failure • Hypercalcemia
- Parathyroidectomy • Thymectomy

Many patients with renal failure present with symptoms associated with chronically elevated levels of phosphate. In particular, the high parathyroid hormone (PTH) levels in patients with renal failure can be a management challenge. Given the unique physiologic state of these patients, their hyperparathyroidism (HPT) warrants special considerations for selecting appropriate medical and surgical management.

Secondary HPT is caused by any condition associated with a chronic depression in the serum calcium level because low serum calcium leads to compensatory overactivity of the parathyroid glands. Renal failure is, by far, the most common cause of secondary HPT, although other diseases, including inadequate dietary calcium intake, steatorrhea, and vitamin D deficiency can also cause this condition. Chronic renal insufficiency is associated with impaired phosphate excretion, which leads to hyperphosphatemia. Elevated serum phosphate directly depresses serum calcium levels and thereby stimulates parathyroid gland activity.

In contrast, tertiary HPT is observed in patients with renal failure that have undergone renal transplantation but still overproduce PTH. This condition is typically observed after successful renal transplantation when asymptomatic elevated calcium levels are observed. Laboratory studies in these patients are similar to patients with primary HPT, namely elevated PTH secondary to over activity of the parathyroid glands.

In renal HPT, the hypercalcemia is observed with elevated synthesis of calcitriol. The persistent hyperphosphatemia, bone resistance, and change in the PTH set point lead to the diffuse hyperplasia of the parathyroid glands. These changes are not limited to a single gland, but affect all of the glands.

University of Chicago Medical Center, 5841 South Maryland Avenue, MC 4052, Chicago, IL 60637, USA
* Corresponding author.
E-mail address: pangelos@surgery.bsd.uchicago.edu

Otolaryngol Clin N Am 43 (2010) 433–440
doi:10.1016/j.otc.2010.01.010
0030-6665/10/$ – see front matter © 2010 Elsevier Inc. All rights reserved.

oto.theclinics.com

It has been reported that 1% to 28% of patients who have hemodialysis develop significant secondary HPT.[1–3] For patients with renal transplant, failure of the resolution of the calcium and phosphate metabolism leading to tertiary HPT has been estimated to occur in 1% to 10%.[4,5]

CALCIUM METABOLISM

Plasma calcium exists in ionized and protein bound phases. Normally about 1gm of calcium in the inorganic form is absorbed daily in the proximal small intestine. Extracellular calcium is constantly being exchanged with that in the bone, intracellular fluid, and glomerular filtrate. Normal kidney can reabsorb 99% of the calcium that is present in the filtrate. Bone is an enormous reservoir of calcium.

The serum calcium level is controlled by the interaction of PTH, calcitonin, and Vitamin D. Vitamin D is not one molecule but a mix of sterols. Active form of Vitamin D results from activity of renal 1a-hydroxylase conversion of 25-Vitamin D to 1,2-dihydroxycholecalciferol, which is the active form of the Vitamin D. The role of the Vitamin D activity in calcium homeostasis is directed at increased intestinal absorption and increased bone resorption. As the glomerular filtration rate decreases, renal production of 1,2-dihydroxycholecalciferol decreases, leading to decreased intestinal calcium absorption to create a negative calcium balance. A compensatory increase in PTH secretion keeps the serum calcium level near normal by mobilizing calcium from bone.

Renal insufficiency with continued decrease in kidney function abrogates Vitamin D effects. Furthermore, chronic elevation of phosphate in renal failure affects parathyroid gland function. With elevated serum phosphate and low active vitamin D levels, serum calcium is low, which triggers development of secondary HPT–hypertrophy of the parathyroid glands. In contrast to what is observed in primary and tertiary HPT, patients with secondary HPT have low serum calcium levels, which lead to elevated levels of PTH.

PARATHYROID HORMONE

Parathyroid hormone is a single-chain polypeptide consisting of 84 amino acids. PTH is synthesized by chief cells of the parathyroid gland. The principal actions of parathyroid hormone include an increase in

- Serum calcium and decrease in serum phosphorus levels
- Bone osteoclast and osteoblast activity
- Gastrointestinal absorption of calcium
- Renal bicarbonate excretion
- Renal hydroxylation of 25-hydroxy Vitamin D3.

The level of serum calcium in humans is under a sensitive feedback-control mechanism. Hypercalcemia reduces parathyroid hormone secretion and the formation of 1,25-dihydroxy vitamin D3 in normal healthy individuals. In cases of secondary HPT, elevated levels of phosphate lead to suppression of the calcium levels and elevation of the PTH in response to low calcium levels.

MEDICAL TREATMENT GOALS

Given that the underlying cause for secondary HPT is overstimulation of the parathyroid glands, medical management is focused on decreasing that stimulation. One of the methods to control serum hyperphosphatemia may be achieved with phosphate binders in conjunction with dietary limits on the phosphate intake. In addition, supplemental calcium and Vitamin D may assist in achieving these goals. Calcium may also be added to patients' dialysate on a regular basis. Despite the best management of hyperphosphatemia, a significant number of patients may develop prominent osteodystrophy. Osteodystrophy is especially common in patients that are on chronic hemodialysis because aluminum accumulates in the bones contributing to osteomalacia. Furthermore, patients may also develop ectopic calcification.

SURGICAL INDICATIONS IN SECONDARY AND TERTIARY HPT

The secondary HPT in the majority of renal patients on hemodialysis may not warrant surgical intervention. Thus, medical management should always be undertaken first. The symptoms that favor surgical intervention are persistent hypercalcemia, uncontrolled hyperphosphatemia, elevated alkaline phosphatase levels, and evidence of significant bone erosion on imaging or development of osteitis fibrosa cystica (OFC). The clinical finding associated with OFC may manifest as worsening bone pain and fractures. Significant discomfort is reported from persistent pruritus and development of the soft tissue calcifications. Several additional clinical findings should be taken into consideration, such as erythropoietin resistant anemia, poorly controlled hypertension, impaired myocardial perfusion, and peripheral neuropathies. Development of significant calciphylaxis (deposition of calcium in skin) should also be taken into consideration when making a decision for surgical intervention. However, elevation of the PTH alone does not warrant surgical intervention.

Table 1 summarizes some of the critical considerations in determining indications for surgery in renal failure. Although many different factors can be examined in deciding whether to operate on patients, calcium levels, alkaline phosphatase levels, and the presence of subperiosteal bone resorption are all important. As patients progress from Stage I to Stage II, they develop relative and then an absolute indication for surgery. Certainly, any patient with a diagnosis of calciphylaxis has an absolute indication for surgery.

In cases of patients that have undergone renal transplantation, additional considerations before surgery should be undertaken. Patients with asymptomatic hypercalcemia should be observed for at least a year with demonstration of persistently elevated levels of calcium before surgery is planned. Patients who develop nephrolithiasis or nephrocalcinosis as a result of the persistent elevated levels of calcium have a clear surgical indication. More urgent surgical exploration should be undertaken if patients have acute hypercalcemia in the immediate posttransplantation period that

Table 1 Indications for surgery			
	Stage I	Stage II	Stage III
Calcium mmol/l Normal range 2.1 to 2.6	<2.6	<2.6	>2.6
Alkaline phosphatase u/l Normal range 50 to 180	<300	>300	Normal or elevated
Hand X ray	Normal	Subperiosteal resorption	Subperiosteal resorption
Surgical indication	None	Relative	Absolute

Adapted from Rothmund M, Wagner PK, Schark C. World J Surg 1991;15:745–50.

is difficult to manage by medical means or symptomatic from hypercalcemia developing muscle weakness, myalgia, mental status changes, nausea, or vomiting.

PREOPERATIVE CONSIDERATIONS

As in cases of primary HPT, noninvasive localization studies may be undertaken to evaluate parathyroid glands. Sestamibi scans provide information about the location of parathyroid glands, especially when in the face of an aberrant location or ectopic parathyroid gland. Alternatively, thallium-technetium scan can be performed although the results with Sestamibi scanning alone seem to be superior. Ultrasound can be helpful in identifying abnormal parathyroid glands in the neck and can also identify thyroid pathology. It is important to identify thyroid pathology preoperatively so that if work-up, such as fine-needle aspiration, is needed before surgery it can be undertaken. Patients can be pretreated with calcitriol for several days preoperatively in an effort to reduce postoperative hypocalcemia. Intraoperative infusion of desmopressin at induction of anesthesia may help to counteract the platelet dysfunction seen in patients with renal failure. Given the complexity of medical problems and frequent significant postoperative hypocalcemia, postoperative intensive care unit management of these patients should also be considered.

OPERATIVE PLAN

In preparation for parathyroidectomy in patients with renal failure, the surgeon should consider several key issues. The control of the symptoms is the goal of the surgery and may be accomplished in several ways:

- Subtotal parathyroidectomy with cervical thymectomy
- Total parathyroidectomy with autotransplantation and cervical thymectomy
- Total parathyroidectomy and cervical thymectomy without autotransplantation.

Each of these surgical approaches has advantages and disadvantages that warrant further evaluation. The incidence of supernumerary parathyroid glands has been reported in the range of 6.5% to 25% and may be the cause of the persistent or recurrent HPT.[6,7] Given that a significant number of supernumerary glands are located in the thymic tissue, the optimal treatment includes resection of the upper portion of the thymus in all operations for secondary HPT. This cervical thymectomy should be considered a standard part of the operation for renal HPT. Furthermore, extra parathyroid glands also can be found in the fatty tissue behind the thyroid along esophagus or along recurrent laryngeal nerves. Niederle and colleagues[8] reported in 1992 that 11.4% of patients had supernumerary parathyroid glands found in the fatty tissue in the neck. These reports point to the importance of thorough evaluation of all thymic tissue and posterior central soft tissue for additional parathyroid glands during any parathyroid operation for secondary HPT.

The choice of whether to perform a subtotal parathyroidectomy (sPTx) or total parathyroidectomy with autotransplantation (tPTx+AT) or just total parathyroidectomy (tPTx) is best made by the individual surgeon based on the prior experience and specific patient issues. If patients have significant calciphylaxis, the mortality rate is so high that total parathyroidectomy without autotransplantation is indicated. In this circumstance, the surgeon should strive to ensure that recurrence rates are absolutely minimized and therefore all parathyroid tissue should be removed. Theoretically, in patients on dialysis who will never receive a kidney transplant, a total parathyroidectomy should also be a reasonable operation. However, because almost every patient on dialysis may be a transplant candidate in the future, the authors advocate either sPTx or tTPx+AT in all patients with secondary HPT in need of parathyroidectomy as long as they do not have life-threatening calciphylaxis. Individual surgeon judgment should be used to make the choice between the two operations as both have pros and cons associated with them.[9,10]

Subtotal parathyroidectomy (sPTx) is thought by some authors to be a less radical procedure with equally effective results.[11] This procedure avoids an incision in the forearm, which may be a difficult location for some patients who have had dialysis access complications. Many surgeons prefer to see a well-vascularized remnant in situ in sPTx rather than depending on autograft function. On the other hand, tPTx+AT has the benefit of making a second operation, if necessary, easier as it can be done under local anesthesia without re-exploration of the neck. Furthermore, some studies have shown a lower recurrence rate with tPTx+AT.[12] With lack of convincing data to support one operation over the other, the authors recommend that the individual surgeon make the choice realizing that to be successful, the operation must be done with meticulous technique and minimal complications.

The subtotal parathyroidectomy with cervical thymectomy should include a careful bilateral exploration of the neck. A critical part of the surgery is to identify all four glands and decide which gland is the most normal looking. This strategy is the opposite of that used for most parathyroidectomies in cases of primary HPT (**Fig. 1**). In primary HPT, the goal is to find the abnormal gland, and frequently when performing a minimally invasive or focused parathyroidectomy, the surgeon will not look at any glands but the abnormal one. In contrast, in patients who have renal failure with HPT, the surgeon must find all the glands and identify the most normal looking gland. If an inferior gland is small and normal looking, it should be preserved. Because inferior glands are more anterior in the neck, it is preferable to preserve an inferior gland if possible. If reoperation is needed in the future, inferior glands are more readily accessible. The gland for preservation should be carefully dissected taking care to protect the vascular pedicle. A vascular clip is then placed across the gland and the distal portion resected leaving the vascularized remnant marked with the clip. The goal is to have a 40 to 80 mg vascularized remnant of the most normal looking gland. It is critical to ensure viability of this remnant before resection of additional glands. As each parathyroid gland is completely dissected, before removing the gland, the remnant is inspected to ensure viability. If at any time the remnant appears nonviable, the surgeon can choose another gland to use for a remnant or the decision can be made to perform a total parathyroidectomy and autotransplant a parathyroid. Tominaga and colleagues[13] have suggested that in choosing the gland to leave as a remnant or for autografting, the least nodular gland should be chosen because the glands with nodular hyperplasia are more likely to grow. In either subtotal parathyroidectomy or total parathyroidectomy with autotransplantation, cryopreservation can be undertaken with close follow-up of patients' calcium status with excellent results achieved with delayed transplantation of the parathyroid tissue.

In cases where total parathyroidectomy with autotransplantation is being undertaken, the surgeon should initially identify all four parathyroid glands. Once this is done, the most normal-appearing and least-nodular gland should be chosen for autotransplantation. The glands for autotransplantation should be minced into approximately 1×2 mm pieces. A pocket should be made in brachioradialis muscle away from arteriovenous fistulae and 20 to 30 pieces of parathyroid should be autotransplanted.[14,15] The autotransplant pocket should be closed with a "figure of 8" stitch and then the knot marked with a vascular clip so that the pocket could be readily found again if needed. Alternatively, parathyroid autografts can be placed in the

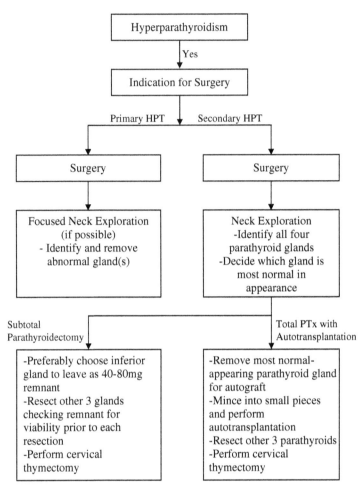

Fig. 1. Differences in surgical algorithms for parathyroidectomy.

subcutaneous fat in the arm. If there is any concern for viability of the transplant, then cryopreservation of at least one parathyroid gland should be performed.

ADDITIONAL PERIOPERATIVE CONSIDERATIONS

At the completion of the parathyroid gland resection, several considerations should be thought through before leaving the operating room. One consideration is the decision about whether to place a cervical drain at the completion of the surgical procedure. Although no data shows that closed tube drainage of the parathyroidectomy wound reduces the likelihood of developing a neck hematoma, the authors continue to use a drain in patients with renal failure undergoing parathyroidectomy because these patients will need hemodialysis in the perioperative period. All such patients will require hemodialysis and they all will get some heparin during dialysis. Patients should be dialyzed with minimum heparin after a parathyroidectomy in the early postoperative period. Drains may be left for close monitoring over the first 24 to 48 hours with removal before the patient is discharged from the hospital. An additional consideration in the operating room is whether parathyroid hormone levels should be checked intra-operatively. A rapid drop in PTH levels intraoperatively is seen in patients after para-thyroidectomy for primary HPT. In patients with renal failure, the speed with which PTH levels drop is reduced and controversy continues to exist at this time regarding how to best interpret the intraoperative PTH results. Nevertheless, most surgeons find knowledge of a significant drop in intraoperative PTH to be valuable in the oper-ating room. Postoperatively, calcium levels are maintained as close as possible to normal range. Patients receive oral supplementation of the calcium and vitamin D, but for refractory cases or patients that experience symptoms of hypocalcemia (perio-ral, hand tingling, numbness) a calcium drip may be initiated. Additionally, arrange-ments are made with hemodialysis services that may provide further assistance with regulation of electrolyte disbalances in renal patients. For example, in patients who are hypocalcemic, hemodialysis is performed with a high calcium bath.

SUMMARY

Treatment of HPT in patients with renal failure is a complex surgical issue. Given the multitude of medical problems that patients with renal failure have, a diligent selection of the patients that should undergo surgical intervention must be undertaken. Further-more, no single optimal approach has been well established and management of these patients requires systematic review of the problems affecting these patients. It appears that strict indication of the surgical intervention with well-documented physical symptoms with laboratory findings provides best guidance for selecting surgical candidates. A meticulous surgical technique, regardless of the method selected to treat these patients, also helps in achieving the best clinical outcomes. It is important to include cervical thymectomy in the surgical plans given high rates of supernumerary of parathyroid gland in patients with renal failure. Finally, patients are best served by surgeons that have gained sufficient surgical experience and clinical expertise in managing these complex patients.

REFERENCES

1. Malberti F, Marcelli D, Conte F, et al. Parathyroidectomy in patients on renal replacement therapy: an epidemiologic study. J Am Soc Nephrol 2001;12: 1242–8.
2. Kestenbaum B, Selinger SL, Gillen DL, et al. Parathyroidectomy rates among United States dialysis patients: 1990–1999. Kidney Int 2004;65:282–8.
3. Foley RN, Li S, Liu J, et al. The fall and rise of parathyroidectomy in U.S. hemo-dialysis patients, 1992 to 2002. J Am Soc Nephrol 2005;16:210–8.
4. D'Alesandro AM, Melzer JS, Pirch JD, et al. Tertiary hyperparathyroidism after renal transplant operation. Surgery 1989;106:1049–55.
5. Kilgo MS, Pirsch JD, Warner TF, et al. Tertiary hyperparathyroidism after renal transplant: surgical strategy. Surgery 1998;124:677–83.
6. Numano S, Tominaga Y, Uchida K, et al. Significance of supernumerary parathy-roid glands in renal hyperparathyroidism. World J Surg 1998;22:1098–103.
7. Pattou FN, Pellissier LC, Noel C, et al. Supernumerary parathyroid glands: frequency and surgical significance in treatment of renal hyperparathyroidism. World J Surg 2000;24:1330–4.
8. Niederle B, Stamn L, Langle F, et al. Primary hyperparathyroidism in Austria: results of an 8 year prospective study. World J Surg 1992;16:777–82.

9. Higgins RM, Richardson AJ, Ratcliffe PJ, et al. Total parathyroidectomy alone or with autograft for renal hyperparathyroidism? New Series. Q J Med 1991;79: 323–32.
10. Richards ML, Wormuth J, Bingener J, et al. Parathyroidectomy in secondary hyperparathyroidism: is there an optimal operative management? Surgery 2006;139:174–80.
11. Gasparri G, Camandona M, Abbona GC, et al. Secondary and tertiary hyperparathyroidism of recurrent disease after 446 parathyroidectomies. Ann Surg 2001; 233:65–9.
12. Rothmund M, Wagner PK, Schark C. Subtotal parathyroidectomy versus total thyroidectomy and autotransplantation in secondary hyperparathyroidism: a randomized trial. World J Surg 1991;15:745–50.
13. Tominaga Y, Numano M, Tanaka Y, et al. Surgical treatment of renal hyperparathyroidism. Semin Surg Oncol 1997;13:87–96.
14. Chon FF, Chan HM, Huang TJ, et al. Autotransplant of parathyroid glands into subcutaneous forearm tissue for renal hyperparathyroidism. Surgery 1998;124: 1–5.
15. Mondrick JM, Bendinelli C, Passero MA Jr, et al. Subcutaneous forearm transplantation of autologous parathyroid tissue in patients with renal hyperparathyroidism. Surgery 1999;126:1152–8.

Parathyroid Carcinoma

W. Cross Dudney, BS[a], Donald Bodenner, MD, PhD[b,c,d],
Brendan C. Stack Jr MD[b,e],*

KEYWORDS

- Parathyroid • Parathyroid carcinoma • Parathyroid cancer
- Parathyroid hormone

Parathyroid carcinoma is an uncommon endocrine malignancy that was first described in 1904 by de Quervain.[1] de Quervain described a metastatic, nonfunctioning parathyroid carcinoma; subsequent descriptions of functioning parathyroid carcinoma were reported in the 1930s.[2] Since that time, only a few hundred cases have been reported in the literature.

The natural history of parathyroid carcinoma is described as slow but progressive. This entity has a tendency for spread to local lymph nodes with eventual metastasis to the lung and less commonly to the liver and bone.[3–5] The majority of tumors are functional (ie, they secrete parathyroid hormone [PTH] with resulting elevated serum calcium levels). Morbidity and mortality usually result from unremitting hypercalcemia and its complications rather than mass effect from tumor burden.[6,7] Nonfunctional tumors present as an expanding neck mass; typically, they are diagnosed at a more advanced stage and subsequently have a generally poorer prognosis. Mortality also is associated with regional disease and metastasis.[8] The cause of parathyroid carcinoma is unknown and at present there are no data describing causal relationships between parathyroid carcinoma and any risk factors.[9]

EPIDEMIOLOGY

The frequency of parathyroid carcinoma is reported as greater than 1% of patients with primary hyperparathyroidism,[10,11] although a higher rate of 5% is reported from Japan.[4,12] It is the least common endocrine malignancy,[10,13–16] with a prevalence of 0.005%[17] of all cancers. According to a report from the National Cancer Data Base,

[a] University of Arkansas for Medical Sciences College of Medicine, 4301 West Markham Street, Little Rock, AR 72205, USA
[b] University of Arkansas for Medical Sciences Thyroid Center, Little Rock, AR 72205, USA
[c] Department of Geriatrics, University of Arkansas for Medical Sciences College of Medicine, 4301 West Markham Street, Little Rock, AR 72205, USA
[d] Central Arkansas Veterans Affairs Healthcare System, Little Rock, Arkansas, USA
[e] Department of Otolaryngology-Head and Neck Surgery, University of Arkansas for Medical Sciences College of Medicine, 4301 West Markham Street #543, Little Rock, AR 72205, USA
* Corresponding author. Department of Otolaryngology-Head and Neck Surgery, University of Arkansas for Medical Sciences College of Medicine, 4301 West Markham Street #543, Little Rock, AR 72205.
E-mail address: BStack@uams.edu

Otolaryngol Clin N Am 43 (2010) 441–453
doi:10.1016/j.otc.2010.01.011
0030-6665/10/$ – see front matter © 2010 Elsevier Inc. All rights reserved.

the estimated incidence is 30 new cases per year in the United States.[17] Most reports indicate an equal gender distribution.[10,17] The typical age at presentation is reported to be from the 40s to the mid-50s, slightly younger than the average age of patients with primary hyperparathyroidism.[3–5,16,17] Parathyroid carcinoma may occur as a sporadic event or as part of a syndrome; relationships are described with hyperparathyroidism–jaw tumor (HPT-JT) syndrome, multiple endocrine neoplasia types 1 and 2A, and familial hypocalciuric hypercalcemia.[18–21]

CASE STUDIES

Case studies can be a helpful tool in expanding understanding of rare diseases seldom encountered in clinical practice. From the surgical experience of the senior author (BCS) with 8 cases, the following 2 cases are presented.

Patient 1

A 50-year-old man was referred to the authors' clinic with a chief complaint of dyspnea of more than 1 year's duration and a right-sided neck mass. Ultrasound (his only preoperative imaging) demonstrated a large, noncystic, right-sided neck mass, which was initially thought a benign colloid goiter. The patient's preoperative calcium level was incidentally noted as 10.6 mg/dL. Hemithyroidectomy was performed; however, operative findings revealed an exceptionally large right inferior parathyroid mass with mediastinal extension just behind and intimately associated with the thyroid lobe. After this discovery, a blood sample was sent and intraoperative measurement of the patient's PTH (ioPTH) was 415 pg/dL (normal range, 10–65 pg/mL). Parathyroidectomy with dissection of the tracheoesophageal groove was undertaken. After dissection, his ioPTH level fell to 86 pg/dL and hypercalcemia normalized postoperatively. Histopathologic examination of surgical specimens revealed extensive necrosis and vascular and perineural invasion, leading to a diagnosis of parathyroid carcinoma.

During the surgery, there was a concern that residual disease might have been left in the mediastinum. A postoperative neck and chest CT scan with contrast was ordered (**Fig. 1**). A right mediastinal lesion was noted. Approximately 1 month later, after the initial surgery, the patient underwent right thoracotomy for excision of a mediastinal mass. Gross findings on thoracotomy included a soft, well-encapsulated mass with necrosis and mustard brown–colored debris that encompassed the right vagus nerve; the involved nerve was sacrificed. Histopathologic examination revealed no evidence of malignancy.

The patient's PTH levels remained elevated for 10 months after surgery (97 to 160 pg/dL, normal range 12 to 88). During this time, his calcium levels were consistently low to low normal (8.2 to 8.9 mg/dL, normal range 8.7 to 10.5); subsequently, a 25-hydroxy (OH) vitamin D level was obtained and was 14 ng/mL (normal range, 30 to 80 ng/mL). The patient was determined to have vitamin D–deficient secondary hyperparathyroidism and he was repleted. On correction of vitamin D levels (44 ng/mL), his calcium and PTH levels normalized (9.0 mg/dL and 68.2 pg/dL, respectively). PTH and chorioembryonic antigen (CEA) levels were used for surveillance of disease recurrence; although PTH levels fluctuated, his CEA levels remained consistently normal (1.3–2.1 ng/mL, normal range 0.5–10). He refused radiation therapy and has since been only sporadically compliant with follow-up.

Patient 2

A 63-year-old man was referred to the authors' clinic for evaluation of a neck mass that had gradually increased in size over a 2-year time period. During this time the patient developed progressive back pain, kyphoscoliosis (**Fig. 2**), a 50-lb weight loss, and

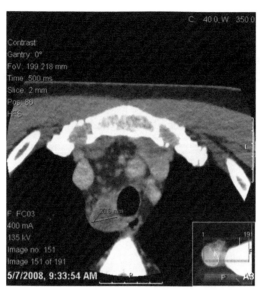

Fig. 1. Mediastinal mass, 2-mm transverse view. Patient 1's parathyroid mass had extended into the mediastinum, requiring thoracotomy.

a pathologic fracture of the left scapula while attempting to start his lawn mower. Initial workup revealed a PTH level of 5578 pg/dL, elevated serum calcium and bone alkaline phosphatase, and decreased activated (25-OH) vitamin D. The findings of a palpable neck mass along with massively elevated PTH led to a high index of suspicion for parathyroid carcinoma. Before his scheduled surgery, he was admitted to the hospital in acute renal failure and his hypercalcemia was treated with aggressive hydration. Results of soft tissue CT scan of the neck with contrast were consistent with a malignant neoplasm arising from the right inferior parathyroid (**Fig. 3**). CT scanning also detected the presence of a mass on the right third rib that was suspicious for a metastasis (**Fig. 4**).

Right-sided inferior parathyroidectomy, hemithyroidectomy, modified neck dissection, and rib resection were performed by a team effort of otolaryngologists and cardiothoracic surgeons. Histopathologic examination of surgical specimens confirmed diagnosis of parathyroid carcinoma with lymphovascular invasion.

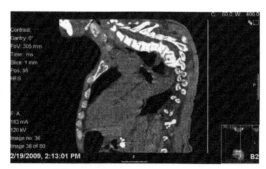

Fig. 2. Kyphoscoliosis due to severe osteoporosis, a late sequela of parathyroid carcinoma. This is also seen in **Fig. 4**.

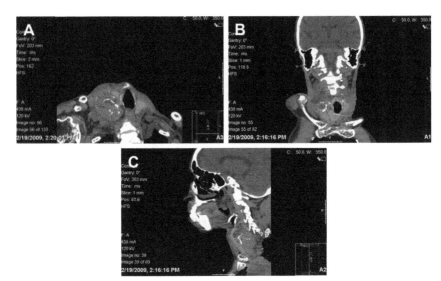

Fig. 3. (A) Neck mass of patient 2, transverse view. (B) Neck mass of patient 2, coronal view. (C) Neck mass of patient 2, sagittal view.

Examination of the rib mass revealed a fibrohistiocytic lesion with abundant giant cells, which, given the context of hypercalcemia, was identified as a brown tumor of hyperparathyroidism. This is a classic association but rarely encountered in clinical practice (**Fig. 5**). After resection, his PTH level normalized but hypocalcemia developed due to severe osteoporosis. Unfortunately, the patient's recovery was complicated by acute tubular necrosis, acute renal failure requiring dialysis, bacteremia, and respiratory insufficiency. Attempts to wean him off the ventilator were unsuccessful. Palliative care was initiated, and he was discharged to hospice care.

PRESENTATION

Parathyroid carcinoma is often misdiagnosed preoperatively as primary hyperparathyroidism due to parathyroid adenoma or hyperplasia. Clinical and laboratory findings may suggest carcinoma, but these findings are nonspecific. At this time, there is no external independent reference standard for the diagnosis of parathyroid carcinoma, and histopathologic diagnosis can be equivocal.[9] A palpable neck mass has been reported in approximately half of patients with parathyroid carcinoma but in less than 1% of patients with primary hyperparathyroidism.[4,22,23] The degree of hypercalcemia is

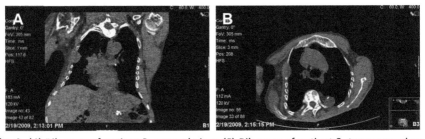

Fig. 4. (A) Rib mass of patient 2, coronal view. (B) Rib mass of patient 2, transverse view.

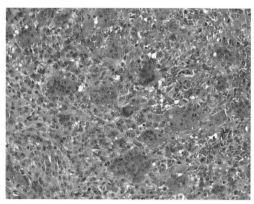

Fig. 5. Brown tumor of hyperparathyroidism, also known as osteitis fibrosa cystica. A rare finding (H and E, original magnification ×200).

often more pronounced in parathyroid carcinoma. Calcium levels above 14 mg/dL (normal, 8.5 to 9.9 mg/dL) are common, in contrast to the elevations of 1 to 2 mg/dL above normal levels typically seen in primary hyperparathyroidism.[22,24,25] PTH levels are frequently 2 to 10 times the normal values in parathyroid carcinoma (normal intact PTH [iPTH], 10 to 65 pg/mL), whereas PTH levels approximately twice the normal range are more commonly seen in primary hyperparathyroidism.[22,24,25] Alkaline phosphatase is also more commonly elevated in parathyroid carcinomas compared with adenomas and hyperplasia; this finding is thought to result from the higher incidence of concomitant bone disease.[25,26] Hypophosphatemia is not a common feature of the disease.[27] Curiously, parathyroid cancers seem to have a predilection for the inferior parathyroid glands, a finding noted by several investigators.[3,28–30]

The most commonly affected organ systems in patients with primary hyperparathyroidism are the renal and skeletal systems.[3,10,24] Parathyroid adenomas and hyperplasia are reported to cause renal impairment (nephrolithiasis, nephrocalcinosis, or impaired glomerular filtration) in fewer than 20% of patients. Renal involvement in parathyroid carcinoma is reported as higher, affecting 32% to 84% of patients.[5,26] Radiologic signs of skeletal abnormalities secondary to hyperparathyroidism (osteitis fibrosa cystica, absent lamina dura, diffuse spinal osteopenia, subperiosteal bone resorption, or salt-and-pepper skull) have been reported in 44% to 91% of patients with parathyroid carcinoma, whereas specific radiologic findings have been reported in less than 10% of patients with benign primary hyperparathyroidism.[4,5,26,31] Patients with parathyroid carcinoma are also at a higher risk for developing complications, such as severe pancreatitis, peptic ulcer disease, and anemia, in other organ systems.[4,5]

None of these findings is specific to the diagnosis of parathyroid carcinoma. For this reason, a high index of preoperative suspicion and the intraoperative recognition of malignant features are of fundamental importance.[32]

OPERATIVE FINDINGS

The appearance of parathyroid carcinoma during surgical resection varies, but the appearance can be different from that of parathyroid adenoma, which typically has a red/brown color, soft texture, and lack of attachments to the surrounding tissue.[3] The classic description of a parathyroid carcinoma is a hard, lobulated mass that is fibrous in texture. The color ranges from tan to grayish.[3,5] The tumor also frequently adheres to the surrounding structures, including the thyroid gland, strap muscles, and recurrent laryngeal nerve.[3,5,12,31] The recurrent laryngeal nerve should be sacrificed only in the case of a locally aggressive tumor.[33] There are several reports of parathyroid carcinoma being indistinguishable from parathyroid adenoma at the time of excision, with diagnosis made after pathologic analysis.[3,13,31]

PATHOLOGY

Shantz and Castleman[34] established a set of criteria for the pathologic diagnosis of parathyroid carcinoma in 1973, which includes

1. Presence of a fibrous capsule or fibrous trabeculae
2. Trabecular or rosette-like cellular architecture
3. Presence of mitotic figures
4. Presence of capsular or vascular invasion.

Subsequent studies have reflected the difficulty of diagnosing parathyroid carcinoma based on histopathologic analysis. McKeown and colleagues[35] indicate that cellular pleomorphism and atypia are not reliable indicators of malignancy in endocrine tumors. Stojadinovic and colleagues[36] described the morphologic features of parathyroid carcinoma as

1. Trabecular growth pattern
2. Thick fibrous bands (**Fig. 6**)
3. Adjacent skeletal muscle invasion by tumor
4. Vascular invasion with tumor attached to vessel wall (**Fig. 7**)
5. Capsular invasion with tongue-like protrusions.

This study found capsular invasion in 92% of patients, vascular invasion in 81%, and perineural invasion in 19%. In their meta-analysis of the parathyroid carcinoma literature, Obara and colleagues[37] stated that the finding of fibrous bands was the most sensitive histopathologic feature, whereas trabecular growth pattern, capsular invasion, and vascular invasion carried the highest specificity. Tumor size does not seem to play a role in prognosis.[17] Currently, no staging system exists for the evaluation of parathyroid carcinoma.

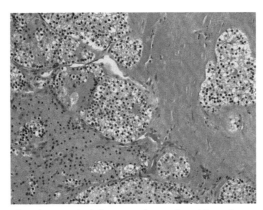

Fig. 6. Thick fibrous bands, a typical feature of parathyroid carcinoma (H and E, original magnification ×200).

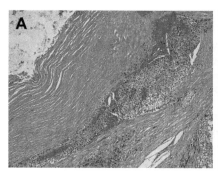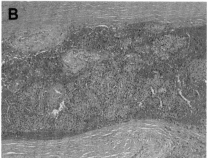

Fig. 7. (*A*) Parathyroid carcinoma exhibiting lymphovascular invasion (H and E, original magnification ×100). (*B*) Parathyroid carcinoma exhibiting lymphovascular invasion (H and E, original magnification ×100).

Nuclear content analysis has also been studied in patients with parathyroid carcinoma. Mean nuclear DNA content is greater, and an aneuploid DNA pattern is more common in parathyroid carcinoma than in parathyroid adenomas. The presence of aneuploidy in parathyroid carcinomas is a poor prognostic indicator.[11,37]

With immunohistochemical staining, several cellular proteins have been determined to occur more commonly in specimens of parathyroid carcinoma than in parathyroid adenoma.[36,38,39] Ki-67 is present in 27% of patients with parathyroid carcinoma in contrast to 2% of those with a parathyroid adenoma.[36] Retinoblastoma (Rb) protein expression is present in most patients with parathyroid adenoma and significantly reduced or entirely absent in patients with parathyroid carcinoma.[36,39] Stojadinovic and colleagues[36] tested several molecular phenotypes and determined that 76% of patients with a parathyroid adenoma and no patients with carcinoma had the phenotype p27(+) bcl-2(−) Ki-67(−) mdm2(+). The phenotypes p27(+) bcl-2(−) Ki-67(+) mdm2(−), p27(−) bcl-2(−) Ki-67(−) mdm2(−), and p27(−) bcl-2(+) Ki-67(+) mdm2(−) were present in 9%, 27%, and 18% of patients with parathyroid carcinoma, respectively, but were not present in any patients with parathyroid adenoma. Although these immunohistochemical markers show potential to discriminate between benign and malignant parathyroid disease, they do not yet exceed the accuracy of surgical findings and conventional histopathology.

GENETICS

Recent genetic research has analyzed possible molecular explanations for tumor development in parathyroid carcinoma. In 2009, Westin and colleagues[40] performed a comprehensive literature review of studies describing the molecular genetics of parathyroid diseases. Of their presented studies, several investigators had determined that somatic HRPT2 mutations with biallelic inactivation are seen in 15% to 100% of sporadic parathyroid carcinomas.[41–45] Parafibromin, the protein product encoded by the HRPT2 gene, is proposed as regulating transcription by interacting with the Wnt/β-catenin and cyclin D1 signaling pathways.[40] Negative immunostaining for parafibromin is considered highly suspicious for parathyroid carcinoma, unless a patient has HPT-JT syndrome.[46,47] The incidence of HRPT2 mutations in parathyroid carcinoma, however, is variable (15% to 100%), and inactivation may also be caused by methylation.[42,43,46–51]

Other molecular associations have been made in the context of parathyroid cancer. Juhlin and colleagues[52] revealed absent immunostaining for the Wnt pathway component adenomatous polyposis coli in 75% of parathyroid carcinomas, indicating that this pathway abnormality may be useful in recognition of parathyroid carcinoma when used alongside immunohistochemisty staining for parafibromin and the proliferation index. A Ki-67 proliferation index greater than 5% may indicate increased risk for cancer in a parathyroid tumor, although a high Ki-67 index can be seen in parathyroid adenomas. A high Ki-67 index may also be associated with a poorer prognosis for patients with parathyroid carcinoma.[53]

Overexpression of cyclin D1 is encountered in up to 90% of parathyroid carcinomas.[44,53] Additionally, allelic loss on chromosome 13q and absent nuclear staining for the Rb protein is found in parathyroid carcinomas but rarely in parathyroid adenomas.[41,44,53] Other allelic losses, including 1q25, 7q13, 10q23, 13q14, and 11p15, are prevalent in these carcinomas, where frequently deleted areas have included HRPT2, PTEN, Rb, HRAS, and p53 genes.[42–44,53,54] Carcinomas show more proximal losses on chromosome 1p than adenomas, and it is suggested that there may be 2 different parathyroid tumor-suppressor genes at this location.[45,54] Research in this field is dynamic, and new findings may offer novel therapeutic modalities for future treatment of parathyroid carcinoma.

DIAGNOSTIC IMAGING

Nuclear medicine studies, including technetium-99m sestamibi and ^{201}thallium, have proved useful in localizing most hyperfunctional parathyroid glands as well as parathyroid carcinomas.[13,55] Ultrasound also is used. Distinguishing features of parathyroid carcinoma on ultrasound include a length/width ratio greater than 1 in 94% of patients, contrasting with 5% of patients with adenoma. An ultrasound scan may also indicate the lobulated appearance and inhomogeneous echogenicity often associated with parathyroid carcinoma.[56] Bone mineral density scans are used to detect significant skeletal abnormalities and, when correlated with grossly abnormal laboratory values of calcium, PTH, and alkaline phosphatase, are helpful in distinguishing patients with parathyroid carcinoma from those with adenoma.[25] In patients with suspected parathyroid carcinoma, MRI with gadolinium and fat suppression is useful in preoperative identification of the tumor.[57] PET has also recently been described in detection of these malignant tumors.[31]

MANAGEMENT

Several reports have stressed the importance of an en bloc resection, including thyroid lobectomy with the isthmus and paratracheal and central neck nodal dissection.[4,5,12,13,31,55] This procedure, when performed as the initial therapeutic step, offers patients the best chance for cure. Unfortunately, the diagnosis of parathyroid carcinoma is frequently made after permanent pathologic review. Controversy exists as to whether or not patients without obvious tumor extension should be taken back to the operating room for ipsilateral thyroidectomy, isthmusectomy, and excision of paratracheal and central neck nodes after the diagnosis is obtained from the pathology report. Some practitioners advocate close observation of calcium levels for evidence of recurrence, holding en bloc excision in reserve in the event of recurrence.[4,11] Most agree that recurrent tumors that can be identified and are amenable to resection should be excised, even multiple times if necessary, for palliative relief from hypercalcemia.[4,5,11,13,24,55] Because parathyroid carcinoma patients are at a relatively high risk of multiple relapses over prolonged time periods, they should be monitored for life using serum calcium and iPTH levels. If elevations of these disease markers are noted, signs of recurrence should be evaluated with localizing imaging studies, such as ultrasonography, CT, MRI, sestamibi scanning, or positron emission tomographic (PET) scanning.[27]

Surveillance for parathyroid carcinoma principally depends on monitoring calcium and iPTH levels. Caution should be used in interpreting modest elevations in iPTH as they may be indicative of secondary hyperparathyroidism due to vitamin D deficiency rather than recurrence.[58,59] If this is of concern, given the widespread prevalence of vitamin D deficiency, a 25-OH vitamin D level should be measured. If deficient, this should be corrected through repletion to a level greater than 30 ng/mL.[58] CEA levels may also be used for surveillance.[58,59]

The role of radiation therapy in the treatment of this disease is described in the literature, albeit with limited data and nondefinitive results.[24] Although parathyroid carcinoma has traditionally been considered a radioresistant tumor, recent retrospective studies have suggested that adjuvant radiotherapy may produce a positive benefit on survival.[33,60] In a 2004 retrospective cohort, Busaidy and colleagues[27] found that adjuvant radiation therapy decreased the risk of localized disease recurrence, although formal statistical analysis was precluded due to the small study population. Additionally, other studies[61,62] have reported that treatment groups receiving adjuvant radiation therapy after surgical excision where margins were positive or close have also shown evidence of possible improvement in preventing recurrence of disease.

Data are limited for the treatment of parathyroid carcinoma with chemotherapy. No defined treatment regimen exists at this time. Dacarbazine alone was shown to provide a brief reduction of a hypercalcemia in 1 report.[63] A remission of hypercalcemia for 13 months has been reported with a regimen of dacarbazine, 5-fluorouracil, and cyclophosphamide.[64] Several other regimens have been tried with poor results.[24]

Profound hypercalcemia can also be a problem for patients with end-stage parathyroid carcinoma. In patients with persistent hypercalcemia and those with unresectable tumors, medical treatment aimed at reducing calcium levels should be implemented. Conservative treatment with saline infusion and loop diuretics is typically not sufficient, and more aggressive medical therapy is usually required.[5] Medications used with some success include pamidronate (bisphosphonates), mithramycin, and calcitonin.[10,64–66]

Schott and colleagues[67] described a case of tumor vaccination with antigen-loaded dendritic cells that demonstrated significant in vitro and in vivo immune responses to the antigens in a patient with disseminated parathyroid carcinoma, although there was no observed clinical improvement. Bradwell and Harvey[68] immunized a metastatic parathyroid carcinoma patient with human and bovine PTH peptides to induce antibodies that block PTH binding to its receptors. This patient showed rapid improvements in serum calcium level and clinical condition. Betea and coworkers[69] reported the long-term hormonal, biochemical, and antitumor effects of anti-PTH immunotherapy in a patient with refractory metastatic parathyroid carcinoma. Further research efforts are needed to elucidate these novel therapeutic techniques.

OUTCOME

Recurrence after surgical excision of parathyroid carcinoma is common, with rates ranging from 33% to 78%.[11,13,24,55] The reported time from surgery to the first recurrence (disease-free interval) varies greatly, from 1 month to 20 years, with the mean most commonly reported as between 2 and 5 years.[11,13,24] Studies reporting statistical estimates of disease-specific survival in patients with parathyroid carcinoma have yielded 5- and 10-year survival rates that range between 20% and 90% and

42% and 86%, respectively. Variation of the survival rates reported in these studies may reflect the differences in histopathologic definitions, the proportions of unequivocal versus equivocal cases, and initial therapeutic interventions used.[9]

SUMMARY

Parathyroid carcinoma is a rare tumor that is prone to recurrence and poor local-regional control. Despite advances in technologies that have shown promise for accurate diagnosis, the mainstay of initial diagnosis remains pathologic analysis and clinical assessment. A surgeon's intraoperative analysis is important in identifying those patients with a high likelihood of parathyroid carcinoma. If parathyroid carcinoma is suspected intraoperatively, a more aggressive surgical strategy should be implemented. As continued advances in diagnosis and treatment develop, medical therapies may provide an alternative to what is currently a surgical disease.

ACKNOWLEDGMENTS

The authors acknowledge the assistance of Dr Chien Chen, Department of Pathology, University of Arkansas for Medical Sciences College of Medicine, and Dr Anil Dewan, Department of Pathology, University of Virginia, in preparation of photomicrographs for this article.

REFERENCES

1. de Quervain F. Parastruma maligna aberrata [Malignant aberrant parathyroid]. Deusche Zeitschr Chir 1904;100:334–52 [in German].
2. Sainton P, Millot J. Malegne d'un adenoma parathyroidiene eosinophile [Malignant eosinophilic parathyroid]. Au cours d'une de Recklinghausen. Ann Anal Pathol 1933;10:813 [in French].
3. Holmes E, Morton D, Ketcham A. Parathyroid carcinoma: a collective review. Ann Surg 1969;169:631–40.
4. Fujimoto Y, Obara T. How to recognize and treat parathyroid carcinoma. Surg Clin North Am 1987;67:343–57.
5. Shane E. Parathyroid carcinoma. J Clin Endocrinol Metab 2001;86:485–93.
6. Iihara M, Okamoto T, Suzuki R, et al. Functional parathyroid carcinoma: long-term treatment outcome and risk factor analysis. Surgery 2007;142:936–43.
7. Obara T, Okamoto T, Ito Y, et al. Surgical and medical management of patients with pulmonary metastasis from parathyroid carcinoma. Surgery 1993;114:1040–9.
8. Giesler G, Beech D. Nonfunctional parathyroid carcinoma. J Natl Med Assoc 2001;93:251–5.
9. Okamoto T, Iihara M, Obara T, et al. Parathyroid carcinoma: diagnosis, etiology, treatment. World J Surg 2009. Available at: http://www.springerlink.com/content/g3h320187l3ru638/. Accessed July 12, 2009.
10. Shane E, Bilezikian J. Parathyroid carcinoma: a review of 62 patients. Endocr Rev 1982;3:218–26.
11. Sandelin K, Auer G, Bondeson L, et al. Prognostic factors in parathyroid cancer: a review of 95 cases. World J Surg 1992;16:724–31.
12. Fujimoto Y, Obara T, Ito Y, et al. Surgical treatment of ten cases of parathyroid carcinoma: importance of an initial en block resection. World J Surg 1984;8:392–400.

13. Favia G, Lumachi F, Polistina F, et al. Parathyroid carcinoma: sixteen new cases and suggestions for correct management. World J Surg 1998;22: 1225–30.

14. Dotzenrath C, Goretzki PE, Sarbia M, et al. Parathyroid carcinoma: problems in diagnosis and the need for radical surgery even in recurrent disease. Eur J Surg Oncol 2001;27:383–9.

15. Hakaim AG, Esselstyn CB Jr. Parathyroid carcinoma: 50-year experience at The Cleveland Clinic Foundation. Cleve Clin J Med 1993;60:331–5.

16. Obara T, Fujimoto Y. Diagnosis and treatment of patients with parathyroid carcinoma: an update and review. World J Surg 1991;15:738–44.

17. Hundahl S, Fleming I, Fremgen A, et al. Two hundred eighty-six cases of parathyroid carcinoma treated in the US between 1985–1995, a national cancer data base report. Cancer 1999;86:538–44.

18. Jenkins P, Satta M, Simmgen M, et al. Metastatic parathyroid carcinoma in the MEN2A syndrome. Clin Endocrinol 1997;41:747–51.

19. Hamill J, Maoate K, Beasley S, et al. Familial parathyroid carcinoma in a child. J Paediatr Child Health 2002;38:314–7.

20. Dionisi S, Minisola S, Pepe J, et al. Concurrent parathyroid adenomas and carcinoma in the setting of multiple endocrine neoplasia type 1: presentation as hypercalcemic crisis. Mayo Clin Proc 2002;77:866–9.

21. Weinstein L, Simonds W. HRPT2, a marker of parathyroid cancer. N Engl J Med 2003;349:1691–2.

22. Cordeiro A, Montenegro F, Kulcsar M, et al. Parathyroid carcinoma. Am J Surg 1998;175:52–5.

23. Levin K, Galante M, Clark O. Parathyroid carcinoma versus parathyroid adenoma in patients with profound hypercalcemia. Surgery 1987;101:647–60.

24. Wynne A, Heerden J, Carney A, et al. Parathyroid carcinoma: clinical and pathologic features in 43 patients. Medicine 1992;71:197–205.

25. Chen Q, Kaji H, Nomura R, et al. Trial to predict malignancy of affected parathyroid glands in primary hyperparathyroidism. Endocr J 2003;50:527–34.

26. Silverberg S, Shane E, Jacobs J, et al. Nephrolithiasis and bone involvement in primary hyperparathyroidism. Am J Med 1990;89:327–34.

27. Busaidy NL, Jimenez C, Habra MA, et al. Parathyroid carcinoma: a 22-year experience. Head Neck 2004;26:716–26.

28. Chon K, Siverman M, Corrado J, et al. Parathyroid carcinoma: the Lahey Clinic experience. Surgery 1985;98:1095–100.

29. Mallette LE, Bilezikian JP, Ketcham AS, et al. Parathyroid carcinoma in familial hyperparathyroidism. Am J Med 1974;57:642–8.

30. Flye MW, Brennan MF. Surgical resection of metastatic parathyroid carcinoma. Ann Surg 1981;193:425–35.

31. Snell S, Gaar E, Stevens S, et al. Parathyroid cancer, a continued diagnostic and therapeutic dilemma: report of four cases and review of the literature. Am Surg 2003;69:711–8.

32. Schoretsanitis G, Daskalakis M, Melissas J, et al. Parathyroid carcinoma: clinical presentation and management. Am J Otol 2009;30:277–80.

33. Clayman GL, Gonzalez HE, El-Naggar A, et al. Parathyroid carcinoma: evaluation and interdisciplinary management. Cancer 2004;100:900–5.

34. Schantz A, Castleman B. Parathyroid carcinoma: a study of 70 cases. Cancer 1973;31:600–5.

35. McKeown P, McGarity W, Sewell C. Carcinoma of the parathyroid gland: is it over diagnosed? A report of three cases. Am J Surg 1984;147:292–7.

36. Stojadinovic A, Hoos A, Nissan A, et al. Parathyroid neoplasms: clinical, histopathological, and tissue microarray-based molecular analysis. Hum Pathol 2003;34:54–64.

37. Obara T, Fujimato Y, Hivayama A, et al. Flow cytometric DNA analysis of parathyroid tumors with special reference to its diagnostic and prognostic value in parathyroid carcinoma. Cancer 1990;65:1789–93.

38. Abbona G, Papotti M, Gasparri G, et al. Proliferative activity in parathyroid tumors as detected by Ki-67 immunostaining. Hum Pathol 1995;26:135–8.

39. Cetani F, Pardi E, Viacava P, et al. A reappraisal of the Rb1 gene abnormalities in the diagnosis of parathyroid cancer. Clin Endocrinol 2004;60:99.

40. Westin G, Bjorklund P, Akerstrom G. Molecular genetics of parathyroid disease. World J Surg 2009. Available at: http://www.springerlink.com/content/a2351831t228j77k/. Accessed July 12, 2009.

41. Tan MH, Morrison C, Wang P, et al. Loss of parafibromin immunoreactivity is a distinguishing feature of parathyroid carcinoma. Clin Cancer Res 2004;10:6629–37.

42. Rogers SE. Perrier ND Parathyroid carcinoma. Curr Opin Oncol 2006;18:16–22.

43. Rawat N, Khetan N, Williams DW, et al. Parathyroid carcinoma. Br J Surg 2005;92: 1345–53.

44. Mittendorf EA, McHenry CR. Parathyroid carcinoma. J Surg Oncol 2005;89: 136–42.

45. Valimaki S, Forsberg L, Farnebo LO, et al. Distinct target regions for chromosome 1p deletions in parathyroid adenomas and carcinomas. Int J Oncol 2002;21: 727–35.

46. Howell VM, Haven CJ, Kahnoski K, et al. HRPT2 mutations are associated with malignancy in sporadic parathyroid tumors. J Med Genet 2003;40: 657–63.

47. Gill AJ, Clarkson A, Gimm O, et al. Loss of nuclear expression of parafibromin distinguishes parathyroid carcinomas and hyperparathyroidism-jaw tumor (HPT-JT) syndrome-related adenomas from sporadic parathyroid adenomas and hyperplasias. Am J Surg Pathol 2006;30:1140–9.

48. Shattuck T, Valimaki S, Obara T, et al. Somatic and germline mutations of PRPT2 gene in sporadic parathyroid carcinoma. N Engl J Med 2003;349:1722–9.

49. Cetani F, Ambrogini E, Viacava P, et al. Should parafibromin staining replace HRPT2 gene analysis as an additional tool for histological diagnosis of parathyroid carcinoma? Eur J Endocrinol 2007;156:547–54.

50. Haven CJ, van Puijenbroek M, Tan MH, et al. Identification of MEN1 and HRPT2 somatic mutations in paraffin embedded (sporadic) parathyroid carcinomas. Clin Endocrinol (Oxf) 2007;67:370–6.

51. Hewitt KM, Sharma PK, Samowitz W, et al. Aberrant methylation of the HRPT2 gene in parathyroid carcinoma. Ann Otol Rhinol Laryngol 2007;116:928–33.

52. Juhlin CC, Haglund F, Villablanca A, et al. Loss of expression for the Wnt pathway components adenomatous polyposis coli and glycogen synthase kinase 3-b in parathyroid carcinomas. Int J Oncol 2009;34:481–92.

53. DeLellis RA. Parathyroid carcinoma: an overview. Adv Anat Pathol 2005;12: 53–61.

54. Hunt JL, Carty SE, Yim IH, et al. Allelic loss in parathyroid neoplasia can help characterize malignancy. Am J Surg Pathol 2005;29:1049–55.

55. Kebebew E, Arici C, Duh Q, et al. Localization and reoperation results for persistent and recurrent parathyroid carcinoma. Arch Surg 2001;136:878–85.

56. Hara H, Igarahi A, Yano Y, et al. Ultrasonographic features of parathyroid carcinoma. Endocr J 2001;48:213–7.

57. Weber A, Randolph G, Aksoy F. The thyroid and parathyroid glands: CT and MR imaging and correlation with pathology and clinic. Radiol Clin North Am 2000;38: 1105–29.

58. Redman C, Bodenner D, Stack B. Role of vitamin D deficiency in continued hyperparathyroidism following parathyroidectomy. Head Neck 2009. Available at: http://www3.interscience.wiley.com/journal/122296749/abstract?CRETRY=1& SRETRY=0. Accessed July 27, 2009.

59. Untch BR, Barfield ME, Dar M. Impact of 25-hydroxyvitamin D deficiency on perioperative parathyroid hormone kinetics and results in patients with primary hyperparathyroidism. Surgery 2007;142:1022–6.

60. Kirkby-Bott J, Lewis P, Harmer CL, et al. One stage treatment of parathyroid cancer. Eur J Surg Oncol 2005;31:78–83.

61. Chow E, Tsang R, Breierley J, et al. Parathyroid carcinoma-the Princess Margaret Hospital experience. Int J Radiat Oncol Biol Phys 1998;41:569–72.

62. Muson N, Foote R, Northcutt R, et al. Parathyroid carcinoma: is there a role for adjuvant radiation therapy? Cancer 2003;98:2378–84.

63. Calandra D, Chejfec G, Foy B, et al. Parathyroid carcinoma: biochemical and pathologic response to DTIC. Surgery 1984;96:1132–7.

64. Bukowski R, Sheller L, Cunningham J, et al. Successful combination chemotherapy for metastatic parathyroid carcinoma. Arch Intern Med 1984;144: 399–400.

65. Newrick P, Braafvedt G, Webd A, et al. Prolonged remission of hypercalcemia due to parathyroid carcinoma with pamidronate. Postgrad Med J 1994;70:231.

66. Singer F, Neer R, Murray T, et al. Mithramycin treatment of intractable hypercalcemia due to parathyroid carcinoma. N Engl J Med 1970;283:634–6.

67. Schott M, Feldkamp J, Schattenberg D, et al. Induction of cellular immunity in parathyroid carcinoma treated with tumor lysate-pulsed dendritic cells. Eur J Endocrinol 2000;142:300–6.

68. Bradwell AR, Harvey TC. Control of hypercalcemia of parathyroid carcinoma by immunisation. Lancet 1999;353:370–3.

69. Betea D, Bradwell AR, Harvey TC, et al. Hormonal and biochemical normalization and tumor shrinkage induced by antiparathyroid hormone immunotherapy in a patient with metastatic parathyroid carcinoma. J Clin Endocrinol Metab 2004; 89:3413–20.

Index

Otolaryngol Clin N Am 43 (2010) 455–460
doi:10.1016/S0030-6665(10)00087-3
0030-6665/10/$ – see front matter © 2010 Elsevier Inc. All rights reserved.

Moving?

Make sure your subscription moves with you!

To notify us of your new address, find your **Clinics Account Number** (located on your mailing label above your name), and contact customer service at:

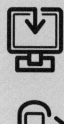

Email: journalscustomerservice-usa@elsevier.com

800-654-2452 (subscribers in the U.S. & Canada)
314-447-8871 (subscribers outside of the U.S. & Canada)

Fax number: 314-447-8029

Elsevier Health Sciences Division
Subscription Customer Service
3251 Riverport Lane
Maryland Heights, MO 63043

*To ensure uninterrupted delivery of your subscription, please notify us at least 4 weeks in advance of move.

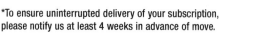

Printed and bound by CPI Group (UK) Ltd, Croydon, CR0 4YY

03/10/2024

01040443-0010